IMMUNOSUPPRESSION: NEW RESEARCH

IMMUNOSUPPRESSION: NEW RESEARCH

CHARLES B. TAYLOR
EDITOR

Nova Biomedical Books
New York

Library of Congress Cataloging-in-Publication Data
Available upon request

ISBN 978-1-60692-102-9

Published by Nova Science Publishers, Inc. ✢ New York

Contents

Preface

Immunosuppression involves an act that reduces the activation or efficacy of the immune system. Some portions of the immune system itself have immuno-suppressive effects on other parts of the immune system, and immunosuppression may occur as an adverse reaction to treatment of other conditions. Deliberately induced immunosuppression is generally done to prevent the body from rejecting an organ transplant, treating graft-versus-host disease after a bone marrow transplant, or for the treatment of auto-immune diseases such as rheumatoid arthritis or Crohn's disease. This is typically done using drugs, but may involve surgery (splenectomy), plasmapharesis, or radiation.

A person who is undergoing immunosuppression, or whose immune system is weak for other reasons (for example, chemotherapy and HIV patients) is said to be immunocompromised. When an organ is transplanted, the immune system of the recipient will most likely recognize it as foreign tissue and attack it. The destruction of the organ will, if untreated, end in the death of the recipient.

In the past, radiation therapy was used to decrease the strength of the immune system, but now immunosuppressant drugs are used to inhibit the reaction of the immune system. The downside is that with such a deactivated immune system, the body is very vulnerable to opportunistic infections, even those usually considered harmless. Also, prolonged use of immunosuppressants increases the risk of cancer.

This new book presents the latest research in the field.

The cost-effectiveness of kidney transplantation over dialysis makes transplantation the treatment of choice for patients with a failing kidney. After decades of use of the first generation immunosuppressives, with their associated increased risks of infections, tumours and other side effects, costimulation blockade was proposed in the nineties as a more specific method of immunosuppression.

As explained in Chapter 1, *in vitro* experiments indicated that costimulation blockade induced a population of anergic cells in mice, humans and in non-human primates. The rediscovery of a suppressor cell population, the naturally occurring regulatory T-cells (Tregs), raised the question whether the anergic cells induced by costimulation blockade were also naturally occurring Tregs and whether Tregs were important for the immunosuppressive effect of costimulation blockade. The effect of costimulation blockade on Tregs is not completely clear, but soon it became evident that costimulation blockade and Tregs can benefit from each other, although they act via different mechanisms. Optimal suppression is only obtained when costimulation blockade and Tregs are both present.

In vivo experiments in rodents demonstrated that costimulation blockade could induce permanent graft survival. When translated to primates, costimulation blockade proved to be less successful for the induction of tolerance. The complicating factor proved to be the presence of memory T-cells induced by viral infections, which crossreact with allo-antigens, the so-called heterologous immunity. Virus-induced T-cells are absent in specific-pathogen free raised mice, whereas primates have substantial numbers of allo-antigen crossreactive memory T-cells. These memory T-cells are less dependent on costimulation blockade compared with the naive T-cells present in specific pathogen free mice.

The focus of tolerance research has therefore shifted to Tregs. Currently, no marker is available that reliably identifies Tregs in humans. FOXP3 seems to be associated with Tregs, but is not exclusively correlated with a regulatory function of the cells in human and non-human primates. Identification of Tregs should therefore be based on functional parameters. Before Tregs can be used for the induction of tolerance in transplant or auto-immune patients, evaluation of the use of Tregs is needed in a relevant pre-clinical model. At the Biomedical Primate Research Centre, the authors have a long-standing experience with treatments that prolong tissue and organ allograft survival. A large number of treatments were evaluated in the rhesus monkey model of kidney and skin transplantation. Recently, the authors have characterized naturally occurring Tregs of the rhesus monkey. This will allow for the evaluation of protocols that either induce Tregs *in vivo*, and of protocols that use *ex vivo* induced and/or expanded Tregs.

Chapter 2 discusses T-cell depletion (TCD), which represents one of the most effective strategies in abrogating the negative effects of severe graft versus host disease (GVHD) due to allogeneic hematopoietic cell transplantation (HCT), particularly for recipients of HLA-mismatched or haploidentical allografts. The past decade has witnessed the development of different graft manipulation strategies, moving from E-rosetting and soybean agglutination, through a combination of negative or positive selection of HSC, to recent one-step positive selection using immunoadsorption columns and monoclonal antibody for ex vivo or in vivo purging. Recent advances with effective T-cell depletion have significantly decreased the early transplant related mortality and risk of severe GVHD, while enabling reliable engraftment, and hence provide encouraging outcomes in both matched or mismatched donor transplantation. However, while they have broadened the array of patients able to be offered immunotherapy to those without a fully matched sibling, post-transplant infections and relapse remain important barriers to overcome. A key challenge is to balance the positive and negative effects of donor T cells to optimize outcome. New directions in the use of adoptive cellular immunity, immunoregulatory T cells, mesenchymal stem cell and selective allodepletion in rapidly reconstituting immunity without GVHD appear promising. The full therapeutic potential of allogeneic HCT will not be realized until approaches to separate GVH and graft versus leukaemia (GVL) are developed.

As presented in Chapter 3, the strong allo-immune response to the transplanted lung necessitates combined pharmacological immunosuppression to prevent graft rejection. Immunosuppressants used to prevent and treat rejection involve several classes of drugs and many target the production of pro-inflammatory cytokines by T cells, monocytes and other immune cells. Although most effective transplantation immunosuppressive strategies are based on interruption of IL-2 signaling by the calcineurin inhibitors cyclosporin A and tacrolimus, intensification of immunosupressive therapies has not led to any improvement in graft survival. Treatment with these drugs is also associated with serious adverse effects including specific organ toxicities, increased risk of developing a range of malignancies and susceptibility to infections. High inter- and intra-individual pharmacokinetic variability of both drugs may mean some patients do not require the high levels of drugs and associated adverse side effects for effective therapeutics. While current assessment of therapeutic drug levels simply involves the empirical measurement of plasma drug concentrations, there is a need for more physiological assessment of combined immunosuppression strategies, particularly at the site of action. Recent research has identified measurement of inflammatory cytokines at the cellular level using novel flow cytometric techniques as a strategy to assess the physiological response to treatment. Intracellular cytokine levels in both peripheral blood and in the airways have been investigated and have highlighted important differences in responses seen at the transplant site versus systemically. While Th1 pro-inflammatory cytokines were significantly reduced in blood T cells from transplant patients, levels of these cytokines in T cells from the airways were significantly greater in transplant patients compared with healthy control subjects. Furthermore, patients undergoing infection or rejection episodes were characterised by significantly decreased or increased Th1 intracellular T cell cytokines in the airways respectively, compared with stable lung transplant patients. To overcome patient inter-individual variability of leucocyte cytokine production, longitudinal monitoring of patient cytokines may be useful in predicting adverse episodes of rejection and/or infection. These techniques may complement or ultimately replace current standard approaches to therapeutic drug monitoring and monitoring by invasive biopsy and have the potential to improve current immunosuppression protocols, optimise individual therapy and possibly provide new therapeutic options to improve the morbidity of lung transplant patients.

The aim of Chapter 3 is to assess our experience with the use and management of m-TORi after liver transplantation .

MATERIAL: From 1988 to 2007, 783 LT were performed in 725 patients. Fifty one patients (7%) received immunosuppression with m-TORi: Rapamicine 36 and Everolimus 15. Mean age was 54.8 years (r: 24-70). Indication of use, time between LT and introduction of m-TORi, efficacy, side effects and survival were analyzed.

RESULTS: Indications were: refractory rejection in the context of renal insufficiency 20 (39%), renal insufficiency 5 (10%), other CNI side effects 6 (12%), extended HCC in the explanted liver 7 (14%), HCC recurrence during follow-up 7 (14%) and de novo tumor 3 (6%). Mean time between LT and m-TORi was 18 ± 29 months with a median of 3 months (r: 10 days-122 months). Mean follow-up after conversion was 14 ± 15 months (r: 0.1-72). In general, half of the patients resolved the event for which the drug was indicated. Refractory rejection was succesfully resolved in half the patients, three required re-LT and six progressed to chronic liver dysfunction with the result of five deaths due to non-resolved rejection and comorbidity. The renal insufficiency at time of conversion resolved in 11 (52%) of the 21 cases. Six out of 7 patients with recurrent HCC died at a mean follow-up of 11.5 months. Three out of 7 patients with extended HCC died at a mean follow-up of 8.2 months. The three cases of de novo tumor were coverted to m-TORi four weeks after surgery and are perfectly healthy. Half of the patients presented m-TORi-related side effects: dyslipemia in 24 (47%), infection in 9 (17.6%); diarrhea in 3 (6%), and hematologic complications in 3 (6%). Six patients (11.7%) developed acute rejection after conversion. Seventeen patients (33.3%) discontinued the drug: 6 due to inefficacy; 5 due to inter-current surgery; 3 due to resolution of the cause; and 3 due to adverse events. Patient actuarial survival was 54%, 46% and 23% at 1, 3 and 5 years post-conversion.

CONCLUSION: m-TORi are indicated in critical and irreversible situations where other immunosuppressants have failed. During the early stage, they are used for refractory rejection or as prophylaxis for recurrence of extended tumors. At any time, but specially in the late period, they are indicated in patients with serious CNI side effects, HCC recurrence, and de novo tumors.

The authors are currently entering a new era of immunosuppressive therapy in liver transplantation (LT), which is discussed in Chapter 5. Since the 1980s, calcineurin inhibitors (CNI) have been the mainstay of both early and late immunosuppressive regimes following LT. The occurrence of significant adverse events with current regimes of CNI combined with tapered corticosteroids, in particular nephrotoxicity, neurotoxicity and hypertension, has been responsible for a changing view of immunosuppression with increased availability of newer potentially less toxic agents.

Combination regimes of various classes of immunosuppressive drugs, the addition of other drug types with reduction or withdrawal of CNI for treatment-related toxicity, or monotherapy with non-CNI agents are increasingly being utilised. Early corticosteroid withdrawal and steroid-free regimens have been successfully used in both children and adults. The use of induction therapy with polyclonal or monoclonal antibodies is now becoming commonplace in patients with renal dysfunction to delay CNI introduction, and to reduce acute rejection episodes. Biological induction agents have also permitted the use of steroid-free regimens and early reduction in CNI dose. Exploitation of the concept of liver tolerance with regimes to induce donor-specific systemic immunological tolerance by recipient pre-treatment, combined with low-dose post-transplant immunosuppression is an exciting and evolving field. Development of innovative immunotherapies that take advantage of natural immunoregulatory mechanisms contributing to immune privilege in the liver may challenge the need for lifelong immunosuppression in the future.

Improvements in the field of transplant immunosuppression have led to a dramatic improvement in long-term survival of liver transplant recipients. The art of immunosuppression involves maintaining a fine balance between optimizing efficacy and minimizing adverse effects. Application of pharmacogenomics in immunotherapy has paved the way towards the concept of individualized therapy. Integrating the knowledge from pharmacogenomics technology with individual factors such as ethnicity and etiology of liver disease may achieve our goals of optimizing immunotherapy. Chapter 6 will discuss the changing landscape of modern immunosuppression and the clinical application of pharmacogenomics in liver transplantation.

Application of photosensitizers (PSs) in medicine [Psoralen+UVA-therapy (PUVA) or Photodynamic Therapy (PDT)] is frequently accompanied by induction of systemic immunosuppression. Taking advantage of this immunosuppressive capacity, PUVA and PDT have been used as immunosuppressive therapies in a variety of diseases. Photosensitized damage of biological targets responsible for immunosuppression can proceed via Type II (singlet oxygen) or Type I (free radicals) mechanisms. Due to the limited lifetime of singlet oxygen or free radical species, the simultaneous exposure to light of both the biological target and the PS is required when Type I or II mechanisms are realized. Exposure to light induces not only the damage of biological targets but also photodegradation of PS molecules with generation of stable PS photooxidation products. Addition of these photoproducts to biosystems in the dark can induce multiple biological effects, including modulation (suppression/activation) of T cell immunity. In Chapter 7, the authors summarize their experimental data on modulation of Delayed Type and Contact Hypersensitivity responses in animals by photooxidation products of psoralens, porphyrins and merocyanine 540 as well as preliminary human clinical studies. Immune mechanisms of immunosuppression caused by PUVA and PDT are compared with those induced by products of PS photooxidation. Development of a new method of photochemotherapy, which is based on application of PS photoproducts to patients without irradiation of their tissues, is discussed.

It has been known for some time that the ultraviolet (UV) component of the solar spectrum is immunosuppressive. This, combined with the DNA damaging properties of UV is the reason why sunlight is such a potent carcinogen. While it is well established that one way UV causes immunosuppression is via the induction of regulatory T cells, recent studies have demonstrated that UV also induces a suppressor B cell population. Furthermore, it has been suggested that inflammatory cytokines and oxidised lipids play a key role in the activation of these regulatory populations. Chapter 8 will review the most recent evidence that elucidate the mechanisms by which UV causes immunosuppression focusing on the activation of regulatory cells and the potential for therapeutic intervention.

Liver transplantation has become the standard treatment for both chronic and acute end-stage liver disease. Because of a progressive increase in the number of patients on waiting list for liver transplant, a number of strategies have been developed in the last few years to increase the donor pool; one of these strategies is adult to adult living-related liver transplantation that showed overall survival similar to deceased donor liver transplantation.

Since adult living-related liver transplantation first became a valuable therapeutic option, the immunosuppressive protocols available to reduce the risk of acute cellular rejection have been continuously changing. Transplanted liver is generally considered immunologically privileged, regardless of the source of donation. Nevertheless, and despite more potential immunological compatibility in living-related transplantation when transplantations are performed between relatives with genetic relationships, acute cellular rejection remains an important risk factor for graft's and patient's loss.

As discussed in Chapter 9, an efficient immunosuppressive protocol, aimed at minimizing potential pharmaceutical side effects and at trying to induce a potential mechanism of tolerance, remains an essential factor for patient's outcome in both deceased donor liver transplantation and living related liver transplantation.

Immunosuppressive therapy based on use of monoclonal antibodies as induction therapy, in combination with calcineurin inhibitor and steroids, or in triple regimen with the addition of azathioprine or mycophenolic acid, results in lower mean acute cellular rejection rates.

In their experience, the authors report that the use of basiliximab, a monoclonal antibody against interleukin-2 receptor, as induction agent in combination with a steroid-and tacrolimus-based regimen in adult to adult living-related liver transplantation, seems to be an efficient immunosuppressive protocol, with low incidence of cellular rejection, side effects, opportunistic infections or malignancies.

Prolonged studies were carried out to elucidate the role of high dose immunosuppression therapy (HDIST) with autologous hematopoietic stem cell transplantation (SCT) in the treatment of severe and refractory autoimmune disease. In Chapter 10, the authors analyzed single center experience of HDIST followed by SCT for refractory SLE.

The 13 patients with SLE, who had disease progression despite previous treatment with pulse Cy intravenous, prednisolone (standard doses and pulse therapy), oral Cy, azathioprine or metotrexate, were enrolled in the clinic of our institution from 1998 to 2007. All patients were seriously ill, with SLE disease activity indices (SLEDAI) of 6-30, including cases with central nervous system lupus, lung vasculitis, carditis, nephritis with nephrotic syndrome and cytopenia. Autologous hematopoietic stem cells were collected from bone marrow (n=4) or mobilized from peripheral blood with Cy (3g/m2/once) and granulocyte colony-stimulating factor (G-CSF) (n=9). Pretransplant conditioning regimens included BEAM ± ATG (n=2), Melphalan 140 mg/m^2 + Etoposid 1600 mg/m^2 (n=2), Cy 200 mg/kg ± ATG (n=2) and Melphalan 120 mg/m^2 (n=1), Cy 140 mg/kg (n=6). Transplanted CD34+ MNC were more than 2x106/kg. Median time to an absolute neutrophil count (ANC) greater than 0.5x10^9 /l and platelet count greater than 50x10^9/l was 11 and 15 days, respectively. Three patients died on days 11, 22 and 63 due to transplant-related complications. All of the patients who died due to transplant-related complications had a long history of corticosteroids treatment, multiple and severe episodes of infections pre-SCT and received more then one anticytostatic drugs or ATG as conditioning regimen. All of the live transplanted patients, who recovered hematopoiesis, showed improvement in disease activity: 8 (CR) and 2 (PR). The median follow up is now 14 months. One patient died due to lung vasculitis progression 8 years after SCT. The authors conclude that HDIST followed by SCT for refractory SLE is feasible and effective, and achievement of prolonged, corticosteroid-free remissions is a reality.

As explained in Chapter 11, transplantation of insulin producing cells in diabetic patients requires technologies to transplant tissues in the absence of immunosuppression since the side effect of immunosuppression can never be an acceptable alternative for insulin therapy. Much effort has been put into the development of immunomodulating technologies to transplant genetically or otherwise modified islet tissue in order to decrease the immunogenicity of the islet tissue. A number of these approaches have been shown to be effective in small rodents and to allow for life-long survival of islet grafts[1,2]. In spite of some successes it has not yet come to clinical application. Another approach is immunoisolation of tissue by encapsulation of pancreatic islets to protect the tissue from the host immune system by an artificial membrane. Basically, there are three major approaches of encapsulation. These include intravascular macrocapsules, which are anastomosed to the vascular system as AV shunt, extravascular macrocapsules, which are mostly diffusion chambers transplanted at different sites, and extravascular microcapsules transplanted in the peritoneal cavity. All systems have been shown to be successful in preclinical studies. These studies also showed that not all approaches meet the technical or physiological requirements for application in men. The extravascular approach provides advantages over the intravascular systems since it is associated with fewer complications such as thrombosis and infection. Microcapsules, due to their spatial characteristics, offer better diffusion capacity than macrocapsules. Recent progress in biocompatibility of microcapsules has brought this technology near clinical application. Critical issues such as limitations in the functional performance and survival are being discussed. The latest results show that both issues can be solved by transplantation of microencapsulated islets near blood vessels in prevascularized solid supports. Also, latest insights will be presented into the composition of the membranes for immuoisolating devices and the associated biocompatibility.

Chapter 12 discusses Graves' ophthalmopathy, which is considered an inflammatory disorder of autoimmune background, and changed reactive oxygen species (ROS) metabolism presumably plays a role in pathogenesis of autoimmune diseases. Corticosteroids and radiotherapy are principal measures of infiltrative ophthalmopathy treatment, and their therapeutic effect is partially connected with influence on ROS generation systems. In this chapter the authors analyse the both therapeutic methods influence on extracellular oxidative stress markers in Graves' ophthalmopathy patients. Plasma indices of free radical generation and scavenging were determined in 20 euthyroid patients with infiltrative Graves' ophthalmopathy initially, after orbital irradiation combined with intensive corticotherapy and off steroid treatment. 24 healthy volunteers and 25 euthyroid Graves' patients without ophthalmopathy served as controls. The changes suggesting peripheral oxidative stress presence (increased hydrogen peroxide, lipid hydroperoxides and ceruloplasmin levels and superoxide dismutase and catalase activities, reduced glutathione peroxidase and glutathione reductase activities) were still found just after radiotherapy, in spite of concurrent corticosteroid treatment. However, longer follow up revealed the ROS metabolism markers normalization in individuals off the therapy. Changed peripheral oxidative stress markers in Graves' ophthalmopathy patients are corrected by the combined immunosuppressive treatment. This effect presumably depends on regression of the orbital inflammatory lesions.

In: Immunosuppression: New Research
Editor: Charles B. Taylor, pp. 1–43

ISBN 978-1-60692-102-9

Chapter 1

Is There a Future for Costimulation Blockade as a Regulatory T-cell Inducing Therapy?

***Krista G. Haanstra*[1], *Bert A. 't Hart*[1], *Frans H.J. Claas*[2] *and Margreet Jonker*[1]**
[1]Biomedical Primate Research Centre, Rijswijk, The Netherlands
[2]Leiden University Medical Centre, Leiden, The Netherlands

Abstract

The cost-effectiveness of kidney transplantation over dialysis makes transplantation the treatment of choice for patients with a failing kidney. After decades of use of the first generation immunosuppressives, with their associated increased risks of infections, tumours and other side effects, costimulation blockade was proposed in the nineties as a more specific method of immunosuppression.

In vitro experiments indicated that costimulation blockade induced a population of anergic cells in mice, humans and in non-human primates. The rediscovery of a suppressor cell population, the naturally occurring regulatory T-cells (Tregs), raised the question whether the anergic cells induced by costimulation blockade were also naturally occurring Tregs and whether Tregs were important for the immunosuppressive effect of costimulation blockade. The effect of costimulation blockade on Tregs is not completely clear, but soon it became evident that costimulation blockade and Tregs can benefit from each other, although they act via different mechanisms. Optimal suppression is only obtained when costimulation blockade and Tregs are both present.

In vivo experiments in rodents demonstrated that costimulation blockade could induce permanent graft survival. When translated to primates, costimulation blockade proved to be less successful for the induction of tolerance. The complicating factor proved to be the presence of memory T-cells induced by viral infections, which cross-react with allo-antigens, the so-called heterologous immunity. Virus-induced T-cells are absent in specific-pathogen free raised mice, whereas primates have substantial numbers of allo-antigen crossreactive memory T-cells. These memory T-cells are less dependent on costimulation blockade compared with the naive T-cells present in specific pathogen free mice.

The focus of tolerance research has therefore shifted to Tregs. Currently, no marker is available that reliably identifies Tregs in humans. FOXP3 seems to be associated with Tregs, but is not exclusively correlated with a regulatory function of the cells in human and non-human primates. Identification of Tregs should therefore be based on functional parameters. Before Tregs can be used for the induction of tolerance in transplant or auto-immune patients, evaluation of the use of Tregs is needed in a relevant pre-clinical model. At the Biomedical Primate Research Centre, we have a long-standing experience with treatments that prolong tissue and organ allograft survival. A large number of treatments were evaluated in the rhesus monkey model of kidney and skin transplantation. Recently, we have characterized naturally occurring Tregs of the rhesus monkey. This will allow for the evaluation of protocols that either induce Tregs *in vivo*, and of protocols that use *ex vivo* induced and/or expanded Tregs.

Introduction

Transplantation as a Treatment for Organ Disease

Transplantation is the only possible cure for the failing organ, without which patients will eventually die. In 1954 the first successful organ replacement therapy was performed when a kidney was transplanted between a set of identical twins [1]. After this first living related kidney transplantation, kidneys from cadaveric non-related donors were increasingly used for transplantation. Immediately it became evident that allotransplantation (transplantation between individuals of the same species) resulted in a vigorous immune response causing graft rejection, which was a boost for transplantation related immunological research. Between 1954 and now, transplantation of organs (heart, lung, liver, pancreas, bone marrow) and tissues (skin, bone) has become a routine procedure .

Studies of Gibson and Medawar in a skin allograft model showed that the acquired immune system was critically involved in the rejection of the grafts [2–4]. An important hallmark in transplantation research was the discovery of the major histocompatibility complex (MHC) [5–7]. The MHC is extremely polymorphic, an evolutionary established feature to ensure the survival of the population. Despite matching for MHC between donor and recipient, rejection still occurs if additional drugs to suppress the immune system of the recipient are not given. First generation drugs such as azathioprine inhibit DNA-synthesis, thereby preventing cell division of recipient lymphocytes. Mycophenolate mofetil (MMF) is a more recently discovered drug in this group of immunosuppressives [8]. A second group of drugs interferes with the activation of lymphocytes. Cyclosporin A (CsA) and FK506 (tacrolimus) inhibit calcineurin, a molecule important for the signal transduction from the T-cell receptor (TCR) to the nucleus [8]. Rapamycin, (sirolimus), interferes with the downstream signalling of the common γ-chain of cytokine receptors. The IL-2 receptor is the most well known receptor using the common γ-chain [9].

Conventional immunosuppressive drugs need to be taken continuously, throughout the life of the recipient. These drugs also affect normal functions of the immune system and are associated with an increased risk of infections and tumours and they cause side effects such as hypertension, atherosclerosis, hirsutism, hyperlipidaemia and myelosuppression. CsA has an additional disadvantage, as it is nephrotoxic. For these reasons, transplantation research has moved into a new era. Mechanisms naturally present in the recipient to prevent autoimmunity are used to create a state of unresponsiveness towards the graft without the need for long-term use of immunosuppressive drugs. Billingham, Brent and Medawar first recognised this possibility, as early as 1953 [10]. This drug-free graft acceptance may be based on anergy or tolerance. Anergy is often used to indicate as state of unresponsiveness without knowing whether this is permanent. Tolerance is the ultimate goal in current transplantation research. It indicates a state of long-term graft acceptance due to active suppression by immune cells or due to clonal deletion of donor-reactive cells without the need for immunosuppression.

Mechanisms of Rejection

Donor MHC molecules are recognised as non-self by the immune system of the recipient (direct recognition). $CD4^+$ T-cells are key players in the recognition of donor MHC class II (MHC-II) [11]. The nature of the peptides presented by donor MHC seems to be less important, although they may be mostly donor-derived MHC peptides, which may also be recognised as non-self [12,13]. The T-cell response to donor antigen presented by self MHC is called indirect recognition. Donor-derived MHC peptides also play an important role in the indirect recognition of non-self [14, 15], but recognised peptides can also be derived from non-MHC polymorphic proteins. This process may resemble an autoimmune process. The relative contributions of the direct and indirect pathway of alloantigen recognition to the rejection process remain to be elucidated. Conceptually, direct recognition takes place early after transplantation, when donor antigen presenting cells (APC) are still present in the donor organ. Direct recognition is held responsible for the acute rejection process, which can manifest within days after transplantation in the absence of immunosuppression, but grafts can be rejected after a period of weeks to months, despite immunosuppressive treatment. Indirect recognition is held responsible for chronic rejection of the graft, although it may also play a role in the acute rejection process [16]. The chronic rejection process may take several months to years to develop and can occur simultaneously with the acute rejection process. Rejection of the kidney is evaluated on the basis of a number of parameters, which together form the international working classification of kidney graft rejection, the Banff 1997 criteria [17]. Two parameters of acute rejection describe the deformation of the vessels and glomeruli, while two additional parameters describe the infiltration of leucocytes into the interstitium (i) and the tubules (t). Infiltration of the tubules is a critical event in the final process leading to failure of the function of the kidney [17]. Chronic rejection is one of the processes leading to allograft loss collectively named chronic allograft nephropathy (CAN). Recently, it was suggested to abandon the indication CAN and to indicate this process as interstitial fibrosis and tubular atrophy (IF/TA) [18].

Both direct and indirect recognition can only lead to an immune response when a second signal, the so-called costimulatory signal coincides with TCR recognition of donor antigen [19]. MHC-TCR recognition (signal 1) leads to the activation and maturation of the professional APC, the dendritic cell (DC). Costimulation molecules are upregulated on the DC and subsequently also on the T-cell, resulting in the activation of the T-cell. This sets in motion a process of further upregulation of positive and negative costimulatory signals (signal 2). In addition, secreted cytokines bind to cytokine receptors (signal 3), leading to further activation of the cells. Activated $CD4^+$ helper T-cells (Th cells) start to proliferate and they provide help to $CD8^+$ T-cells and B-cells (discussed below); B-cells are activated and start to produce donor-specific antibodies. $CD8^+$ T-cells can reject donor MHC-I mismatched skin grafts directly [20], but the most important pathway of $CD8^+$ T-cell activation includes help from $CD4^+$ T-cells, upon which the $CD8^+$ T-cells become functional effector cells, the cytotoxic T-lymphocytes (CTLs). CTLs migrate back to the kidney. Tissue homing receptors are upregulated on the cells and CTLs eventually invade the tubules of the kidney. The secretion of inflammatory mediators further recruits macrophages and natural killer (NK)-cells to the graft, which all contribute to the graft destruction.

Alloantigen Recognition and Costimulatory Pathways

Recipient T-cells recognising non-self MHC, will only be fully activated when accompanied by a second signal of costimulation ligand-receptor interaction. The two most important and well-known pathways of costimulation are the CD28-B7 pathway and the CD40-CD40L (CD154) pathway (Fig. 1). TCR signalling leads to the upregulation of CD40L on T-cells. CD40L can interact with constitutively expressed CD40 on the APC. CD40 engagement activates the APC and induces the upregulation of APC surface expression of the costimulatory molecules CD80 and CD86, previously known as the B7 molecules B7-1 and B7-2, respectively [21,22]. CD80 and CD86 can interact with constitutively expressed CD28. Binding of CD40L and CD28 on the T-cell leads to its full activation. Activation of the T-cell includes further upregulation of CD40L and CD28, as well as secretion of cytokines (signal 3) [23,24]. Activation of CD28 induces upregulation of negative regulators that will downregulate the immune response, such as the costimulatory molecule cytotoxic T lymphocyte-associated antigen-4 (CTLA-4; CD152). Expression of CTLA-4 is induced several hours after CD28 upregulation. The ligands for CTLA-4 are the same as for CD28, the B7 molecules.

B7 and CD40 signalling are both important to provide T-cell help to B-cells for immunoglobulin (Ig) class switching [23]. Differentiation of $CD8^+$ T-cells into CTLs is largely dependent on CD28 signalling [25]. Ridge et al. have shown that indeed both the B7-CD28 and CD40-CD40L pathways are needed for the induction of CTLs. Expression of the B7 molecules on APC does not induce CTLs, unless APCs were first activated and had upregulated CD40. Once activated, CD28 signalling is needed to propagate the CD40-CD40L induced CTL activation [26].

The roles of the CD40-CD40L and B7-CD28/CTLA-4 costimulatory pathways have been studied in rodent models of transplantation, using antibodies to block the ligands and receptors of these pathways. These experiments indicate that TCR engagement without a second signal leads to anergy of recipient T-cells. This dogma was first discovered *in vitro* [27], but has been extensively investigated *in vivo*.

Blockade of the CD28-B7 pathway is achieved through several strategies. Antibod-

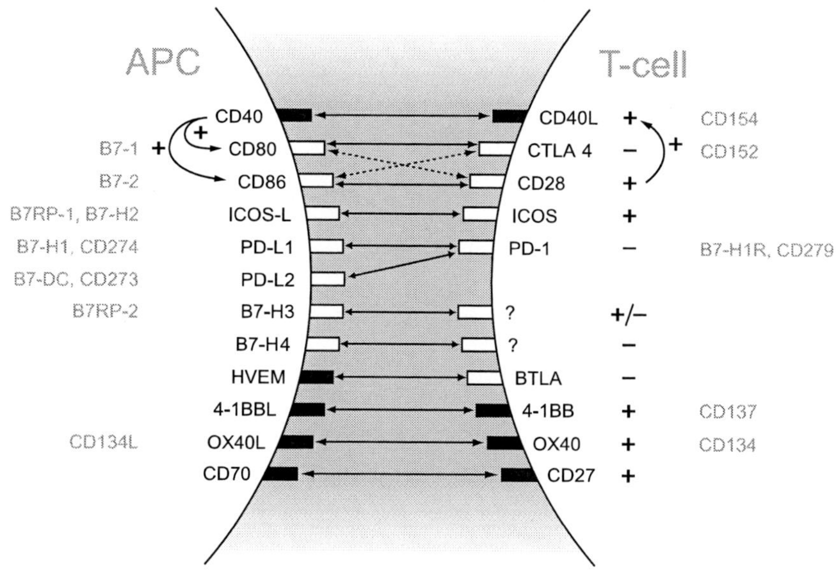

Figure 1. Costimulation ligand-receptor pairs. Alternative names for some of the molecules are indicated in grey. Molecules indicated in black are members of the TNF-TNFR family and molecules indicated in white are members of the Ig superfamily.

ies against CD80, CD86, and CD28 have been described. In addition, blockade of both CD80 and CD86 is achieved by using the CTLA-4 molecule fused to the Fc part of an immunoglobulin G (IgG) molecule (CTLA4-Ig). However, the timed expression of CD28 and CTLA-4, together with the different binding avidity and dissociation rates of CD80 and CD86 with CD28 and CTLA-4, have indicated that CD86 may preferentially bind and activate CD28, while CD80 may preferentially bind and activate CTLA-4 [28,29], enabling downregulation of the immune response. This concept was tested by several groups. Blockade of CD86 prolongs allograft survival in mice [30], whereas blockade of CD80 has no effect [31] or even enhanced graft rejection [32, 33]. Blockade of CTLA-4 with an anti-CD152 monoclonal antibodies (mAb) prevented vascularised mouse heart allograft survival [30, 32, 33]. However, blockade of both CD80 and CD86 had a synergistic effect in other models [31, 34].

In addition to the major costimulatory pathways CD40-CD40L and B7-CD28/ CTLA-4, several other costimulatory pathways have been described. Some act, like the CD86-CTLA-4 pair, to downregulate immune responses, but most pairs act to stimulate T-cells. The transmembrane glycoprotein Ig superfamily, of which the CD28-B7 molecules are members, further includes the stimulatory inducible costimulator (ICOS) on the T-cell and its ligand ICOS-L (also named B7RP-1, B7h, B7-H2, see Figure 1) which is expressed at a low level on resting APCs, B-cells and endothelial cells, but is rapidly induced after activation [35, 36]. The ICOS-ICOS-L pathway is particularly important for the signalling of memory $CD4^+$ and $CD8^+$ T-cells [37]. ICOS blockade enhanced rejection when given immediately post transplant, but it prolonged graft survival when initiation of treatment was delayed [38]. The CD28-B7 family also includes the negative signalling pathway programmed death-1 (PD-1, CD279) expressed on T-cells, B-cells, NK cells and macrophages and its ligands PD-L1 (B7-H1, CD274) and PD-L2 (B7-DC, CD273) expressed on activated APC [39,40]. Three more recently discovered members of the family are the B7-like molecules, B7-homologue 3 (B7-H3), B7-H4 and B and T lymphocyte attenuator (BTLA). B7-H3 binds to an unknown ligand on the T-cell and is expressed on non-lymphoid tissues where it is upregulated after activation of the tissues and can be induced on DC [41]. Whether it is a negative or a positive stimulator is currently unknown. B7-H4 is expressed on tubular renal epithelial cells and may activate tubular epithelium [42]. BTLA is a receptor for herpes virus entry mediator (HVEM) and may downregulate T-cells [43,44]. Interestingly, HVEM is a tumour necrosis factor (TNF)-TNF receptor (TNFR) family member, which makes the BTLA-HVEM pathway the only currently known pathway where members of the Ig superfamily and the TNF-TNFR superfamilies interact.

The TNF-TNFR superfamily, with its members CD40 and CD40L, further consists of the positive signalling pathways 4-1BB (CD137)/4-1BBL, OX40 (CD134)/OX40L (CD134L), and CD27/CD70. 4-1BB is expressed on activated T-cells and NK cells [45]. It binds to 4-1BBL, which is expressed on the APC [46]. OX40 is induced upon activation of T-cells [47] and its ligand OX40L is expressed on activated APC [48]. This pathway primarily promotes effector and memory T-cell function [49]. CD27 is expressed on T-cells, B-cells and NK-cells and activation of CD27 is important for B-cell function [50]. CD27 binds to CD70, which is expressed on DCs and on activated T and B-cells. Its expression is reciprocally regulated with CD27 [51]. Whether CD70 only serves as a ligand for CD27 or whether itself also induces DC or T-cell activation remains a matter of debate [52].

The complex system of positive and negative costimulation pathways possesses a certain level of redundancy. However, each pathway is dedicated to a specific function. Some pathways are involved in the signalling of naive T-cells, while others are more involved in the signalling of memory T-cells, as indicated above. This becomes apparent when certain pathways are blocked to prevent allograft rejection in experimental animal models.

Costimulation Blockade

Costimulation Blockade Therapy to Prevent Kidney Graft Rejection, Preclinical and Clinical

In view of the redundancy of the costimulation system, it is remarkable that long-term graft acceptance can be achieved in rodents with CTLA4-Ig, which blocks only one pathway [53, 54]. However, more stringent models, such as skin transplantation indicate that blocking both the CD40-CD40L and B7-CD28 pathways can induce tolerance in mice, whereas blocking only one of these pathways is not sufficient to achieve this [55]. The importance of the CD40-CD40L and B7-CD28 pathways is further illustrated by the fact that blockade of the other members of the family of costimulation molecules only prolongs graft survival when the major costimulatory pathways CD40-CD40L and B7-CD28 are blocked or knocked out [56–59]. These data already indicate that the focus of using costimulation blockade to induce tolerance in higher animal models lies on blocking the major costimulatory pathways, since little effect is to be expected from blocking other pathways without simultaneous blockade of the major pathways. Antibodies against both major costimulatory pathways have been tested in non-human primates (NHP) models. The effect of costimulation blockade in a number of NHP models is summarised in a review by Kean et al. [60].

Tested strategies in the NHP kidney allograft model can be divided into blocking CD28-B7 interactions, CD40-CD40L interactions, or blocking both pathways. Untreated or control (intravenous immunoglobulin (IVIG) or albumin) treated monkeys consistently reject their kidney allograft within five to seven days in this model [34, 61–67].

Blocking only CD80 or CD86 without additional treatment prolongs graft survival compared to untreated animals, but is not sufficient to prevent rejection during treatment [64]. Combined blockade of CD80 and CD86, using either anti-CD80 + anti-CD86 mAb has the potency to prevent rejection for the duration of the treatment [34, 64, 66, 68–70]. About 50% of animals survive for more than two months after cessation of treatment, provided that treatment duration and mAb levels are sufficient. Antibodies directed against CD28 have not (yet) been tested in a preclinical kidney transplantation setting.

CTLA4-Ig is a molecule with a CTLA-4 domain coupled to an IgG domain, resulting in a soluble construct that binds CD80 and CD86, thereby preventing interaction with both CD28 and CTLA-4. CTLA4-Ig (abatacept) was tested in a limited number of NHP kidney transplant studies, either as a monotherapy, or in addition to treatment with anti-CD40, anti-CD40L or conventional immunosuppression [62, 65, 70]. CTLA4-Ig monotherapy for two weeks is unable to prolong graft survival [65, 70], and no effects of the addition of CTLA4-Ig treatment on treatment with CD40 or CD40L blocking antibodies was observed [62, 65]. Abatacept seemed to be unable to completely prevent T-cell activation through CD28, possibly because of the poor binding properties to CD86 [71]. Abatacept is registered as a treatment for rheumatoid arthritis. A CTLA4-Ig construct with superior binding affinity to CD86 was made by changing two amino acid residues in the CD80 and CD86 binding region. This construct, LEA29Y or belatacept, resulted in higher serum levels and far better kidney graft survival as compared to abatacept [70]. With the improved *in vivo* effects of belatacept, the first trials investigating belatacept as a treatment for kidney transplantation indicate that it is equally effective as CsA when added to the standard regimen of anti-IL-2R mAb induction therapy, MMF and steroids. Belatacept prevents biopsy proven acute rejection at 6 months equally well as CsA, but without the nephrotoxic side effects of CsA [72].

Blockade of the CD40-CD40L pathway can be achieved using antibodies against either CD40 or against CD40L. Four different antibodies directed against CD40L have been tested, (hu)5C8, ABI793, IDEC-131 and H106; of which the latter has only been tested in combination with CTLA4-Ig [65]. IDEC-131 was tested in combination with sirolimus and donor-specific blood transfusions [73]. Although this approach was rather successful, the mechanism may be different from costimulation blockade combined with conventional immunosuppressive drugs, because it relies on the deletion of donor-reactive cells [74]. It is therefore difficult to compare this treatment with other costimulation blocking antibodies. Monotherapy with either hu5C8, IDEC-131 or ABI793 can prolong graft survival, with a clear dose and duration dependent effect [61, 62, 73, 75, 76]. CD40L blocking mAb have been tested in combination with several different conventional immunosuppressive drugs and with other costimulation blocking antibodies. Combining anti-CD40L therapy with other immunosuppressive drugs does not lead to better graft survival than anti-CD40L monotherapy, and may even have adverse effects [63, 73, 77, 78]. Hu5C8 was also tested in human kidney transplant recipients, but trials were halted due to thromboembolic complications [79]. In addition, the effects of hu5C8 treatment on allograft survival were disappointing after the success of this treatment in the NHP kidney allograft model [76]. Thromboembolic effects observed in human patients were subsequently also recognised in NHP Experiments in NHP treated with anti-CD40L antibodies showed that microthrombi formed due to the aggregation of activated platelets that express CD40L, which was bound by the antibody, not only the hu5C8 antibody, but also by other anti-CD40L antibodies [61, 75]. Although this effect could be blocked by the use of anti-coagulation factors [80], scientists have changed their strategy to blocking the receptor at the side of the APC using antibodies directed against CD40.

Effects of antibodies binding CD40 can be either agonistic or antagonistic. Agonistic anti-CD40 mAb are used to stimulate immune reactions, but have also been shown to be effective in preventing NHP kidney allograft survival [65]. One aspect of such an agonistic anti-CD40 mAb, Chi220, is an almost complete depletion of peripheral B-cells, which lasts until 20 days after cessation of dosing. Treatment with Chi220 either alone, or in combination with CTLA4-Ig prevents rejection but when antibody administration was stopped after day 14, no long-term graft survival was observed. The effect of Chi220 on graft survival is unlikely to be due solely to the depletion of B-cells, since rejection can occur in B-cell deficient mice [81]. Recently, a fully human antagonistic anti-CD40 mAb, 4D11, was tested at dosages of 1, 5, 10, and 20 μg/kg, for a total of 180 days. Due to neutralisation of the anti-CD40 antibody, only a few animals of the groups receiving the two highest dosages maintained high levels of circulating antibody and could maintain their graft beyond the treatment period [67]. When combined with Rapamycin, the 5 μg/kg dose was considerably more effective [82]. Our lab has investigated the use of CD40-CD40L blockade with a chimeric anti-human anti-CD40 mAb clone ch5D12, as a possible way to induce tolerance. When anti-CD40 treatment resulted in high serum trough levels, it was found to prolong graft survival after cessation of treatment for 30 to 150 days. When serum concentrations were low during maintenance therapy, grafts were rejected during treatment [83]. A remarkable finding was the absence of significant levels of anti-donor antibodies in monkeys receiving ch5D12 [83]. Blockade of CD40 prevented activation of B-cells and inhibited T-cell dependent immunoglobulin production *in vitro* [84, 85]. The ch5D12 antibody prevented the production of donor-specific antibodies even until after the treatment was stopped. The agonistic anti-CD40 mAb Chi220 did not have this effect and the antagonistic mAb 4D11 only prevented anti-donor antibody formation during treatment [65, 67].

Although blockade of either costimulatory pathway alone is efficient for preventing rejection in most studies, the synergistic effect of blocking both pathways was investigated as well. Addition of CTLA4-Ig to 5C8 treatment is equally effective as hu5C8 monotherapy, although combined treatment with high dosages of both agents induced graft survival more than 150 days in two animals [62]. Combination of hu5C8 with antibodies directed against CD80 and CD86 leads to increased survival over therapy with antibodies against CD80 and CD86, but is not different from graft survival induced by hu5C8 monotherapy [86]. However, the combination is superior to blocking only one pathway with regard to prevention of development of donor-specific antibodies. The addition of anti-CD86 mAb (chFun-1) to the treatment with anti-CD40, clone ch5D12 tested in our lab, overcame the need for high anti-CD40 mAb serum levels. All animals treated with both antibodies survived the treatment period, although in some animals signs of rejection were seen already during treatment [83]. Addition of anti-CD86 to the treatment lowered the amount of infiltrating cells in the interstitium and tubules in day 21 biopsies, and even more in day 42 biopsies. Since the animals treated with both costimulation blocking antibodies had shorter graft survival than animals treated with only anti-CD40 mAb, we hypothesised that the infiltrates seen on day 42 may have a beneficial, regulatory function. However, treatment of patients with subclinical rejection resulted in improvement of graft survival as opposed to when subclinical infiltrates were not treated. These results indicated that at least in patients treated with conventional immunosuppressive drugs there is no evidence to support the possibility of benign graft infiltrates [87]. Whether the same holds true for subclinical infiltrates seen during treatment with costimulation blockade needs to be investigated further.

Several animals survived more than one year after high dose 181- or 365-day hu5C8 therapy [76]. No other costimulation blockade therapy was tested for the same duration at which hu5C8 was tested. Kidney graft survival in animals treated with hu5C8 for shorter periods was comparable to kidney graft survival in animals treated with other costimulation blocking reagents. Almost all animals that are able to maintain their graft drug-free for prolonged periods eventually loose their graft because of chronic rejection. Chronic rejection / CAN / IF/TA is a poorly understood process that seems to be less sensitive to immunosuppressive drugs or costimulation blockade.

Costimulation blockade as a single treatment is not a realistic option for clinical application. Any new therapy willl first be combined with conventional immunosuppressive drugs. For costimulation blockade, addition of conventional immunosuppressive drugs seems to add little effect on graft survival compared to costimulation blockade alone in experimental models. Caution is needed with the type of conventional immunosuppressive drugs. Initially, calcineurin inhibitors were shown not to interfere with anergy induction by costimulation blockade *in vitro* [88], but in the mouse skin transplant model, the calcineurin inhibitor CsA abolished the tolerogenic effect of CTLA4-Ig and anti-CD40L [55], although CsA contributed to skin graft survival when only CTLA4-Ig was given [89]. In NHP conventional immunosuppressive drugs were shown to have a negative impact on graft survival induced by hu5C8 therapy [63]. Rapamycin, a conventional immunosuppressive drug that prevents signalling through the common γ-chain of cytokine receptors, the receptor used by cytokines such as IL-2 and IL-15, may be a better candidate for combination with costimulation blockade [90,91], possibly because it allows initial activation of the cells via the TCR and allowing subsequent activation induced cell death (AICD) [90, 92]. *In vitro*, combination of anti-CD40 plus anti-CD86 costimulation blockade with tacrolimus or Rapamycin did not induce tolerance/anergy, while combination with CsA did [88]. However, CsA is a nephrotoxic drug. To allow for an initial conventional immunosuppressive drug-free period, combined anti-CD40 plus anti-CD86 costimulation blockade with a delayed onset (day 42) of CsA treatment was tested [93]. On day 42, none of the anti-CD40 plus anti-CD86 treated animals had started to reject, so CsA was given as supplementary immunosuppression and not as anti-rejection treatment. CsA was given at tapering dosages until day 126 after which all immunosuppression was stopped. This treatment prevented the graft rejection immediately after costimulation blockade withdrawal. However, two animals rejected after cessation of CsA treatment, one on day 140 and one in a more delayed fashion on day 231. Two animals lived more than six years after cessation of all treatment. Eventually, both animals had a slowly deteriorating kidney function, evidenced by increased serum creatinine levels and signs of CAN (IF/TA), in kidney biopsies. This outcome of chronic renal failure is very similar to what has been observed in NHP treated with hu5C8. A number of animals survived beyond the treatment period, but in the end, all developed CAN [94]. IF/TA is a poorly understood process. Attempts to reverse acute and chronic rejection with hu5C8 rescue therapy in monkeys initially treated with hu5C8, but drug-free for periods ranging from 8 to 395 days, were only partially successful [94]. Acute rejection after initial hu5C8 treatment could be reversed, but acute rejection after initial conventional immunosuppressive drugs and hu5C8 treatment could not be reversed. In addition, graft failure could not be reversed by the hu5C8 rescue therapy in monkeys with IF/TA.

Tolerance induction protocols based on mixed chimerism induction do not seem to be influenced by the addition of conventional immunosuppressive drugs such as the calcineurin inhibitors CsA and tacrolimus, Rapamycin, steroids or MMF [95].

Costimulation Blockade and Regulatory T-cells

In the early eighties, it was recognised that some cells of the immune system, so called suppressor cells, were able to downregulate T-effector cell function [96]. Failure to isolate the cells for further characterisation and clinical application led to a general disbelief that they existed [97]. The rediscovery by Sakaguchi et al. of a suppressor cell, the naturally occurring, thymus-derived CD25 expressing $CD4^+$ T-cell that prevented autoimmune diseases [98] put these so called regulatory T-cells (Tregs) back on the map. They could be isolated from the spleens of mice and from human peripheral blood by selecting $CD25^+$ cells (IL-2 receptor positive cells), enabling their *in vitro*, *in vivo* and *ex vivo* characterisation.

Mixed lymphocyte cultures/reactions (MLCs/MLRs) of recipient (responder) cells with irradiated donor (stimulator) cells are used to study rejection processes *in vitro*. MLCs in the presence of costimulation blockade induce a population of anergic cells in mice [99], humans [100] and also in NHP [101]. The anergic population can suppress an allogeneic (responder and stimulatory cells from different individuals) primary MLR. This raised the question whether the costimulation blockade induced anergic cells are natural Tregs and whether natural Tregs are important for the immunosuppressive effect of costimulation blockade. When $CD4^+$ T-cells are cultured with allogeneic stimulators in the presence of costimulation blockade by CD40L or anti-CD80 plus anti-CD86, the resulting population is only anergic and suppressive in the mouse graft-versus-host disease (GVHD) model when $CD4^+CD25^+$ cells are present from the start of the culture [102]. This was confirmed *in vitro* using mouse MLRs. Costimulation blockade by anti-CD86 and anti-CD40L was more effective in the presence of Tregs [103].

Despite the well-established beneficial effect of costimulation blockade on graft survival and in autoimmune models, the effect of costimulation blockade on the induction and actions of natural Tregs is much less clear. Costimulation blockade and Tregs have synergistic effects. Costimulation blockade can suppress effector T-cells (Teff) and with Tregs present, the balance between Teff and Tregs shifts in favour of Tregs [103]. Possibly, costimulation blockade and Tregs work on different arms of the immune system, with both components needed for optimal downregulation of the immune response.

CTLA-4 is expressed at high levels in naturally occurring Tregs. However, the effect of blocking CTLA-4 on the function of Tregs remains a matter of debate. CTLA-4 blockade *in vitro* did not inhibit suppression mediated by Tregs, rather, it affected Teff directly. Costimulation blockade (anti-CD86 + anti-CD40L) induced inhibition of $CD8^+$ T-cell division was abrogated by CTLA-4 blockade [104]. In contrast, CTLA-4 blockade abrogates Treg mediated suppression of colitis by targeting Tregs directly. CTLA-4 deficient $CD8^+$ effector T-cell mediated colitis is inhibited by Tregs and this suppression is inhibited by anti-CTLA-4 mAb [105].

In conclusion, most evidence points towards separate functions of costimulation blockade and natural Tregs in the mechanism of suppression. They can benefit from each other, but each can act separate from the other.

Regulatory T-Cells

Phenotype of Human Naturally Occurring Regulatory T-cells *ex vivo*

Shortly after the rediscovery of regulatory cells in mice by Sakaguchi and colleagues [98], and the *in vitro* analysis of mouse $CD4^+CD25^+$ cells, a homologous CD25 expressing Treg population was isolated from human blood. Mouse $CD4^+CD25^+$ T-cells have a rather homogeneous CD25 expression. About 10% of resting $CD4^+$ T-cells express CD25 and this entire CD25 expression population is regulatory [98]. CD25 expression can be detected on up to 46% of all $CD4^+$ human T-cells in the peripheral blood [106, 107]. However only the population with the highest CD25 expression and a somewhat lower CD4 expression as compared to Th cells displays regulatory function. $CD25^{high}$ cells comprise around 1-3% of total $CD4^+$ T-cells [107–110]. Tregs were not only identified in peripheral blood, but also in cord blood, thymus, lymph node and spleen [107, 109, 111]. Initially, no specific marker for Tregs was available to facilitate analysis of Tregs. Tregs are identified by a combination of phenotypic and functional analyses.

In addition to high CD25 and lower CD4 expression, natural Tregs differ from Th cells with regard to the expression of a number of other markers. $CD4^+CD25^{high}$ cells are mainly of a memory phenotype ($CD45RO^+CD45RA^-$) [108], although Tregs with a naive, intermediate CD25 expression ($CD25^{int}$) phenotype have also been described [109, 112]. CD25 expressing cells in cord blood are mainly of the naive phenotype [107, 109]. With ageing and encounter of antigens, a population of $CD25^{high}$, memory Tregs emerges, explaining the presence of naive as well as memory Tregs. Although it was initially thought that Tregs are generated as a separate lineage from the thymus [113], Vukmanovic-Stejic et al. show that indeed $CD25^{high}$ expressing cells are more likely to be generated in the periphery, as they showed a rapid turnover [110]. Some $CD25^{int}$ naive Tregs are still present in adult peripheral blood [109, 112]. This population is missed when gating on $CD25^{high}$ cells and is not analysed in most reports.

Natural $CD25^{high}$ Tregs express activation markers such as HLA-DR and CD122 (IL-2Rβ) [107, 108, 114] and the lymph node homing markers CD62L and CCR7 [108, 112].

Furthermore, expression of a number of markers associated with downregulation of the immune response, such as CTLA-4 and GITR is significantly higher on Tregs as compared to $CD25^{int}$ or $CD25^{-}CD4^{+}$ T-cells [107, 114].

An important functional property of Tregs is the absence of a proliferative response after polyclonal or allogeneic stimulation [108, 112, 114]. Polyclonal stimulation is usually done with plate-bound anti-CD3, which stimulates T-cells via the TCR, without the need for costimulation. Increasing the amount of plate-bound anti-CD3 and adding soluble anti-CD28 increases the signal strength. Addition of IL-2 can even further enhance the strength of the stimulus. Natural Tregs are resistant to activation by polyclonal stimulation only to a certain level. When a threshold is reached, Tregs start to proliferate and they (temporarily) loose their suppressive capacity [108, 112, 114]. This feature can be exploited to expand Tregs. Not only do Tregs not proliferate when stimulated (below the threshold level), they also do not produce cytokines such as IFN-γ, IL-2 and IL-13 [108, 112, 114], although some IL-4 and IL-10 may be produced [112, 114].

The first most important functional feature however, is the capacity of Tregs to down regulate responses by $CD4^{+}CD25^{-}$ cells. Tregs can suppress responses of $CD4^{+}CD25^{-}$ cells in a dose-dependent and cell-cell contact dependent manner [108, 112]. The cell-cell contact dependent suppression may act via CTLA-4 and/or membrane-bound TGF-β1, since antibodies directed against these molecules abrogated suppression by $CD4^{+}CD25^{+}$ thymocytes [111].

Therapeutic applicability of Tregs would greatly benefit from the identification of a marker that is specific for Tregs and that is preferentially expressed on the cell surface. No definitive marker has been found thus far and therefore we can only identify Tregs on the basis of their functional suppressive activity. By correlating functional activity with expression of phenotypic markers on these cells, these markers can then be used to identify putative suppressive cells. One such marker seems to be FOXP3.

FOXP3

Since 1949 an inbred mouse strain was studied which was called the scurfy mouse, because of scaling of its skin. It had a number of immune related problems that resembled graft-versus host disease [115]. A mutation in a X-linked gene was responsible for this phenotype and sequence analysis of the gene revealed that it encoded a novel member of the forkhead/winged-helix family of transcriptional regulators, Foxp3 [116]. Very soon thereafter it was recognised that many patients with the immunodysregulation, polyendocrinopathy, enteropathy X-linked syndrome (IPEX), a syndrome very similar to the scurfy mouse, also had mutations in the transcription factor gene encoding FOXP3 [117–122]. Not all IPEX patients have mutations in the FOXP3 gene, but they may have mutations in other genes that interact with FOXP3. It was immediately recognised that FOXP3 was mainly expressed intracellularly in naturally occurring $CD4^{+}CD25^{+}$ Tregs [123, 124]. Ectopic Foxp3 expression can convert $CD25^{-}$ cells into regulatory cells [125, 126] and targeted disruption of the Foxp3 gene leads to reduced activity of Tregs [123].

A population of $CD4^{+}CD25^{+}FOXP3^{+}$ T-cells is also present in humans [127]. However, unlike in mice, low level FOXP3 expression can be detected in $CD4^{+}CD25^{-}$ and $CD8^{+}$ cells [123, 128, 129]. $CD4^{+}CD25^{+}FOXP3^{+}$ cells are not a uniform population, as both naive and memory $CD4^+$ cells express FOXP3 [127]. Two FOXP3 isoforms can be found in human Tregs, an ortholog to the mouse Foxp3 and an isoform lacking exon 2 [130, 131]. Human $FOXP3^+$ Tregs have similar functions as mouse $Foxp3^+$ Tregs; they are anergic and can suppress immune responses [108, 124]. An even more striking difference between mice and humans is the induction of FOXP3 expression in activated cells [124, 128, 129, 132–136]. Some reports indicate that these induced $FOXP3^+$ cells become regulatory [124, 132, 133, 136], but others indicate that this is not the case [128, 134]. Ectopic expression of either isoform of FOXP3 induced an anergic, but not a suppressive phenotype [130]. Possibly, sustained FOXP3 expression after activation is needed for the induction of a regulatory cell type, while transient expression of FOXP3 is not representative of a regulatory phenotype [137].

Expression of FOXP3 is facilitated by the integrated signalling of the TCR, CD28 and the common γ-chain receptor [138, 139]. TCR signalling mediates activation of calcineurin, which in turn dephosphorylates nuclear factor of activated T-cells (NFAT). Activated NFAT is translocated to the nucleus. NFAT is a transcription factor for many genes, including FOXP3 [135, 140] and IL-2. CsA is an inhibitor of calcineurin. It has been used for over 25 years in transplantation to inhibit TCR mediated IL-2 production, thereby preventing graft rejection. More recently, it was shown that CsA also inhibits FOXP3 expression [135, 141].

FOXP3 is very important for the function of Tregs. However, it does not fulfil the criteria as definitive, clinically applicable marker for Tregs. It is not expressed on the cell surface, and thus far, no Treg specific, cell surface expressed products of FOXP3 mediated transcription have been identified. Furthermore, it is not only expressed on natural Tregs, but can also be induced on $CD4^+CD25^-$ T-cells. Whether cells with induced FOXP3 are suppressive in all circumstances remains a matter of debate.

TGF-β

One of the side effects of long-term CsA treatment is fibrosis of kidney tissue, not only of transplanted kidneys, but also of native kidneys [142–144]. This effect of CsA is mediated by the cytokine transforming growth factor-β (TGF-β) [145]. CsA inhibits calcineurin, which leads to increased expression of TGF-β [146]. TGF-β enhances extracellular matrix remodelling and wound healing, hence its profibrotic reputation [147].

Besides its profibrotic effects, TGF-β is also known for its anti-inflammatory and antiproliferative effects. TGF-β knockout mice suffer from multi-organ inflammatory diseases [148, 149]. TGF-β1 can downregulate IL-2 induced proliferation [150], thereby acting directly on responder cells. TGF-β also suppresses IFN-γ production by NK-cells, which prevents Th1 development [151]. Intravenous injection of an adenoviral vector encoding human active TGF-β can restore self-tolerance in the non-obese diabetic (NOD) mouse, a mouse model for diabetes [152]. Furthermore, TGF-β is implicated in upregulation of CD25 and FOXP3 after activation of $CD4^+CD25^-$ cells, leading to the subsequent acquisition of a regulatory function of these cells [133, 153–155]. After activation, these $CD4^+CD25^-$ cells also upregulate CD103 [153], which may link them to the $CD25^-CD103^+$ regulatory cells that are found in tonsils and which also upregulate CD25 after allogeneic stimulation in the presence of endogenous TGF-β [156]. They may start to produce TGF-β themselves and they can inhibit naive cells [153]. Suppression is mostly cell-cell contact dependent, although inhibition of IL-10 and TGF-β may decrease suppression [154].

TGF-β is secreted as an inactive, latent complex, which is held in an inactive conformation by its own propeptide, the latency-associated peptide (LAP). Thrombospondin can convert the latent TGF-β into active TGF-β, by dissociating LAP from the complex. In mice, LAP is a positive marker for yet another type of regulatory $CD4^+$ T-cell population [157]. In humans, LAP^+ immature DC promote down-regulation of the immune responses by suppressing Th1 differentiation [158].

Possible mechanisms by which TGF-β may act to induce FOXP3 expression is that FOXP3 increases its own expression via the positive feedback loop via SMAD7 (short for mothers against decapentaplegic homologue 7), on $CD4^+CD25^-$ cells. SMAD7 normally inhibits TGF-β mediated signalling. FOXP3 expression inhibits the expression of SMAD7, thereby increasing TGF-β mediated FOXP3 induction [133]. In mice, the presence of IL-2 is required for the TGF-β mediated upregulation of Foxp3 [159].

In conclusion, TGF-β is an important cytokine in the anti-inflammatory immune response. Although the mechanism remains elusive, one possibility is that it is expressed on immature DC and thereby induces FOXP3 in T-cells. This process can be mimicked *in vitro* by the exogenous addition of TGF-β to the cultures, thereby using the suppressive properties of this cytokine.

Treg Targets; DC versus T-cell

The mechanism of suppression by natural Tregs remains largely unknown, although some key elements were identified, such as intact FOXP3 expression and cell-cell contact. It is clear that Tregs can suppress $CD4^+CD25^-$ cells, as demonstrated by numerous *in vitro* experiments. Annunziato et al. showed that CTLA-4 and membrane bound TGF-β1 may be involved [111], although this was not confirmed by Jonuleit et al. [160]. Furthermore, IL-2 seems to play an important role. Uptake of IL-2 by the $CD4^+CD25^+$ cells also seems to depend on cell-cell contact [161]. As discussed above, the strength and type of the activation signal determines whether Tregs remain unresponsive and suppressive. Addition of a high concentration of IL-2 is one way to alter responsiveness and capacity to suppress [108,112]. Possibly, Tregs suppress immune responses by taking up IL-2, before the IL-2 can activate responder cells in an autocrine mechanism. This would be in accordance with the finding that responder cells do not upregulate CD25 in the presence of Tregs [111]. Once IL-2 levels reach a threshold, Tregs can no longer take up all IL-2 present, the remaining IL-2 can then activate responder cells and Tregs to start proliferating, producing cytokines and upregulate CD25. In addition to the uptake of IL-2, Tregs also suppress the cytokine production of Teff directly, mediated by Foxp3. Foxp3 binds to the transcription factors NFAT and nuclear factor κB (NF-κB), which prevents the NFAT and NF-κB mediated transcription of cytokine genes [162].

Experiments in mice show that Tregs express glucocorticoid-induced T-cell receptor (GITR) [163]. Activation of Tregs through soluble GITR ligand (sGITR-L) induces GITR dependent NF-κB activation. Activation of $CD4^+CD25^-$ cells through sGITR-L induced IL-2 production by $CD25^-$ cells. IL-2 and sGITR-L together induce proliferation of $CD25^+$ Tregs [164], further stressing the importance of IL-2 as a modulator of suppressive activity of Tregs.

Suppression of $CD4^+CD25^-$ cells does not seem to be the only mechanism by which Tregs can downregulate immune responses, they also affect DC maturation. Tregs prevent the maturation of myeloid DC, but not of plasmacytoid DC, induced by stimulation of several toll-like receptors (TLRs). This mechanism is, like T-cell suppression, cell-cell contact dependent [165]. Further evidence for Treg mediated modulation of DC comes from the observation that DC co-cultured with autologous anti-CD3 stimulated T-cells or allogeneic T-cells, acquire a semimature phenotype when the T-cells are Tregs. When the T-cells are naive cells or memory cells, DC acquire a mature phenotype [166]. Mechanisms of suppression, as described above, have thus far only been studied as isolated events; an integrated view has not emerged yet. Knowledge of this process is very important to be able to move application of Tregs as a therapy towards the clinic.

Towards Clinical Application of Tregs: *in vivo* Manipulation of Tregs

Natural Tregs are present only at low numbers in the peripheral blood. The amount is too low for isolation and direct clinical application. Tregs will need to be manipulated before it will be possible to use them for therapeutic purposes. Two ways of manipulation are currently investigated: *in vitro* or *in vivo*. *In vivo* enhancement of Tregs is a successful method in the treatment of autoimmune diseases. Treatment with an anti-CD3 mAb prevents further progression of diabetes in new-onset diabetes patients [167]. The anti-CD3 mAb induces $Foxp3^+$ Tregs from $CD4^+CD25^-$ peripheral T-cells in the NOD mouse [168]. Treatment with anti-CD3 mAb has not been tested in the setting of allotransplantation yet. In human recent onset diabetes anti-CD3 treatment is a promising treatment that reverses diabetes [169]. Whether Tregs are responsible for the success of the treatment needs to be established. A second mechanism of *in vivo* manipulation is transplantation under the cover of costimulation blockade. Activation of responder cells in a mouse MLR was inhibited by costimulation blockade by anti-CD86 and anti-CD40L. Inhibition was more effective in the presence of Tregs, possibly by shifting the balance between Teff and Tregs in favour of Tregs [103]. The effect of costimulation blockade on Tregs *in vivo* is more difficult to demonstrate.

In vivo induction of Tregs was demonstrated in a patient with severe combined immune deficiency (SCID) who developed tolerance to a stem-cell allograft [170]. These IL-10 producing Tregs were called Tr1 cells and are discussed further below.

Towards Clinical Application of Tregs: *in vitro* Induction or Expansion of Regulatory $CD4^+$ T-cells

Two *in vitro* approaches are investigated to obtain larger numbers of Tregs. One approach is to isolate natural Tregs and expand them, either by culturing them with a polyclonal stimulus in the presence of growth factors such as IL-2 and/or IL-15 [171], or by culturing them with donor cells in the presence of growth factors [172, 173]. Expanded $CD4^+CD25^+$ cells can become regulatory after polyclonal stimulation without addition of modulatory agents; as long as the starting population is $CD4^+CD25^+CD45RA^+$ [171]. Suppressive activity may vary according to type of polyclonal stimulus [124]. The expansion with donor cells leads to a lower number of Tregs after the same number of expansion rounds when compared to expansion with beads. However, antigen-specific expanded Tregs can suppress responder cells at lower responder cell to regulator cell ratios in an antigen-specific mechanism [172, 174, 175]. Isolation of Tregs with high suppressive capacity may be further enhanced by including or excluding cells on the basis of certain markers. Highly suppressive Tregs are included in the $CD27^+$ subset of expanded Tregs [172] and/or in the $CD127^-$ subset [176].

The second approach to obtain larger numbers of Tregs is to culture $CD4^+CD25^-$ cells, which are present in much higher numbers in the peripheral blood, under conditions that favour the conversion into $CD4^+CD25^+$ cells with regulatory capacity. An example of such a Treg inducing condition is to culture in the presence of TGF-β [133, 153–155]. In addition to TGF-β, also other mechanisms have been described to induce regulatory cells from total $CD4^+$ or $CD4^+CD25^-$ cells. Prostaglandin E_2 is secreted by several tumour cells and may suppress anti-tumour responses [177]. A possible explanation for the suppression of immune responses against the tumour is the induction of cells with a regulatory phenotype from $CD4^+CD25^-$ cells by Prostaglandin E_2 [132]. Stimulation with DC can also induce regulatory cells. Verhasselt et al. report that the DC need to be mature, whereas Jonuleit et al. report that immature DC are needed to obtain cells with regulatory function [136, 178]. The stimulation of naive $CD4^+$ T-cells with immature DC results in an IL-10 producing, anergic and suppressive population. IL-10 producing suppressive cells induced after alloantigen stimulation are collectively called T regulatory type 1 (Tr1) cells. Tr1 cells also produce low level IFN-γ [179]. They differ from natural Tregs in that they do not express CD25 at high levels and they do not require cell-cell contact for suppression, since the mode of action is mainly through IL-10. A cell-cell contact dependent mechanism is not completely excluded, though. Tr1 cells do not constitutively express FOXP3, although FOXP3 will be upregulated upon activation, as in activated $CD4^+CD25^-$ cells (for a complete review of the features of Tr1 cells see Battaglia et al. and Roncarolo et al. [180, 181]). The clear evidence of an *in vivo* role for Tr1 cells in SCID patients has already led to the first clinical trials exploiting the regulatory capacity of these cells. Donor cells are tolerised against the host *in vitro*, by culturing them in the presence of IL-10. The tolerised cells are then transfused into the myeloablated host, together with donor stem cells in a Human Leukocyte Antigen (HLA) haploidentical setting [180].

Tr1 cells can also be induced when $CD4^+CD25^-$ cells are cultured with natural Tregs [178, 182]. Tr1 cells may also secrete TGF-β and an important feature for their induction seems to be the presence of IL-10 [183]. However, culturing of $CD4^+CD25^-$ cells with natural Tregs may also lead to the induction of another type of Treg, the Th3 cell, which primarily produces TGF-β, although distinction between Th3 and Tr1 is difficult, since they have many overlapping features. Th3 cells can also be induced *in vivo* after oral exposure to the specific antigen.

Other Types of Regulatory T-cells

Several types of non-$CD4^+$ Tregs have been described, in virtually every main lymphocyte subset. $CD8^+CD28^-$ T-cells have been described by Sucia-Foca and colleagues. $CD8^+CD28^-$ T-cells induce the expression of immunoglobulin-like transcript 3 (ILT3) and

ILT4 on monocytes and DCs, rendering them tolerogenic and unable to stimulate $CD4^+$ T-cells [184]. $CD3^+CD4^-CD8^-$ T-cells were first identified in the mouse skin transplantation model [185], but may also play a role in humans [186]. The NKT-cell subset also has its regulatory subpopulation. They were also first identified in mice, but were later implicated in human autoimmune diseases (reviewed by Jiang et al. [187]). Regulatory NKT-cells may also play a role in transplantation [188]. The existence of regulatory B-cells was first suggested in 1996 [189]. They seem to play a role in autoimmune and infectious disease models. The main mechanism of suppression is via production of IL-10, but the clinical relevance of regulatory B-cells needs to be established further [190].

It is clear that nature has found several ways to regulate immune responses. Without such regulatory mechanisms, infections of any kind would lead to an excessive immune response. To make use of these types of regulatory cells for the induction of transplantation tolerance, is clearly a challenge for future research.

Regulatory T-cells in Non-human Primates

Costimulation blockade can increase the number of Tregs over effector T-cells *in vitro*, when stimulated with allogeneic cells [103]. The resulting anergic T-cell population can suppress alloantigen responses [100, 103]. This was tested both *in vitro* and *in vivo* using NHP. Costimulation blockade using anti-CD80 + anti-CD86 was used to render *ex vivo* cultured alloreactive T-cells anergic [101]. These cells were unresponsive towards donor antigens, but not towards 3rd party antigens in culture. The number of CD25 and CTLA-4 expressing cells was increased amongst anergic cells.

Subsequently, these cells were tested *in vivo*. On the day of allogeneic kidney transplantation, a culture of recipient cells with donor or 3rd party cells was initiated with or without costimulation blockade using antibodies against CD80 and/or CD86. Recipients were treated with cyclophosphamide and CsA for 13 days, after which cultured cells were infused. Cultured cells were anergic *in vitro* and recipients treated with cells stimulated with donor cells in the presence of both anti-CD80 + anti-CD86 showed prolonged graft survival. Kidney graft survival of control monkeys in which cells cultured with 3rd party cells or cells cultured with donor cells plus only one of the antibodies were infused was significantly shorter.

Natural Tregs and Tr1 cells were characterised in normal monkeys as well as in tolerant kidney graft recipient monkeys [191, 192]. As in other species, monkey natural Tregs exhibit a memory phenotype and can suppress polyclonally activated $CD4^+CD25^-$ responder cells. Analysis of Tregs in tolerant monkeys reveals that they have significantly more $CD4^+$ $CD25^+$ cells in the periphery and significantly more IL-10 in the circulation. However, these latter results cannot be valued to its full extent, because the original article describing the tolerance induction [191] in these monkeys has been retracted [193]. Natural Tregs in NHP have also been identified and expanded [192, 194, 195]. All three describe a protocol for expansion of the cells using anti-CD3/anti-CD28 coated beads. Anderson et al. [194] subsequently sort on the $CD25^+CD127^{low/-}$ population, which generated a highly suppressive population.

Evidence for induced Tregs *in vivo* in NHP also comes from the observation that TGF-β^+ cells could be found in kidney biopsies from tolerant and long-term drug-free rhesus monkeys [196]. TGF-β was found to be responsible for the (down) regulation of the donor-specific response.

Involvement of TGF-β, IL10, FOXP3 and natural Tregs was also established in another NHP model. African green monkeys (agm) are natural hosts for simian immunodeficiency virus (SIV), and the SIV viruses are normally non-pathogenic in their natural hosts. Infection of African green monkeys with SIVagm is accompanied by an immediate anti-inflammatory response [197]. The number of $CD4^+CD25^+$ cells in the periphery is increased and TGF-β, IL-10, and FOXP3 expression are upregulated.

Human Tregs are characterized by higher expression of CD25 and lower expression of CD4 as compared to Th cells. Up to 46% of total $CD4^+$ cells may be positive for CD25, but only 1-3% are $CD25^{high}$. Mouse Tregs have a more uniform CD25 expression and all $CD25^+$ cells have a regulatory function [107–110]. Rhesus monkey $CD4^+$ cells have a uniform expression of CD25 as described by us and others [101, 191, 195, 198]. This expression pattern resembles more the CD25 expression pattern as found in mice, and in human cord blood [109]. Mouse and cord blood $CD4^+CD25^+$ cells are immunologically naive, but rhesus monkey $CD4^+CD25^+$ are not immunologically naive, as indicated by the low percentage of $CD45RA^+CCR7^+$ cells in this population [198]. The difference in CD25 staining pattern between human and rhesus monkey $CD25^+$ cells is most likely due to the species difference, but a difference in binding kinetics of the CD25 antibody cannot be excluded. Arbitrary separation of the $CD4^+CD25^+$ population into a $CD4^+CD25^{int}$ population and a $CD4^+CD25^{high}$ population indicates that both populations express CTLA-4 and FOXP3 at higher levels as compared to $CD4^+CD25^-$ cells, and that highest expression can be found in the $CD4^+CD25^{high}$ population. In conclusion, rhesus monkey $CD4^+CD25^+$ share phenotypical characteristics with human $CD4^+CD25^{high}$ cells, although Th cells may be included in the rhesus monkey $CD4^+CD25^+$ population.

Isolation of the $CD4^+CD25^+$ cells selectively enriched for the $CD4^+$ cells expressing CD25 at high levels. Functional analysis of this population revealed that this population was anergic and suppressed the activity of $CD4^+CD25^-$ cells. $CD4^+CD25^+$ cells did not respond to polyclonal ConA stimulation, plate-bound anti-CD3 or allogeneic stimulation, although individual variation was detected [198]. Furthermore, rhesus monkey $CD25^+$ cells inhibited $CD25^-$ cells stimulated with plate-bound anti-CD3 or allogeneic cells. Inhibition was demonstrated at the level of proliferation as well as IL-2 and IFN-γ production. The mechanism of suppression depended on cell-cell contact and suppression was not inhibited by the addition of antibodies against the suppressive cytokines TGF-β and IL-10. To conclude, rhesus monkey $CD4^+CD25^+$ have a comparable functional phenotype as human Tregs [108, 114].

In conclusion, Tregs, TGF-β, and IL-10 are present in NHP, and they have similar effects in NHP as in mice and humans. These results warrant further development of the rhesus monkey model as model to study the induction of tolerance by Tregs. The low amount of naturally occurring Tregs in the periphery necessitates enlargement of the number of Tregs before therapeutic application of Tregs is feasible. Enlargement of the number of Tregs can be achieved either by induction of Tregs from non-regulatory $CD4^+CD25^-$ cells, or by expansion of the naturally occurring Treg population. Knowledge of the phenotype and functional suppressive capacities of naturally occurring Tregs in NHP will guide the evaluation of the phenotype and function of NHP induced or expanded Tregs.

Characterization of Graft-Infiltrating Cells

Transplantation research would benefit from the identification of a marker or set of markers that would indicate whether it is safe to withdraw immunosuppression in long-term stable patients. The monkey model of transplantation provides a unique opportunity to study markers inside the graft that may be indicative of tolerance because immunosuppressive treatment is always withdrawn at some point, in all studies. The survival and function of the graft after drug withdrawal can then be related to immune parameters prior to drug withdrawal. We studied expression profiles of leucocyte subset markers and Treg markers inside the graft in a number of animals, which were grouped according to the presence or absence of rejection and the type of immunosuppression [199].

Nodular infiltrates develop over time, when the tissues are rejected, forming structures resembling lymphoid follicles with clear T-cell and B-cell areas. These structures are called tertiary lymphoid organs and can be found in a variety of chronic inflammatory conditions [200]. The lymphoid-like structures suggest that antigen presentation takes place in these structures. The composition of nodular infiltrates differs considerably from the composition of diffuse infiltrates; higher percentages of $CD4^+$ T-cells, $CD20^+$ B-cells and $CD83^+$ DCs, and lower percentages $CD68^+$ macrophages were present in the nodular infiltrates. In addition, the composition of the infiltrates also differs considerably in rejected versus non-rejected grafts. Rejected grafts had higher percentages of $CD20^+$ cells in nodular infiltrates; furthermore they had higher percentages of $CD4^+$ cells, $CD20^+$ cells, $CD68^+$ cells and $CD83^+$ cells in diffuse infiltrates.

Rejected and non-rejected kidney speciments were each subdivided according to the type of immunosuppression, e.g. costimulation blockade, CsA, no immunosuppression. For non-rejected tissues the additional category no immunosuppression and graft survival for more than six months without immunosuppression, the long-term survivors (LTS) was defined. We observed that the type of immunosuppression was generally of little influence on the composition of the infiltrates.

Differences between rejected and non-rejected tissues and influence of the type or the absence of immunuosuppression were studied. It was hypothesized that non-rejected tissues and in particular in tissues from animals without immunosuppression may have higher percentages of Treg marker positive cells in the grafts. Currently, FOXP3, a nuclear transcription factor, is the most specific marker for Tregs. Suppressive natural $CD4^+$ T-cells express FOXP3, but in humans, non-suppressive cells may also (temporarily) express FOXP3, which makes them anergic, but not suppressive [128, 134, 137]. Other markers expressed on Tregs such as CD25, CTLA-4, CD103 and GITR were also investigated, although these markers can also be expressed on activated cells.

The percentage $FOXP3^+$ cells is higher in nodular infiltrates than in diffuse infiltrates. In both nodular and diffuse infiltrates percentages $FOXP3^+$ cells are higher in samples from rejected than from non-rejected kidneys. Percentages of $CD25^+$ and CTLA-4^+ cells followed this same pattern. The percentages $GITR^+$ cells were also higher in nodular infiltrates, but no differences were found between rejected and non-rejected tissues. High percentages of $CD103^+$ cells were found in diffuse infiltrates of rejected tissues, but even more in tubular infiltrates. $CD8^+$ T-cells were found in tubular infiltrates of rejected tissues in similar numbers as $CD103^+$ cells, indicating that these were most likely $CD8^+CD103^+$

CTLs infiltrating the tubules [201].

The observation that higher percentages of FOXP3$^+$, CD25$^+$ and CTLA-4$^+$ T-cells were associated with rejection was further strengthened by the observation that only low percentages of cells positive for these markers were found in four animals in the LTS group. Percentages of cells expressing FOXP3, CD25 and CTLA-4 did not significantly differ between the other subgroups defined by type of immunosuppression.

Veronese et al. have investigated the presence of FOXP3$^+$ cells in tissues with acute cellular and humoral rejection [202]. Although they did not compare this with non-rejected tissues, they also found increased numbers of FOXP3$^+$ cells in patients with shorter graft survival. Their observation that the majority (96%) of FOXP3$^+$ cells are CD4$^+$ T-cells is also consistent with our findings. Interestingly, they found FOXP3$^+$ cells in tubuli, which was not confirmed in our study. This discrepancy could be due to differences between humans and NHP, the antibodies used or the fact that they investigated tissues which had been rejected in the presence of immunosuppression, whereas most of our rejected tissue samples came from animals without immunosuppression.

We conclude that high percentages of the Treg markers FOXP3, CD25 and CTLA-4 are not indicative for acceptance of the graft, as percentages of cells positive for these markers were significantly higher in nodular infiltrates of rejected tissues. Two not mutually-exclusive explanations may account for the presence of regulatory markers inside rejected grafts. Either, these markers are not representative for a regulatory function of these cells, as was shown *in vitro* [128,134,137], or regulatory cells expressing CD25, FOXP3 and CTLA-4 represent a failed counter-active mechanism, limiting immune activation. When during rejection the number of effector T-cells increases, the number of regulatory T-cells, already present in healthy and diseased individuals, is also increased (Fig. 2). This process occurs in the absence of immunosuppression, when no long-term drug free survival is achieved, but may also occur in the presence of immunosuppression, when the immunosuppressive treatment is unable to prevent an anti-donor response in the graft.

Memory T-cells and the Barrier to Induce Tolerance in Memory T-cells

Considering the available markers to monitor regulatory cells and the long-term graft survival after costimulation blockade in rodents, costimulation blockade in higher primates has been disappointingly unsuccessful. Of the twelve strategies known to induce tolerance in rodents, only four work partially in NHP models of transplantation, or in a clinical setting [203]. One reason for this discrepancy may be the different levels of antigen-experienced cells between rodents and primates. Mice used for transplantation studies are kept in a specific pathogen-free (SPF) environment. Costimulation blockade can easily induce tolerance in these SPF, and thus immunologically naive mice. If however, mice go through a viral infection, tolerance can no longer be induced, by the various tolerance inducing protocols, including costimulation blockade [204,205]. It is now believed that virus induced memory cells can cross-react with donor antigens after transplantation, a process named heterologous immunity. In addition to viral antigen-induced allospecific T-cells, patients often also have allo-reactive memory cells induced by prior transplants, pregnancy, or blood transfusions [206]. In patients with high pre-transplant anti-donor reactivity, as measured by IFN-γ Elispot, an increased incidence of rejection is observed [207,208].

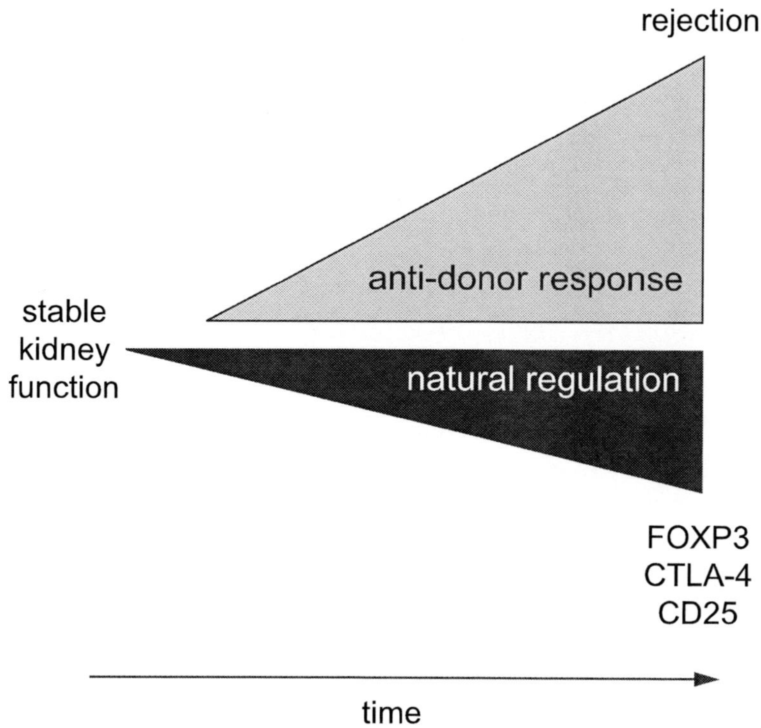

Figure 2. Hypothetical representation of the immune response in the graft. In case of stable transplant function, there is little need for the presence of active immune regulation in the graft. Upon anti-donor T-cells entrance in the graft, regulatory T-cells might also enter the graft, explaining the presence of high numbers of cells with regulatory T-cell markers in rejected tissues.

The presence of memory T-cells is a complication when one considers costimulation blockade as an anti-rejection treatment. Memory T-cells have a lower activation threshold and are less dependent on costimulation via CD28 or CD40L for full activation [209–212]. Unlike naive T-cells, memory T-cells circulate through, and can mount an immune response in peripheral non-lymphoid tissues [213, 214].

Donor antigen recognition by memory T-cells is difficult to be inhibited by costimulation blockade of the B7-CD28 and CD40-CD40L pathways, since these pathways are more important in the activation of naive cells.

Zhai et al. showed, that allo-antigen primed $CD8^+$ T-cells do not depend on CD154 signalling to mediate rejection [215]. Also memory $CD4^+$ T-cells were shown to be resistant to CD154 blockade in a mouse heart allograft model using donor-specific transfusion [216]. Significance of cross-reactive viral antigen-specific T-cells in humans was demonstrated by the fact that Epstein-Barr virus (EBV)-specific $CD4^+$ or $CD8^+$ T-cell clones recognise alloantigens and respond by killing dendritic cells expressing MHC molecules commonly found in the population [217, 218]. Cytomegalovirus (CMV)-specific $CD8^+$ T-cells cross-react with allogeneic cells, although no cytotoxic killing of the target cells could be demonstrated [219].

Special attention needs to be addressed to the fact that homeostatic expansion of peripheral cells leads to induction of a population of cells with a memory phenotype [220], a process also seen in human transplant patients treated with the T-cell depleting agents alemtuzumab (anti-CD52, a common T-cell antigen) or rabbit anti-thymocyte globulin (ATG) [221]. Without low-dose immunosuppression, patients experience rejection indicating the sustained presence of allo-reactive cells [221–223]. In addition, T-cells undergoing homeostatic expansion cannot be tolerised by costimulation blockade as was shown in a mouse heart allograft model [224], which is not surprising, given the inability of costimulation blockade to effectively block memory T-cell responses [209–212]. Interestingly, Tregs seem to be spared and/or preferentially expanded after ATG treatment [225], a phenomenon that is further enhanced by sirolimus, but not CsA maintenance therapy [226]. In mice, experiments to investigate whether or not Tregs are spared and preferentially expanded after lymphocyte depletion yielded contradictory results [227, 228]. However, adoptive transfer of Tregs or blocking homeostatic expansion provide a possible strategy to overcome the problems of homeostatic expansion [228].

The detrimental effects of memory T-cells on costimulation blockade induced survival became apparent when we combined ATG treatment, to reduce circulating heterologous immune cells with costimulation blockade. Although delayed CsA treatment had an additive effect on costimulation blockade treatment in our model, it was insufficient to prevent rejection in two of the four animals [93]. We therefore hypothesised that induction therapy with ATG would remove alloreactive cells present in the normal repertoire, leaving a population that could be more easily tolerised by costimulation blockade [204, 215, 229]. CsA treatment was initiated on day 42. Surprisingly, two out of five ATG treated animals experienced rejection during these first 42 days (days 21 and 38), while none of the nine non-ATG treated animals rejected their kidneys in this period [230]. Rejections were defined as a 50% rise of the serum creatinine levels within three to four days. First rejections in the ATG treated animals were treated with steroids if they occurred after day 42, and all animals received high dose CsA from day 42 onwards. However, this did not reverse the ongoing rejection process, leading to shorter graft survival times as compared to costimulation blockade plus CsA treated animals. It appeared that our first assumption was not correct. $CD4^+$ and $CD8^+$ T-cells were analyzed for the naive subset $CD95^{low}/CD11a^{low}$. Memory T-cells were defined as the remaining non-naive $CD4^+$ and $CD8^+$ T-cells. We found a reduction in absolute numbers of naive $CD4^+$ and $CD8^+$ T-cells in the peripheral blood of ATG-treated animals and significantly lower ratios of naive to memory T-cell populations were present in ATG-treated animals. This process of reappearance of memory T-cells in a lymphopenic environment, termed homeostatic proliferation, could explain our observations [228, 231–233]. Experiments in mice demonstrated that cells undergoing homeostatic proliferation are not susceptible to tolerance induction by costimulation blockade [224]. Memory cells also have an intrinsic lower activation threshold, reducing the requirements for costimulation [209–212]. $CD4^+$ memory T-cells can provide help to $CD8^+$ cells even in the presence of costimulation blockade [216] and they can provide help to B-cells for isotype switching, which may be responsible for the presence of donor-specific alloantibodies in ATG-treated animals, whereas they are absent in costimulation blockade treated animals.

Conclusion

Non-human Primates as a Valid Preclinical Model of Transplant Tolerance

The lack of natural infections and the consequent absence of immunological memory in SPF rodent models is a pitfall for studying tolerance-inducing therapies [204,224]. As a consequence, rodent models are a poor predictor for the success of tolerance inducing therapies in primates [203]. NHP have been used to study rejection and tolerance mechanisms since the 1960s and are in many cases the model of choice for testing new drugs for several reasons. 1) The NHP immune system is more closely related to humans. 2) NHP acquire immunological memory as happens in humans. Rhesus monkeys were shown to have increasing frequencies of memory T-cells with age, similar to the acquisition of memory in humans [234]. 3) Many biological therapeutics target human proteins. These biologicals may not always cross-react with homologs of the protein in rodent or other large mammal species such as dogs or pigs. 4) Tools to monitor the immune response during testing of a new treatment may not always work in dogs or pigs.

The Biomedical Primate Research Centre (BPRC) has had a long-standing interest in treatments that prolong tissue and organ allograft survival [235–238]. In order to study the effect of MHC matching, a breeding colony was established and this colony provided the basis for the research on MHC matching in transplantation as well as for the research on the MHC of the rhesus monkey [239,240]. The research has provided important insights in the graft survival prolonging effects of MHC matching, blood transfusions, anti-lymphocyte polyclonal antibodies, monoclonal anti-T-cell antibodies, costimulation blockade, as well as number of other treatments [34,241–245]. A therapy of three random blood transfusions and a 12-month treatment with CsA resulted in prolonged graft survival in a number of rhesus monkeys, of which one survived more than 25 years without immunosuppression [246,247].

The NHP model of transplantation may have its limitations, such as the absence of organ failure due to recurrence of disease, as occurs in humans. In addition, monitoring tools in NHP need to be refined further. The advantages outweigh the shortcommings, which can be solved. Even with the limitations, NHP are still very important for the evaluation of new therapies [60].

Testing of costimulation blockade in NHP models has demonstrated that costimulation is not suited for the induction of tolerance in primates. No evidence was found that costimulation blockade induces Tregs. Rodent models demonstrate that tolerance can be induced via the use of Tregs. Bone marrow transplantation may provide the best opportunity to test the use of Tregs in patients, because of the limited amount of effector cells present. For solid organ transplantation, graft survival in the presence of Tregs in combination with low level conventional immunosuppressive drugs should be compared with graft survival in the presence of clinically relevant doses of immunosuppression. This is ethically not justified in patients without testing it first in NHP. When graft survival in NHP would be similar, or possibly even better, when using Tregs, with a concurrent reduction of the side effects associated with conventional immunosuppressive drugs, Treg treatment becomes a promising and powerfull alternative for the current clinical practice of immunosuppression.

References

[1] Merrill JP, Murray JE, Harrison JH, Guild WR. Successful homotransplantation of the human kidney between identical twins. *J Am Med Assoc* 1956;160(4):277–82.

[2] Gibson T, Medawar PB. The fate of skin homografts in man. *J Anat* 1943;77(Pt 4):299–310 4.

[3] Medawar PB. The behaviour and fate of skin autografts and skin homografts in rabbits: A report to the War Wounds Committee of the Medical Research Council. *J Anat* 1944;78(Pt 5):176–199.

[4] Medawar PB. A second study of the behaviour and fate of skin homografts in rabbits: A Report to the War Wounds Committee of the Medical Research Council. *J Anat* 1945;79(Pt 4):157–176 4.

[5] Dausset J. [Iso-leuko-antibodies.]. *Acta Haematol* 1958;20(1-4):156–66.

[6] Payne R, Tripp M, Weigle J, Bodmer W, Bodmer J. A New Leukocyte Isoantigen System in Man. *Cold Spring Harb Symp Quant Biol* 1964;29:285–95.

[7] Van Rood JJ, Van Leeuwen A. Leukocyte Grouping. a Method and Its Application. *J Clin Invest* 1963;42:1382–90.

[8] Samaniego M, Becker BN, Djamali A. Drug insight: maintenance immunosuppression in kidney transplant recipients. *Nat Clin Pract Nephrol* 2006;2(12):688–99.

[9] Augustine JJ, Bodziak KA, Hricik DE. Use of sirolimus in solid organ transplantation. *Drugs* 2007;67(3):369–91.

[10] Billingham RE, Brent L, Medawar PB. Actively acquired tolerance of foreign cells. *Nature* 1953;172(4379):603–6.

[11] Krieger NR, Yin DP, Fathman CG. CD4+ but not CD8+ cells are essential for allorejection. *J Exp Med* 1996;184(5):2013–8.

[12] Benichou G, Takizawa PA, Olson CA, McMillan M, Sercarz EE. Donor major histocompatibility complex (MHC) peptides are presented by recipient MHC molecules during graft rejection. *J Exp Med* 1992;175(1):305–8.

[13] Gould DS, Auchincloss Jr H. Direct and indirect recognition: the role of MHC antigens in graft rejection. *Immunol Today* 1999;20(2):77–82.

[14] Ciubotariu R, Liu Z, Colovai AI, Ho E, Itescu S, Ravalli S, et al. Persistent allopeptide reactivity and epitope spreading in chronic rejection of organ allografts. *J Clin Invest* 1998;101(2):398–405.

[15] Vella JP, Spadafora-Ferreira M, Murphy B, Alexander SI, Harmon W, Carpenter CB, et al. Indirect allorecognition of major histocompatibility complex allopeptides in human renal transplant recipients with chronic graft dysfunction. *Transplantation* 1997;64(6):795–800.

[16] Auchincloss Jr H, Lee R, Shea S, Markowitz JS, Grusby MJ, Glimcher LH. The role of "indirect" recognition in initiating rejection of skin grafts from major histocompatibility complex class II-deficient mice. *Proc Natl Acad Sci U S A* 1993;90(8):3373–7.

[17] Racusen LC, Solez K, Colvin RB, Bonsib SM, Castro MC, Cavallo T, et al. The Banff 97 working classification of renal allograft pathology. *Kidney Int* 1999;55(2):713–23.

[18] Solez K, Colvin RB, Racusen LC, Sis B, Halloran PF, Birk PE, et al. Banff '05 Meeting Report: differential diagnosis of chronic allograft injury and elimination of chronic allograft nephropathy ('CAN'). *Am J Transplant* 2007;7(3):518–26.

[19] Bretscher P, Cohn M. A theory of self-nonself discrimination. *Science* 1970;169(950):1042–9.

[20] Rosenberg AS, Mizuochi T, Sharrow SO, Singer A. Phenotype, specificity, and function of T cell subsets and T cell interactions involved in skin allograft rejection. *J Exp Med* 1987;165(5):1296–315.

[21] Ranheim EA, Kipps TJ. Tumor necrosis factor-alpha facilitates induction of CD80 (B7-1) and CD54 on human B cells by activated T cells: complex regulation by IL-4, IL-10, and CD40L. *Cell Immunol* 1995;161(2):226–35.

[22] Roy M, Aruffo A, Ledbetter J, Linsley P, Kehry M, Noelle R. Studies on the interdependence of gp39 and B7 expression and function during antigen-specific immune responses. *Eur J Immunol* 1995;25(2):596–603.

[23] de Boer M, Kasran A, Kwekkeboom J, Walter H, Vandenberghe P, Ceuppens JL. Ligation of B7 with CD28/CTLA-4 on T cells results in CD40 ligand expression, interleukin-4 secretion and efficient help for antibody production by B cells. *Eur J Immunol* 1993;23(12):3120–5.

[24] Jenkins MK, Taylor PS, Norton SD, Urdahl KB. CD28 delivers a costimulatory signal involved in antigen-specific IL-2 production by human T cells. *J Immunol* 1991;147(8):2461–6.

[25] Harding FA, Allison JP. CD28-B7 interactions allow the induction of CD8+ cytotoxic T lymphocytes in the absence of exogenous help. *J Exp Med* 1993;177(6):1791–6.

[26] Ridge JP, Di Rosa F, Matzinger P. A conditioned dendritic cell can be a temporal bridge between a CD4+ T-helper and a T-killer cell. *Nature* 1998;393(6684):474–8.

[27] Schwartz RH. A cell culture model for T lymphocyte clonal anergy. *Science* 1990;248(4961):1349–56.

[28] Ikemizu S, Gilbert RJ, Fennelly JA, Collins AV, Harlos K, Jones EY, et al. Structure and dimerization of a soluble form of B7-1. *Immunity* 2000;12(1):51–60.

[29] Pentcheva-Hoang T, Egen JG, Wojnoonski K, Allison JP. B7-1 and B7-2 selectively recruit CTLA-4 and CD28 to the immunological synapse. *Immunity* 2004;21(3):401–13.

[30] Judge TA, Wu Z, Zheng XG, Sharpe AH, Sayegh MH, Turka LA. The role of CD80, CD86, and CTLA4 in alloimmune responses and the induction of long-term allograft survival. *J Immunol* 1999;162(4):1947–51. frame.html.

[31] Lenschow DJ, Zeng Y, Hathcock KS, Zuckerman LA, Freeman G, Thistlethwaite JR, et al. Inhibition of transplant rejection following treatment with anti-B7-2 and anti-B7-1 antibodies. *Transplantation* 1995;60(10):1171–8.

[32] Hancock WW, Sayegh MH, Zheng XG, Peach R, Linsley PS, Turka LA. Costimulatory function and expression of CD40 ligand, CD80, and CD86 in vascularized murine cardiac allograft rejection. *Proc Natl Acad Sci U S A* 1996;93(24):13967–72.

[33] Yamada A, Kishimoto K, Dong VM, Sho M, Salama AD, Anosova NG, et al. CD28-independent costimulation of T cells in alloimmune responses. *J Immunol* 2001;167(1):140–6.

[34] Ossevoort MA, Ringers J, Kuhn EM, Boon L, Lorre K, van den Hout Y, et al. Prevention of renal allograft rejection in primates by blocking the B7/CD28 pathway. *Transplantation* 1999;68(7):1010–8.

[35] Beier KC, Hutloff A, Dittrich AM, Heuck C, Rauch A, Buchner K, et al. Induction, binding specificity and function of human ICOS. *Eur J Immunol* 2000;30(12):3707–17.

[36] Coyle AJ, Lehar S, Lloyd C, Tian J, Delaney T, Manning S, et al. The CD28-related molecule ICOS is required for effective T cell-dependent immune responses. *Immunity* 2000;13(1):95–105.

[37] Khayyamian S, Hutloff A, Buchner K, Grafe M, Henn V, Kroczek RA, et al. ICOS-ligand, expressed on human endothelial cells, costimulates Th1 and Th2 cytokine secretion by memory CD4+ T cells. *Proc Natl Acad Sci U S A* 2002;99(9):6198–203.

[38] Harada H, Salama AD, Sho M, Izawa A, Sandner SE, Ito T, et al. The role of the ICOS-B7h T cell costimulatory pathway in transplantation immunity. *J Clin Invest* 2003;112(2):234–43.

[39] Freeman GJ, Long AJ, Iwai Y, Bourque K, Chernova T, Nishimura H, et al. Engagement of the PD-1 immunoinhibitory receptor by a novel B7 family member leads to negative regulation of lymphocyte activation. *J Exp Med* 2000;192(7):1027–34.

[40] Latchman Y, Wood CR, Chernova T, Chaudhary D, Borde M, Chernova I, et al. PD-L2 is a second ligand for PD-1 and inhibits T cell activation. *Nat Immunol* 2001;2(3):261–8.

[41] Chapoval AI, Ni J, Lau JS, Wilcox RA, Flies DB, Liu D, et al. B7-H3: a costimulatory molecule for T cell activation and IFN-gamma production. *Nat Immunol* 2001;2(3):269–74.

[42] Chen Y, Yang C, Xie Z, Zou L, Ruan Z, Zhang X, et al. Expression of the novel co-stimulatory molecule B7-H4 by renal tubular epithelial cells. *Kidney Int* 2006;70(12):2092–9.

[43] Sedy JR, Gavrieli M, Potter KG, Hurchla MA, Lindsley RC, Hildner K, et al. B and T lymphocyte attenuator regulates T cell activation through interaction with herpesvirus entry mediator. *Nat Immunol* 2005;6(1):90–8.

[44] Wang XF, Chen YJ, Wang Q, Ge Y, Dai Q, Yang KF, et al. Distinct expression and inhibitory function of B and T lymphocyte attenuator on human T cells. *Tissue Antigens* 2007;69(2):145–53.

[45] Pollok KE, Kim YJ, Zhou Z, Hurtado J, Kim KK, Pickard RT, et al. Inducible T cell antigen 4-1BB. Analysis of expression and function. *J Immunol* 1993;150(3):771–81.

[46] DeBenedette MA, Shahinian A, Mak TW, Watts TH. Costimulation of CD28- T lymphocytes by 4-1BB ligand. *J Immunol* 1997;158(2):551–9.

[47] Durkop H, Latza U, Himmelreich P, Stein H. Expression of the human OX40 (hOX40) antigen in normal and neoplastic tissues. *Br J Haematol* 1995;91(4):927–31.

[48] Ohshima Y, Tanaka Y, Tozawa H, Takahashi Y, Maliszewski C, Delespesse G. Expression and function of OX40 ligand on human dendritic cells. *J Immunol* 1997;159(8):3838–48.

[49] Gramaglia I, Jember A, Pippig SD, Weinberg AD, Killeen N, Croft M. The OX40 costimulatory receptor determines the development of CD4 memory by regulating primary clonal expansion. *J Immunol* 2000;165(6):3043–50.

[50] Kobata T, Jacquot S, Kozlowski S, Agematsu K, Schlossman SF, Morimoto C. CD27-CD70 interactions regulate B-cell activation by T cells. *Proc Natl Acad Sci U S A* 1995;92(24):11249–53.

[51] Orengo AM, Cantoni C, Neglia F, Biassoni R, Ferrini S. Reciprocal expression of CD70 and of its receptor, CD27, in human long term-activated T and natural killer (NK) cells: inverse regulation by cytokines and role in induction of cytotoxicity. *Clin Exp Immunol* 1997;107(3):608–13.

[52] Brugnoni D, Airo P, Marino R, Notarangelo LD, van Lier RA, Cattaneo R. CD70 expression on T-cell subpopulations: study of normal individuals and patients with chronic immune activation. *Immunol Lett* 1997;55(2):99–104.

[53] Lenschow DJ, Zeng Y, Thistlethwaite JR, Montag A, Brady W, Gibson MG, et al. Long-term survival of xenogeneic pancreatic islet grafts induced by CTLA4lg. *Science* 1992;257(5071):789–92.

[54] Linsley PS, Wallace PM, Johnson J, Gibson MG, Greene JL, Ledbetter JA, et al. Immunosuppression in vivo by a soluble form of the CTLA-4 T cell activation molecule. *Science* 1992;257(5071):792–5.

[55] Larsen CP, Elwood ET, Alexander DZ, Ritchie SC, Hendrix R, Tucker-Burden C, et al. Long-term acceptance of skin and cardiac allografts after blocking CD40 and CD28 pathways. *Nature* 1996;381(6581):434–8.

[56] DeBenedette MA, Wen T, Bachmann MF, Ohashi PS, Barber BH, Stocking KL, et al. Analysis of 4-1BB ligand (4-1BBL)-deficient mice and of mice lacking both 4-1BBL and CD28 reveals a role for 4-1BBL in skin allograft rejection and in the cytotoxic T cell response to influenza virus. *J Immunol* 1999;163(9):4833–41.

[57] Kosuge H, Suzuki J, Gotoh R, Koga N, Ito H, Isobe M, et al. Induction of immunologic tolerance to cardiac allograft by simultaneous blockade of inducible co-stimulator and cytotoxic T-lymphocyte antigen 4 pathway. *Transplantation* 2003;75(8):1374–9.

[58] Vu MD, Amanullah F, Li Y, Demirci G, Sayegh MH, Li XC. Different costimulatory and growth factor requirements for CD4+ and CD8+ T cell-mediated rejection. *J Immunol* 2004;173(1):214–21.

[59] Yuan X, Salama AD, Dong V, Schmitt I, Najafian N, Chandraker A, et al. The role of the CD134-CD134 ligand costimulatory pathway in alloimmune responses in vivo. *J Immunol* 2003;170(6):2949–55.

[60] Kean LS, Gangappa S, Pearson TC, Larsen CP. Transplant tolerance in non-human primates: progress, current challenges and unmet needs. *Am J Transplant* 2006;6(5 Pt 1):884–93.

[61] Kanmaz T, Fechner Jr J J, Torrealba J, Kim HT, Dong Y, Oberley TD, et al. Monotherapy with the novel human anti-CD154 monoclonal antibody ABI793 in rhesus monkey renal transplantation model. *Transplantation* 2004;77(6):914–20.

[62] Kirk AD, Harlan DM, Armstrong NN, Davis TA, Dong Y, Gray GS, et al. CTLA4-Ig and anti-CD40 ligand prevent renal allograft rejection in primates. *Proc Natl Acad Sci U S A* 1997;94(16):8789–94.

[63] Kirk AD, Burkly LC, Batty DS, Baumgartner RE, Berning JD, Buchanan K, et al. Treatment with humanized monoclonal antibody against CD154 prevents acute renal allograft rejection in nonhuman primates. *Nat Med* 1999;5(6):686–93.

[64] Kirk AD, Tadaki DK, Celniker A, Batty DS, Berning JD, Colonna JO, et al. Induction therapy with monoclonal antibodies specific for CD80 and CD86 delays the onset of acute renal allograft rejection in non-human primates. *Transplantation* 2001;72(3):377–84.

[65] Pearson TC, Trambley J, Odom K, Anderson DC, Cowan S, Bray R, et al. Anti-CD40 therapy extends renal allograft survival in rhesus macaques. *Transplantation* 2002;74(7):933–40.

[66] Boulday G, Ashton-Chess J, Bernard P, Karam G, Vie H, Moreau A, et al. Association of rapamycin and co-stimulation blockade using anti-B7 antibodies in renal allotransplantation in baboons. *Nephrol Dial Transplant* 2004;19(7):1752–60.

[67] Imai A, Suzuki T, Sugitani A, Itoh T, Ueki S, Aoyagi T, et al. A novel fully human anti-CD40 monoclonal antibody, 4D11, for kidney transplantation in cynomolgus monkeys. *Transplantation* 2007;84(8):1020–8.

[68] Hausen B, Klupp J, Christians U, Higgins JP, Baumgartner RE, Hook LE, et al. Coadministration of either cyclosporine or steroids with humanized monoclonal antibodies against CD80 and CD86 successfully prolong allograft survival after life supporting renal transplantation in cynomolgus monkeys. *Transplantation* 2001;72(6):1128–37.

[69] Birsan T, Hausen B, Higgins JP, Hubble RW, Klupp J, Stalder M, et al. Treatment with humanized monoclonal antibodies against CD80 and CD86 combined with sirolimus prolongs renal allograft survival in cynomolgus monkeys. *Transplantation* 2003;75(12):2106–13.

[70] Larsen CP, Pearson TC, Adams AB, Tso P, Shirasugi N, Strobertm E, et al. Rational development of LEA29Y (belatacept), a high-affinity variant of CTLA4-Ig with potent immunosuppressive properties. *Am J Transplant* 2005;5(3):443–53.

[71] Linsley PS, Greene JL, Brady W, Bajorath J, Ledbetter JA, Peach R. Human B7-1 (CD80) and B7-2 (CD86) bind with similar avidities but distinct kinetics to CD28 and CTLA-4 receptors. *Immunity* 1994;1(9):793–801.

[72] Vincenti F, Larsen C, Durrbach A, Wekerle T, Nashan B, Blancho G, et al. Costimulation blockade with belatacept in renal transplantation. *N Engl J Med* 2005;353(8):770–81.

[73] Preston EH, Xu H, Dhanireddy KK, Pearl JP, Leopardi FV, Starost MF, et al. IDEC-131 (anti-CD154), sirolimus and donor-specific transfusion facilitate operational tolerance in non-human primates. *Am J Transplant* 2005;5(5):1032–41.

[74] Kurtz J, Lie A, Griffith M, Eysaman S, Shaffer J, Anosova N, et al. Lack of role for CsA-sensitive or Fas pathways in the tolerization of CD4 T cells via BMT and anti-CD40L. *Am J Transplant* 2003;3(7):804–16.

[75] Schuler W, Bigaud M, Brinkmann V, Di Padova F, Geisse S, Gram H, et al. Efficacy and safety of ABI793, a novel human anti-human CD154 monoclonal antibody, in cynomolgus monkey renal allotransplantation. *Transplantation* 2004;77(5):717–26.

[76] Xu H, Elster E, Batty D, Berning J, Burkly L, Kampen R, et al. Effects of dose and duration of anti-CD154 antibody therapy in preventing renal allograft rejection in a nonhuman primate model. *Transplant Proc* 2001;33(1-2):223–4.

[77] Xu H, Elster EA, Blair PJ, Burkly LC, Tadaki DK, Harlan DM, et al. Effects of Combined Treatment with CD25- and CD154-Specific Monoclonal Antibodies in Non-Human Primate Allotransplantation. *Am J Transplant* 2003;3(11):1350–1354.

[78] Cho CS, Burkly LC, Fechner Jr J H, Kirk AD, Oberley TD, Dong Y, et al. Successful conversion from conventional immunosuppression to anti-CD154 monoclonal antibody costimulatory molecule blockade in rhesus renal allograft recipients. *Transplantation* 2001;72(4):587–97.

[79] Knechtle SJ, Hamawy MM, Hu H, Fechner Jr J H, Cho CS. Tolerance and near-tolerance strategies in monkeys and their application to human renal transplantation. *Immunol Rev* 2001;183:205–13.

[80] Koyama I, Kawai T, Andrews D, Boskovic S, Nadazdin O, Wee SL, et al. Thrombophilia associated with anti-CD154 monoclonal antibody treatment and its prophylaxis in nonhuman primates. *Transplantation* 2004;77(3):460–2.

[81] Brandle D, Joergensen J, Zenke G, Burki K, Hof RP. Contribution of donor-specific antibodies to acute allograft rejection: evidence from B cell-deficient mice. *Transplantation* 1998;65(11):1489–93.

[82] Uno M, Suzuki T, Aoyagi T, Sugitani A, Goto R, Yamashita K, et al. Immunosuppression by a Novel Anti-CD40 mAb, 4D11, Is Not Abrogated by Combined Treatment with Tacrolimus for Renal Transplantation in Cynomolgus Monkeys. In: *American Transplant Congress*. vol. Abstract 213. San Francisco; 2007. Q.

[83] Haanstra KristaG, Ringers Jan, Sick EllaA, Ramdien-Murli Seema, Kuhn EvaMaria, Boon Louis, et al. Prevention of kidney allograft rejection using anti-CD40 and anti-CD86 in primates. *Transplantation* 2003;75(5):637–43.

[84] Kwekkeboom J, De Boer M, Tager JM, De Groot C. CD40 plays an essential role in the activation of human B cells by murine EL4B5 cells. *Immunology* 1993;79(3):439–44.

[85] Kwekkeboom J, de Rijk D, Kasran A, Barcy S, de Groot C, de Boer M. Helper effector function of human T cells stimulated by anti-CD3 mAb can be enhanced by co-stimulatory signals and is partially dependent on CD40-CD40 ligand interaction. *Eur J Immunol* 1994;24(3):508–17.

[86] Montgomery SP, Xu H, Tadaki DK, Celniker A, Burkly LC, Berning JD, et al. Combination induction therapy with monoclonal antibodies specific for CD80, CD86, and CD154 in nonhuman primate renal transplantation. *Transplantation* 2002;74(10):1365–9.

[87] Nankivell BJ, Chapman JR. The significance of subclinical rejection and the value of protocol biopsies. *Am J Transplant* 2006;6(9):2006–12.

[88] Koenen HJ, Fasse E, Joosten I. Cyclosporine preserves the anergic state of human T cells induced by costimulation blockade in vitro. *Transplantation* 2005;80(4):522–9.

[89] Hale DA, Gottschalk R, Maki T, Monaco AP. Use of CTLA4-Ig in combination with conventional immunosuppressive agents to prolong allograft survival. *Transplantation* 1997;64(6):897–900.

[90] Li Y, Li XC, Zheng XX, Wells AD, Turka LA, Strom TB. Blocking both signal 1 and signal 2 of T-cell activation prevents apoptosis of alloreactive T cells and induction of peripheral allograft tolerance. *Nat Med* 1999;5(11):1298–302.

[91] Li Y, Zheng XX, Li XC, Zand MS, Strom TB. Combined costimulation blockade plus rapamycin but not cyclosporine produces permanent engraftment. *Transplantation* 1998;66(10):1387–8.

[92] Wells AD, Li XC, Li Y, Walsh MC, Zheng XX, Wu Z, et al. Requirement for T-cell apoptosis in the induction of peripheral transplantation tolerance. *Nat Med* 1999;5(11):1303–7.

[93] Haanstra KristaG, Sick EllaA, Ringers Jan, Wubben JacquelineAM, Kuhn EvaMaria, Boon Louis, et al. Costimulation blockade followed by a 12-week period of cyclosporine A facilitates prolonged drug-free survival of rhesus monkey kidney allografts. *Transplantation* 2005;79(11):1623–6.

[94] Xu H, Tadaki DK, Elster EA, Burkly LC, Berning JD, Cruzata F, et al. Humanized anti-CD154 antibody therapy for the treatment of allograft rejection in nonhuman primates. *Transplantation* 2002;74(7):940–3.

[95] Adams AB, Shirasugi N, Jones TR, Williams MA, Durham MM, Ha J, et al. Conventional immunosuppression is compatible with costimulation blockade-based, mixed chimerism tolerance induction. *Am J Transplant* 2003;3(7):895–901.

[96] Dorf ME, Benacerraf B. Suppressor cells and immunoregulation. *Annu Rev Immunol* 1984;2:127–57.

[97] Moller G. Do suppressor T cells exist? *Scand J Immunol* 1988;27(3):247–50.

[98] Sakaguchi S, Sakaguchi N, Asano M, Itoh M, Toda M. Immunologic self-tolerance maintained by activated T cells expressing IL-2 receptor alpha-chains (CD25). Breakdown of a single mechanism of self-tolerance causes various autoimmune diseases. *J Immunol* 1995;155(3):1151–64.

[99] Blazar BR, Taylor PA, Noelle RJ, Vallera DA. CD4(+) T cells tolerized ex vivo to host alloantigen by anti-CD40 ligand (CD40L:CD154) antibody lose their graft-versus-host disease lethality capacity but retain nominal antigen responses. *J Clin Invest* 1998;102(3):473–82.

[100] Koenen HJ, Joosten I. Blockade of CD86 and CD40 induces alloantigen-specific immunoregulatory T cells that remain anergic even after reversal of hyporesponsiveness. *Blood* 2000;95(10):3153–61.

[101] Bashuda H, Kimikawa M, Seino K, Kato Y, Ono F, Shimizu A, et al. Renal allograft rejection is prevented by adoptive transfer of anergic T cells in nonhuman primates. *J Clin Invest* 2005;115(7):1896–902.

[102] Taylor PA, Noelle RJ, Blazar BR. CD4(+)CD25(+) immune regulatory cells are required for induction of tolerance to alloantigen via costimulatory blockade. *J Exp Med* 2001;193(11):1311–8.

[103] Coenen JJ, Koenen HJ, van Rijssen E, Hilbrands LB, Joosten I. Tolerizing effects of co-stimulation blockade rest on functional dominance of CD4+CD25+ regulatory T cells. *Transplantation* 2005;79(2):147–56.

[104] Coenen JJ, Koenen HJ, van Rijssen E, Boon L, Joosten I, Hilbrands LB. CTLA-4 engagement and regulatory CD4+CD25+ T cells independently control CD8+-mediated responses under costimulation blockade. *J Immunol* 2006;176(9):5240–6.

[105] Read S, Greenwald R, Izcue A, Robinson N, Mandelbrot D, Francisco L, et al. Blockade of CTLA-4 on CD4+CD25+ regulatory T cells abrogates their function in vivo. *J Immunol* 2006;177(7):4376–83.

[106] Baan CC, van der Mast BJ, Klepper M, Mol WM, Peeters AM, Korevaar SS, et al. Differential effect of calcineurin inhibitors, anti-CD25 antibodies and rapamycin on the induction of FOXP3 in human T cells. *Transplantation* 2005;80(1):110–7.

[107] Wing K, Ekmark A, Karlsson H, Rudin A, Suri-Payer E. Characterization of human CD25+ CD4+ T cells in thymus, cord and adult blood. *Immunology* 2002;106(2):190–9.

[108] Baecher-Allan C, Brown JA, Freeman GJ, Hafler DA. CD4+CD25high regulatory cells in human peripheral blood. *J Immunol* 2001;167(3):1245–53.

[109] Seddiki N, Santner-Nanan B, Tangye SG, Alexander SI, Solomon M, Lee S, et al. Persistence of naive CD45RA+ regulatory T cells in adult life. *Blood* 2006;107(7):2830–8.

[110] Vukmanovic-Stejic M, Zhang Y, Cook JE, Fletcher JM, McQuaid A, Masters JE, et al. Human CD4+ CD25hi Foxp3+ regulatory T cells are derived by rapid turnover of memory populations in vivo. *J Clin Invest* 2006;116(9):2423–33.

[111] Annunziato F, Cosmi L, Liotta F, Lazzeri E, Manetti R, Vanini V, et al. Phenotype, localization, and mechanism of suppression of CD4(+)CD25(+) human thymocytes. *J Exp Med* 2002;196(3):379–87.

[112] Valmori D, Merlo A, Souleimanian NE, Hesdorffer CS, Ayyoub M. A peripheral circulating compartment of natural naive CD4 Tregs. *J Clin Invest* 2005;115(7):1953–62.

[113] Shevach EM. CD4+ CD25+ suppressor T cells: more questions than answers. *Nat Rev Immunol* 2002;2(6):389–400.

[114] Stephens LA, Mottet C, Mason D, Powrie F. Human CD4(+)CD25(+) thymocytes and peripheral T cells have immune suppressive activity in vitro. *Eur J Immunol* 2001;31(4):1247–54.

[115] Godfrey VL, Rouse BT, Wilkinson JE. Transplantation of T cell-mediated, lymphoreticular disease from the scurfy (sf) mouse. *Am J Pathol* 1994;145(2):281–6.

[116] Brunkow ME, Jeffery EW, Hjerrild KA, Paeper B, Clark LB, Yasayko SA, et al. Disruption of a new forkhead/winged-helix protein, scurfin, results in the fatal lymphoproliferative disorder of the scurfy mouse. *Nat Genet* 2001;27(1):68–73.

[117] Bennett CL, Christie J, Ramsdell F, Brunkow ME, Ferguson PJ, Whitesell L, et al. The immune dysregulation, polyendocrinopathy, enteropathy, X-linked syndrome (IPEX) is caused by mutations of FOXP3. *Nat Genet* 2001;27(1):20–1.

[118] Gambineri E, Torgerson TR, Ochs HD. Immune dysregulation, polyendocrinopathy, enteropathy, and X-linked inheritance (IPEX), a syndrome of systemic autoimmunity caused by mutations of FOXP3, a critical regulator of T-cell homeostasis. *Curr Opin Rheumatol* 2003;15(4):430–5.

[119] Kobayashi I, Shiari R, Yamada M, Kawamura N, Okano M, Yara A, et al. Novel mutations of FOXP3 in two Japanese patients with immune dysregulation, polyendocrinopathy, enteropathy, X linked syndrome (IPEX). *J Med Genet* 2001;38(12):874–6.

[120] Ochs HD, Ziegler SF, Torgerson TR. FOXP3 acts as a rheostat of the immune response. *Immunol Rev* 2005;203:156–64.

[121] Owen CJ, Jennings CE, Imrie H, Lachaux A, Bridges NA, Cheetham TD, et al. Mutational analysis of the FOXP3 gene and evidence for genetic heterogeneity in the immunodysregulation, polyendocrinopathy, enteropathy syndrome. *J Clin Endocrinol Metab* 2003;88(12):6034–9.

[122] Wildin RS, Ramsdell F, Peake J, Faravelli F, Casanova JL, Buist N, et al. X-linked neonatal diabetes mellitus, enteropathy and endocrinopathy syndrome is the human equivalent of mouse scurfy. *Nat Genet* 2001;27(1):18–20.

[123] Fontenot JD, Gavin MA, Rudensky AY. Foxp3 programs the development and function of CD4+CD25+ regulatory T cells. *Nat Immunol* 2003;4(4):330–6.

[124] Walker MR, Kasprowicz DJ, Gersuk VH, Benard A, Van Landeghen M, Buckner JH, et al. Induction of FoxP3 and acquisition of T regulatory activity by stimulated human CD4+CD25- T cells. *J Clin Invest* 2003;112(9):1437–43.

[125] Albert MH, Liu Y, Anasetti C, Yu XZ. Antigen-dependent suppression of alloresponses by Foxp3-induced regulatory T cells in transplantation. *Eur J Immunol* 2005;35(9):2598–607.

[126] Khattri R, Kasprowicz D, Cox T, Mortrud M, Appleby MW, Brunkow ME, et al. The amount of scurfin protein determines peripheral T cell number and responsiveness. *J Immunol* 2001;167(11):6312–20.

[127] Banham AH, Powrie FM, Suri-Payer E. FOXP3+ regulatory T cells: Current controversies and future perspectives. *Eur J Immunol* 2006;36(11):2832–6.

[128] Morgan ME, van Bilsen JH, Bakker AM, Heemskerk B, Schilham MW, Hartgers FC, et al. Expression of FOXP3 mRNA is not confined to CD4+CD25+ T regulatory cells in humans. *Hum Immunol* 2005;66(1):13–20.

[129] Roncador G, Brown PJ, Maestre L, Hue S, Martinez-Torrecuadrada JL, Ling KL, et al. Analysis of FOXP3 protein expression in human CD4+CD25+ regulatory T cells at the single-cell level. *Eur J Immunol* 2005;35(6):1681–91.

[130] Allan SE, Passerini L, Bacchetta R, Crellin N, Dai M, Orban PC, et al. The role of 2 FOXP3 isoforms in the generation of human CD4+ Tregs. *J Clin Invest* 2005;115(11):3276–84.

[131] Smith EL, Finney HM, Nesbitt AM, Ramsdell F, Robinson MK. Splice variants of human FOXP3 are functional inhibitors of human CD4+ T-cell activation. *Immunology* 2006;119(2):203–11.

[132] Baratelli F, Lin Y, Zhu L, Yang SC, Heuze-Vourc'h N, Zeng G, et al. Prostaglandin E2 induces FOXP3 gene expression and T regulatory cell function in human CD4+ T cells. *J Immunol* 2005;175(3):1483–90.

[133] Fantini MC, Becker C, Monteleone G, Pallone F, Galle PR, Neurath MF. Cutting edge: TGF-beta induces a regulatory phenotype in CD4+CD25- T cells through Foxp3 induction and down-regulation of Smad7. *J Immunol* 2004;172(9):5149–53.

[134] Gavin MA, Torgerson TR, Houston E, DeRoos P, Ho WY, Stray-Pedersen A, et al. Single-cell analysis of normal and FOXP3-mutant human T cells: FOXP3 expression without regulatory T cell development. *Proc Natl Acad Sci U S A* 2006;103(17):6659–64.

[135] Mantel PY, Ouaked N, Ruckert B, Karagiannidis C, Welz R, Blaser K, et al. Molecular mechanisms underlying FOXP3 induction in human T cells. *J Immunol* 2006;176(6):3593–602.

[136] Verhasselt V, Vosters O, Beuneu C, Nicaise C, Stordeur P, Goldman M. Induction of FOXP3-expressing regulatory CD4pos T cells by human mature autologous dendritic cells. *Eur J Immunol* 2004;34(3):762–72.

[137] Wang J, Ioan-Facsinay A, van der Voort EI, Huizinga TW, Toes RE. Transient expression of FOXP3 in human activated nonregulatory CD4+ T cells. *Eur J Immunol* 2007;37(1):129–38.

[138] Tai X, Cowan M, Feigenbaum L, Singer A. CD28 costimulation of developing thymocytes induces Foxp3 expression and regulatory T cell differentiation independently of interleukin 2. *Nat Immunol* 2005;6(2):152–62.

[139] Zheng Y, Rudensky AY. Foxp3 in control of the regulatory T cell lineage. *Nat Immunol* 2007;8(5):457–62.

[140] Wu Y, Borde M, Heissmeyer V, Feuerer M, Lapan AD, Stroud JC, et al. FOXP3 controls regulatory T cell function through cooperation with NFAT. *Cell* 2006;126(2):375–87.

[141] Segundo DS, Ruiz JC, Izquierdo M, Fernandez-Fresnedo G, Gomez-Alamillo C, Merino R, et al. Calcineurin inhibitors, but not rapamycin, reduce percentages of CD4+CD25+FOXP3+ regulatory T cells in renal transplant recipients. *Transplantation* 2006;82(4):550–7.

[142] Klintmalm G, Bohman SO, Sundelin B, Wilczek H. Interstitial fibrosis in renal allografts after 12 to 46 months of cyclosporin treatment: beneficial effect of low doses in early post-transplantation period. *Lancet* 1984;2(8409):950–4.

[143] Myers BD, Ross J, Newton L, Luetscher J, Perlroth M. Cyclosporine-associated chronic nephropathy. *N Engl J Med* 1984;311(11):699–705.

[144] Palestine AG, Austin 3rd H A, Balow JE, Antonovych TT, Sabnis SG, Preuss HG, et al. Renal histopathologic alterations in patients treated with cyclosporine for uveitis. *N Engl J Med* 1986;314(20):1293–8.

[145] Wolf G, Thaiss F, Stahl RA. Cyclosporine stimulates expression of transforming growth factor-beta in renal cells. Possible mechanism of cyclosporines antiproliferative effects. *Transplantation* 1995;60(3):237–41.

[146] Gooch JL, Roberts BR, Cobbs SL, Tumlin JA. Loss of the alpha-isoform of calcineurin is sufficient to induce nephrotoxicity and altered expression of transforming growth factor-beta. *Transplantation* 2007;83(4):439–47.

[147] Ignotz RA, Massague J. Transforming growth factor-beta stimulates the expression of fibronectin and collagen and their incorporation into the extracellular matrix. *J Biol Chem* 1986;261(9):4337–45.

[148] Kulkarni AB, Huh CG, Becker D, Geiser A, Lyght M, Flanders KC, et al. Transforming growth factor beta 1 null mutation in mice causes excessive inflammatory response and early death. *Proc Natl Acad Sci U S A* 1993;90(2):770–4.

[149] Shull MM, Ormsby I, Kier AB, Pawlowski S, Diebold RJ, Yin M, et al. Targeted disruption of the mouse transforming growth factor-beta 1 gene results in multifocal inflammatory disease. *Nature* 1992;359(6397):693–9.

[150] Kehrl JH, Wakefield LM, Roberts AB, Jakowlew S, Alvarez-Mon M, Derynck R, et al. Production of transforming growth factor beta by human T lymphocytes and its potential role in the regulation of T cell growth. *J Exp Med* 1986;163(5):1037–50.

[151] Laouar Y, Sutterwala FS, Gorelik L, Flavell RA. Transforming growth factor-beta controls T helper type 1 cell development through regulation of natural killer cell interferon-gamma. *Nat Immunol* 2005;6(6):600–7.

[152] Luo X, Yang H, Kim IS, Saint-Hilaire F, Thomas DA, De BP, et al. Systemic transforming growth factor-beta1 gene therapy induces Foxp3+ regulatory cells, restores self-tolerance, and facilitates regeneration of beta cell function in overtly diabetic nonobese diabetic mice. *Transplantation* 2005;79(9):1091–6.

[153] Rao PE, Petrone AL, Ponath PD. Differentiation and expansion of T cells with regulatory function from human peripheral lymphocytes by stimulation in the presence of TGF-beta. *J Immunol* 2005;174(3):1446–55.

[154] Zheng SG, Gray JD, Ohtsuka K, Yamagiwa S, Horwitz DA. Generation ex vivo of TGF-beta-producing regulatory T cells from CD4+CD25- precursors. *J Immunol* 2002;169(8):4183–9.

[155] Zheng SG, Wang JH, Stohl W, Kim KS, Gray JD, Horwitz DA. TGF-beta requires CTLA-4 early after T cell activation to induce FoxP3 and generate adaptive CD4+CD25+ regulatory cells. *J Immunol* 2006;176(6):3321–9.

[156] Allakhverdi Z, Fitzpatrick D, Boisvert A, Baba N, Bouguermouh S, Sarfati M, et al. Expression of CD103 identifies human regulatory T-cell subsets. *J Allergy Clin Immunol* 2006;118(6):1342–9.

[157] Oida T, Zhang X, Goto M, Hachimura S, Totsuka M, Kaminogawa S, et al. CD4+CD25- T cells that express latency-associated peptide on the surface suppress CD4+CD45RBhigh-induced colitis by a TGF-beta-dependent mechanism. *J Immunol* 2003;170(5):2516–22.

[158] Gandhi R, Anderson DE, Weiner HL. Cutting Edge: Immature human dendritic cells express latency-associated peptide and inhibit T cell activation in a TGF-beta-dependent manner. *J Immunol* 2007;178(7):4017–21.

[159] Davidson TS, DiPaolo RJ, Andersson J, Shevach EM. Cutting Edge: IL-2 is essential for TGF-beta-mediated induction of Foxp3+ T regulatory cells. *J Immunol* 2007;178(7):4022–6.

[160] Jonuleit H, Schmitt E, Kakirman H, Stassen M, Knop J, Enk AH. Infectious tolerance: human CD25(+) regulatory T cells convey suppressor activity to conventional CD4(+) T helper cells. *J Exp Med* 2002;196(2):255–60.

[161] Field EH, Kulhankova K, Dailey ME, Rouse T, Nasr ME. Visualizing IL-2: CD25 Interactions on CD4+CD25+ Regulatory Cells. *Immunol Res* 2007;39(1-3):62–78.

[162] Bettelli E, Dastrange M, Oukka M. Foxp3 interacts with nuclear factor of activated T cells and NF-kappa B to repress cytokine gene expression and effector functions of T helper cells. *Proc Natl Acad Sci U S A* 2005;102(14):5138–43.

[163] Shimizu J, Yamazaki S, Takahashi T, Ishida Y, Sakaguchi S. Stimulation of CD25(+)CD4(+) regulatory T cells through GITR breaks immunological self-tolerance. *Nat Immunol* 2002;3(2):135–42.

[164] Ji HB, Liao G, Faubion WA, Abadia-Molina AC, Cozzo C, Laroux FS, et al. Cutting edge: the natural ligand for glucocorticoid-induced TNF receptor-related protein abrogates regulatory T cell suppression. *J Immunol* 2004;172(10):5823–7.

[165] Houot R, Perrot I, Garcia E, Durand I, Lebecque S. Human CD4+CD25high regulatory T cells modulate myeloid but not plasmacytoid dendritic cells activation. *J Immunol* 2006;176(9):5293–8.

[166] Bayry J, Triebel F, Kaveri SV, Tough DF. Human dendritic cells acquire a semimature phenotype and lymph node homing potential through interaction with CD4+CD25+ regulatory T cells. *J Immunol* 2007;178(7):4184–93.

[167] Keymeulen B, Vandemeulebroucke E, Ziegler AG, Mathieu C, Kaufman L, Hale G, et al. Insulin needs after CD3-antibody therapy in new-onset type 1 diabetes. *N Engl J Med* 2005;352(25):2598–608.

[168] You S, Leforban B, Garcia C, Bach JF, Bluestone JA, Chatenoud L. Adaptive TGF-beta-dependent regulatory T cells control autoimmune diabetes and are a privileged target of anti-CD3 antibody treatment. *Proc Natl Acad Sci U S A* 2007;104(15):6335–40.

[169] Chatenoud L, Bluestone JA. CD3-specific antibodies: a portal to the treatment of autoimmunity. *Nat Rev Immunol* 2007;7(8):622–32.

[170] Bacchetta R, Bigler M, Touraine JL, Parkman R, Tovo PA, Abrams J, et al. High levels of interleukin 10 production in vivo are associated with tolerance in SCID patients transplanted with HLA mismatched hematopoietic stem cells. *J Exp Med* 1994;179(2):493–502.

[171] Hoffmann P, Eder R, Boeld TJ, Doser K, Piseshka B, Andreesen R, et al. Only the CD45RA+ subpopulation of CD4+CD25high T cells gives rise to homogeneous regulatory T-cell lines upon in vitro expansion. *Blood* 2006;108(13):4260–7.

[172] Koenen HJ, Fasse E, Joosten I. CD27/CFSE-based ex vivo selection of highly suppressive alloantigen-specific human regulatory T cells. *J Immunol* 2005;174(12):7573–83.

[173] Levings MK, Sangregorio R, Roncarolo MG. Human cd25(+)cd4(+) t regulatory cells suppress naive and memory T cell proliferation and can be expanded in vitro without loss of function. *J Exp Med* 2001;193(11):1295–302.

[174] Koenen HJ, Joosten I. Antigen-specific regulatory T-cell subsets in transplantation tolerance regulatory T-cell subset quality reduces the need for quantity. *Hum Immunol* 2006;67(9):665–75.

[175] Masteller EL, Tang Q, Bluestone JA. Antigen-specific regulatory T cells–ex vivo expansion and therapeutic potential. *Semin Immunol* 2006;18(2):103–10.

[176] Seddiki N, Santner-Nanan B, Martinson J, Zaunders J, Sasson S, Landay A, et al. Expression of interleukin (IL)-2 and IL-7 receptors discriminates between human regulatory and activated T cells. *J Exp Med* 2006;203(7):1693–700.

[177] Huang M, Sharma S, Mao JT, Dubinett SM. Non-small cell lung cancer-derived soluble mediators and prostaglandin E2 enhance peripheral blood lymphocyte IL-10 transcription and protein production. *J Immunol* 1996;157(12):5512–20.

[178] Jonuleit H, Schmitt E, Schuler G, Knop J, Enk AH. Induction of interleukin 10-producing, nonproliferating CD4(+) T cells with regulatory properties by repetitive stimulation with allogeneic immature human dendritic cells. *J Exp Med* 2000;192(9):1213–22.

[179] Bacchetta R, Sartirana C, Levings MK, Bordignon C, Narula S, Roncarolo MG. Growth and expansion of human T regulatory type 1 cells are independent from TCR activation but require exogenous cytokines. *Eur J Immunol* 2002;32(8):2237–45.

[180] Battaglia M, Gregori S, Bacchetta R, Roncarolo MG. Tr1 cells: from discovery to their clinical application. *Semin Immunol* 2006;18(2):120–7.

[181] Roncarolo MG, Gregori S, Battaglia M, Bacchetta R, Fleischhauer K, Levings MK. Interleukin-10-secreting type 1 regulatory T cells in rodents and humans. *Immunol Rev* 2006;212:28–50.

[182] Dieckmann D, Bruett CH, Ploettner H, Lutz MB, Schuler G. Human CD4(+)CD25(+) regulatory, contact-dependent T cells induce interleukin 10-producing, contact-independent type 1-like regulatory T cells [corrected]. *J Exp Med* 2002;196(2):247–53.

[183] Groux H, O'Garra A, Bigler M, Rouleau M, Antonenko S, de Vries JE, et al. A CD4+ T-cell subset inhibits antigen-specific T-cell responses and prevents colitis. *Nature* 1997;389(6652):737–42.

[184] Chang CC, Ciubotariu R, Manavalan JS, Yuan J, Colovai AI, Piazza F, et al. Tolerization of dendritic cells by T(S) cells: the crucial role of inhibitory receptors ILT3 and ILT4. *Nat Immunol* 2002;3(3):237–43.

[185] Zhang ZX, Yang L, Young KJ, DuTemple B, Zhang L. Identification of a previously unknown antigen-specific regulatory T cell and its mechanism of suppression. *Nat Med* 2000;6(7):782–9.

[186] Ling E, Shubinsky G, Press J. Increased proportion of CD3+CD4-CD8- double-negative T cells in peripheral blood of children with Behcet's disease. *Autoimmun Rev* 2007;6(4):237–40.

[187] Jiang S, Lechler RI. Regulatory T cells in the control of transplantation tolerance and autoimmunity. *Am J Transplant* 2003;3(5):516–24.

[188] Jiang X, Kojo S, Harada M, Ohkohchi N, Taniguchi M, Seino KI. Mechanism of NKT Cell-Mediated Transplant Tolerance. *Am J Transplant* 2007;7(6):1482–1490.

[189] Wolf SD, Dittel BN, Hardardottir F, Janeway Jr C A. Experimental autoimmune encephalomyelitis induction in genetically B cell-deficient mice. *J Exp Med* 1996;184(6):2271–8.

[190] Mizoguchi A, Bhan AK. A case for regulatory B cells. *J Immunol* 2006;176(2):705–10.

[191] Asiedu CK, Goodwin KJ, Balgansuren G, Jenkins SM, Le Bas-Bernardet S, Jargal U, et al. Elevated T regulatory cells in long-term stable transplant tolerance in rhesus macaques induced by anti-CD3 immunotoxin and deoxyspergualin. *J Immunol* 2005;175(12):8060–8.

[192] Porter CM, Horvath-Arcidiacono JA, Singh AK, Horvath KA, Bloom ET, Mohiuddin MM. Characterization and expansion of baboon CD4+CD25+ Treg cells for potential use in a non-human primate xenotransplantation model. *Xenotransplantation* 2007;14(4):298–308.

[193] Thomas JM, Eckhoff DE, Contreras JL, Thomas FT, Neville Jr D M, Lobashevsky A, et al. Retraction: Durable donor-specific T and B cell tolerance in rhesus macaques induced with peritransplantation anti-CD3 immunotoxin and deoxyspergualin: absence of chronic allograft nephropathy. *Transplantation* 2006;82(4):577.

[194] Anderson AR, Kean L, Stempora L, Gangappa S, Larsen C. Expanded nonhuman primate tregs exhibit a unique gene expression signature and potently downregulate alloimmune responses. *Am J Transplant*2008;8(11):2252–64

[195] Gansuvd B, Asiedu CK, Goodwin J, Jargal U, Deckard LA, Andrades P, et al. Expansion of CD4(+)CD25(+) suppressive regulatory T cells from rhesus macaque peripheral blood by FN18/antihuman CD28-coated Dynal beads. *Hum Immunol*2007;68(6):478–90.

[196] Torrealba JR, Katayama M, Fechner Jr J H, Jankowska-Gan E, Kusaka S, Xu Q, et al. Metastable tolerance to rhesus monkey renal transplants is correlated with allograft TGF-beta 1+CD4+ T regulatory cell infiltrates. *J Immunol* 2004;172(9):5753–64.

[197] Kornfeld C, Ploquin MJ, Pandrea I, Faye A, Onanga R, Apetrei C, et al. Antiinflammatory profiles during primary SIV infection in African green monkeys are associated with protection against AIDS. *J Clin Invest* 2005;115(4):1082–91.

[198] Haanstra KristaG, van der Maas MartinJ, 't Hart BertA, Jonker Margreet. Characterisation of naturally occurring $CD4^{+}CD25^{+}$ regulatory T-cells in rhesus monkeys. *Transplantation* 2008;85(8):1185–92.

[199] Haanstra KG, Wubben JAM, Korevaar SS, Kondova I, Baan CC, Jonker M. Expression patterns of regulatory T-cell markers in accepted and rejected nonhuman primate kidney allografts. *Am J Transplant* 2007;7(10):2236–46.

[200] Drayton DL, Liao S, Mounzer RH, Ruddle NH. Lymphoid organ development: from ontogeny to neogenesis. *Nat Immunol* 2006;7(4):344–53.

[201] Hadley GA, Charandee C, Weir MR, Wang D, Bartlett ST, Drachenberg CB. CD103+ CTL accumulate within the graft epithelium during clinical renal allograft rejection. *Transplantation* 2001;72(9):1548–55.

[202] Veronese F, Rotman S, Smith RN, Pelle TD, Farrell ML, Kawai T, et al. Pathological and Clinical Correlates of FOXP3(+) Cells in Renal Allografts during Acute Rejection. *Am J Transplant* 2007;7(4):914–22.

[203] Sachs DH. Tolerance: of mice and men. *J Clin Invest* 2003;111(12):1819–21.

[204] Adams AB, Williams MA, Jones TR, Shirasugi N, Durham MM, Kaech SM, et al. Heterologous immunity provides a potent barrier to transplantation tolerance. *J Clin Invest* 2003;111(12):1887–95.

[205] Williams MA, Onami TM, Adams AB, Durham MM, Pearson TC, Ahmed R, et al. Cutting edge: persistent viral infection prevents tolerance induction and escapes immune control following CD28/CD40 blockade-based regimen. *J Immunol* 2002;169(10):5387–91.

[206] Kupiec-Weglinski JW. Graft rejection in sensitized recipients. *Ann Transplant* 1996;1(1):34–40.

[207] Augustine JJ, Siu DS, Clemente MJ, Schulak JA, Heeger PS, Hricik DE. Pretransplant IFN-gamma ELISPOTs are associated with post-transplant renal function in African American renal transplant recipients. *Am J Transplant* 2005;5(8):1971–5.

[208] Heeger PS, Greenspan NS, Kuhlenschmidt S, Dejelo C, Hricik DE, Schulak JA, et al. Pretransplant frequency of donor-specific, IFN-gamma-producing lymphocytes is a manifestation of immunologic memory and correlates with the risk of posttransplant rejection episodes. *J Immunol* 1999;163(4):2267–75.

[209] Bachmann MF, Barner M, Viola A, Kopf M. Distinct kinetics of cytokine production and cytolysis in effector and memory T cells after viral infection. *Eur J Immunol* 1999;29(1):291–9.

[210] Garcia S, DiSanto J, Stockinger B. Following the development of a CD4 T cell response in vivo: from activation to memory formation. *Immunity* 1999;11(2):163–71.

[211] Rogers PR, Dubey C, Swain SL. Qualitative changes accompany memory T cell generation: faster, more effective responses at lower doses of antigen. *J Immunol* 2000;164(5):2338–46.

[212] Veiga-Fernandes H, Walter U, Bourgeois C, McLean A, Rocha B. Response of naive and memory CD8+ T cells to antigen stimulation in vivo. *Nat Immunol* 2000;1(1):47–53.

[213] Chalasani G, Dai Z, Konieczny BT, Baddoura FK, Lakkis FG. Recall and propagation of allospecific memory T cells independent of secondary lymphoid organs. *Proc Natl Acad Sci U S A* 2002;99(9):6175–80.

[214] Masopust D, Vezys V, Marzo AL, Lefrancois L. Preferential localization of effector memory cells in nonlymphoid tissue. *Science* 2001;291(5512):2413–7.

[215] Zhai Y, Meng L, Gao F, Busuttil RW, Kupiec-Weglinski JW. Allograft rejection by primed/memory CD8+ T cells is CD154 blockade resistant: therapeutic implications for sensitized transplant recipients. *J Immunol* 2002;169(8):4667–73.

[216] Chen Y, Heeger PS, Valujskikh A. In vivo helper functions of alloreactive memory CD4+ T cells remain intact despite donor-specific transfusion and anti-CD40 ligand therapy. *J Immunol* 2004;172(9):5456–66.

[217] Burrows SR, Khanna R, Burrows JM, Moss DJ. An alloresponse in humans is dominated by cytotoxic T lymphocytes (CTL) cross-reactive with a single Epstein-Barr virus CTL epitope: implications for graft-versus-host disease. *J Exp Med* 1994;179(4):1155–61.

[218] Landais E, Morice A, Long HM, Haigh TA, Charreau B, Bonneville M, et al. EBV-specific CD4+ T cell clones exhibit vigorous allogeneic responses. *J Immunol* 2006;177(3):1427–33.

[219] Gamadia LE, Remmerswaal EB, Surachno S, Lardy NM, Wertheim-van Dillen PM, van Lier RA, et al. Cross-reactivity of cytomegalovirus-specific CD8+ T cells to allo-major histocompatibility complex class I molecules. *Transplantation* 2004;77(12):1879–85.

[220] Kieper WC, Jameson SC. Homeostatic expansion and phenotypic conversion of naive T cells in response to self peptide/MHC ligands. *Proc Natl Acad Sci U S A* 1999;96(23):13306–11.

[221] Pearl JP, Parris J, Hale DA, Hoffmann SC, Bernstein WB, McCoy KL, et al. Immunocompetent T-cells with a memory-like phenotype are the dominant cell type following antibody-mediated T-cell depletion. *Am J Transplant* 2005;5(3):465–74.

[222] Kirk AD, Hale DA, Mannon RB, Kleiner DE, Hoffmann SC, Kampen RL, et al. Results from a human renal allograft tolerance trial evaluating the humanized CD52-specific monoclonal antibody alemtuzumab (CAMPATH-1H). *Transplantation* 2003;76(1):120–9.

[223] Swanson SJ, Hale DA, Mannon RB, Kleiner DE, Cendales LC, Chamberlain CE, et al. Kidney transplantation with rabbit antithymocyte globulin induction and sirolimus monotherapy. *Lancet* 2002;360(9346):1662–4.

[224] Wu Z, Bensinger SJ, Zhang J, Chen C, Yuan X, Huang X, et al. Homeostatic proliferation is a barrier to transplantation tolerance. *Nat Med* 2004;10(1):87–92.

[225] Lopez M, Clarkson MR, Albin M, Sayegh MH, Najafian N. A novel mechanism of action for anti-thymocyte globulin: induction of CD4+CD25+Foxp3+ regulatory T cells. *J Am Soc Nephrol* 2006;17(10):2844–53.

[226] Noris M, Casiraghi F, Todeschini M, Cravedi P, Cugini D, Monteferrante G, et al. Regulatory T cells and T cell depletion: role of immunosuppressive drugs. *J Am Soc Nephrol* 2007;18(3):1007–18.

[227] Minamimura K, Gao W, Maki T. CD4+ regulatory T cells are spared from deletion by antilymphocyte serum, a polyclonal anti-T cell antibody. *J Immunol* 2006;176(7):4125–32.

[228] Neujahr DC, Chen C, Huang X, Markmann JF, Cobbold S, Waldmann H, et al. Accelerated memory cell homeostasis during T cell depletion and approaches to overcome it. *J Immunol* 2006;176(8):4632–9.

[229] Valujskikh A, Pantenburg B, Heeger PS. Primed allospecific T cells prevent the effects of costimulatory blockade on prolonged cardiac allograft survival in mice. *Am J Transplant* 2002;2(6):501–9.

[230] Haanstra KristaG, Sick EllaA, Ringers Jan, Wubben JacquelineAM, Kuhn Eva-Maria, 't Hart BertA, et al. No synergy between ATG induction and costimulation blockade induced kidney allograft survival in rhesus monkeys. *Transplantation* 2006;82(9):1194–201.

[231] Almeida AR, Borghans JA, Freitas AA. T cell homeostasis: thymus regeneration and peripheral T cell restoration in mice with a reduced fraction of competent precursors. *J Exp Med* 2001;194(5):591–9.

[232] Ge Q, Hu H, Eisen HN, Chen J. Different contributions of thymopoiesis and homeostasis-driven proliferation to the reconstitution of naive and memory T cell compartments. *Proc Natl Acad Sci U S A* 2002;99(5):2989–94.

[233] Tanchot C, Le Campion A, Martin B, Leaument S, Dautigny N, Lucas B. Conversion of naive T cells to a memory-like phenotype in lymphopenic hosts is not related to a homeostatic mechanism that fills the peripheral naive T cell pool. *J Immunol* 2002;168(10):5042–6.

[234] Pitcher CJ, Hagen SI, Walker JM, Lum R, Mitchell BL, Maino VC, et al. Development and homeostasis of T cell memory in rhesus macaque. *J Immunol* 2002;168(1):29–43.

[235] Balner H. Skin grafting in monkeys and apes. *Transplantation* 1969;8(2):206–9.

[236] van Bekkum DW. Bone marrow transplantation. *Transplant Proc* 1977;9(1):147–54.

[237] van Bekkum DW. The rhesus monkey as a preclinical model for bone marrow transplantation. *Transplant Proc* 1978;10(1):105–11.

[238] van Vreeswijk W, Balner H. Major histocompatibility complex matching and other factors influencing skin allograft survival in related and unrelated rhesus monkeys. *Transplantation* 1980;30(3):196–202.

[239] Balner H, Dersjant H, Van Roodj. A Method to Relate Leukocyte Antigens and Transplantation Antigens in Monkeys. *Transplantation* 1965;3:230–4.

[240] Balner H, Dersjant H, Van Roodj. Leukoagglutinating Isoantibodies in Rhesus Monkeys. *Transplantation* 1965;3:402–22.

[241] Balner H, Eysvoogel VP, Cleton FJ. Testing of anti-human lymphocyte sera in chimpanzees and lower primates. *Lancet* 1968;1(7532):19–22.

[242] Balner H, Yron I, Dersjant H, Zaalberg O, Betel I. ALG treatment of Rhesus monkeys. Attempts to reduce complications by the induction of tolerance. *Transplantation* 1970;10(5):416–24.

[243] Jonker M, Goldstein G, Balner H. Effects of in vivo administration of monoclonal antibodies specific for human T cell subpopulations on the immune system in a rhesus monkey model. *Transplantation* 1983;35(6):521–6.

[244] van Es AA, Balner H. Serological matching for D locus antigens improves kidney allograft survival in rhesus monkeys. *Transplantation* 1978;26(3):187–90.

[245] van Es AA, Marquet RL, van Rood JJ, Kalff MW, Balner H. Blood-transfusions induce prolonged kidney allograft survival in rhesus monkeys. *Lancet* 1977;1(8010):506–9.

[246] Jonker M, van de Hout Y, Neuhaus P, Ringers J, Kuhn EM, Bruijn JA, et al. Complete withdrawal of immunosuppression in kidney allograft recipients: a prospective study in rhesus monkeys. *Transplantation* 1998;66(7):925–7.

[247] Leonard AA, Jonker M, Lagaaij EL. Complete withdrawal of immunosuppression in allograft recipients. A study in rhesus monkeys. *Transplantation* 1996;61(11):1648–51.

In: Immunosuppression: New Research
Editor: Charles B. Taylor, pp. 45-88
ISBN: 978-1-60692-102-9

Chapter 2

Strategies for T Cell Depletion to Prevent Graft versus Host Disease

Liang-Piu Koh[1, 2] ***and David A. Rizzieri***[1]
[1]Adult Bone Marrow and Stem Cell Transplantation Program
Duke University Medical Center, Durham, North Carolina.
[2] Stem Cell Transplant Program, Department of Hematology-Oncology, National University Hospital, Singapore

Abstract

T-cell depletion (TCD) represents one of the most effective strategies in abrogating the negative effects of severe graft versus host disease (GVHD) due to allogeneic hematopoietic cell transplantation (HCT), particularly for recipients of HLA-mismatched or haploidentical allografts. The past decade has witnessed the development of different graft manipulation strategies, moving from E-rosetting and soybean agglutination, through a combination of negative or positive selection of HSC, to recent one-step positive selection using immunoadsorption columns and monoclonal antibody for ex vivo or in vivo purging. Recent advances with effective T-cell depletion have significantly decreased the early transplant related mortality and risk of severe GVHD, while enabling reliable engraftment, and hence provide encouraging outcomes in both matched or mismatched donor transplantation. However, while they have broadened the array of patients able to be offered immunotherapy to those without a fully matched sibling, post-transplant infections and relapse remain important barriers to overcome. A key challenge is to balance the positive and negative effects of donor T cells to optimize outcome. New directions in the use of adoptive cellular immunity, immunoregulatory T cells, mesenchymal stem cell and selective allodepletion in rapidly reconstituting immunity without GVHD appear promising. The full therapeutic potential of allogeneic HCT will not be realized until approaches to separate GVH and graft versus leukaemia (GVL) are developed.

Introduction

Graft-versus-host disease (GvHD) remains one of the major impediments to long term remission of hematological disorders following allogeneic hematopoietic cell transplantation (HCT), causing significant morbidity and mortality even when the donor and recipient are allele level matched at the major human-leukocyte-antigen (HLA) loci. GVHD occurs in 30-50% of unmanipulated HLA-identical sibling transplant recipients and in more than 60% of mismatched or unrelated donor transplants. [1,2] In its acute and chronic forms, GVHD has an important impact on survival and the recipient's quality of life.[3] As therapy for active GVHD is often disappointing, the ability to prevent GVHD, i.e. the application of successful prophylaxis, is crucial and remains suboptimal . This review presents current techniques for T cell depletion as a means of prophylaxis and discusses the recent successes and persistent challenges.

Acute GVHD results from the activation of donor-derived T cells, which recognize host-specific alloantigens.[4] The T-cell response to these antigenic differences results in the clinical syndrome of acute GVHD. In its most severe forms, GVHD may be largely refractory to immunosuppressive therapy, leading directly or indirectly to the patient's death. On the other hand, the presence of GVHD is not entirely a negative event. GVHD has been reported to be associated with a graft-versus-leukaemia (GVL) effect, because of widely distributed histocompatibility antigens of the recipient not shared by the donor. In the context of transplantation for the treatment of haematological malignancies, GVHD-associated GVL effect results in a decreased relapse incidence.[5] Thus, the goal of any approach for prophylaxis of GvHD is not only to effectively control GvHD but also simultaneously preserve the anti-malignancy as well as anti-pathogen effects.

Improved understanding of the pathophysiology of GVHD has led to rational approaches to both prophylaxis and therapy. To diminish the risk of GVHD, all patients are either given immunosuppressive agents that impair T-cell functions or allografts that have been depleted of T cells, the putative cells causing this side effect. To diminish the risk of GVHD, all patients are either given immunosuppressive agents that impair T-cell functions or allografts that have been depleted of T cells, the putative cells causing this side effect. Early attempts in mismatched bone marrow transplant has shown that a 3-log T cell depletion of the donor bone marrow can be achieved using soybean agglutination and E-rosetting technique.[6]This approach, while contributing substantially to the control of GvHD, has been associated with negative consequences though. First, the use of pharmacological agents for immunosuppression is associated with several undesirable adverse effects. Secondly, the immunosuppression achieved with rigorous T cell depletion (TCD) greatly enhances the risk of graft rejection and leukemia relapse, as well as impairs the immune reconstitution, with a consequent increased risk of viral and fungal infections, and Epstein-Barr virus associated post transplant lymphoproliferative disorders (PTLD). [7, 8, 9]

Despite the problems associated with T-cell depletion (TCD), great interest remains in developing this technology due to the negative effects of severe GVHD, particularly for recipients of HLA-mismatched or haploidentical allografts. The past decade has witnessed the development of different graft manipulation strategies, moving from E-rosetting and soybean agglutination, through a combination of negative or positive selection of HSC, to the current method of one-step positive selection using immunoadsorption columns and monoclonal antibody for ex vivo or in vivo purging. The rapid progress in this area has resulted in effective prophylaxis of GVHD and broadened the application of allogeneic transplant to individuals who do not have an HLA-matched related or unrelated donor, making the hapoidentical or mismatched transplant feasible for these patients. Issues of disease relapse and infection still persist though.

This chapter will provide an overview of different strategies of T cell depletion with an emphasis on the non-pharmacological approach. GVHD prevention using pharmacological agents such as calcineurine inhibitor is largely beyond the scope of this chapter. However, the topic will be briefly discussed on under the following subsection.

Pharmacological Intervention

Current approaches for the prevention and treatment of GvHD involve direct blockade of T-cell function. These include down-regulation of T lymphocytes by inhibiting cellular proliferation (methotrexate), inhibition of de novo purine synthesis (mycophenolate mofetil), suppression of IL-2 secretion by blocking calcineurin activity (cyclosporine, tacrolimus), interfering downstream growth signaling pathways (sirolimus), reduction of T-cell responsiveness by blocking IL-2 receptor (daclizumab). The combination of cyclosporin and short course of methotrexate is a standard for GvHD prevention as randomized studies showed less grade III-IV GvHD and improvement of overall survival in patients with leukemia and aplastic anemia compared to adding steroids to further improve prophylaxis.[10, 11, 12, 13, 14, 15] But despite the use of these agents, acute GVHD occurs after 35% to 50% of matched-related donor (MRD) transplantation and occurs even more frequently after unrelated donor (URD) transplantation.[16] One-year transplantation-related mortality after MRD transplantation ranges from 27% to 37% [17,18] and is higher after URD transplantation, in large part due to GVHD or the immunosuppression associated in part with its treatment. [19,20, 21]

Alternative regimens, such as substituting with another calcineurin inhibitors like tacrolimus and other newer agents such as sirolimus and mycophenolate mofetil (MMF) are recently being evaluated in clinical studies with encouraging results in GvHD prevention.[22, 23,24, 25, 26, 27, 28,29, 30,31] Tacrolimus, a calcineurin inhibitor with similar mechanism as cyclosporine (CsP) but with higher potency on an equimolar basis, has been used in combination with methotrexate (MTX) in several clinical studies. In both related HLA-identical sibling HCT and matched unrelated donor HCT, the combination of tacrolimus and MTX resulted in significantly reduced incidence of GvHD when compared with CsP/MTX and comparable renal toxicity and relapse rate, suggesting tacrolimus as an appropriate alternative to CsP, [22,23] although the superior effect seemed to be clearer in unrelated donor HCT in other analyses.[24]

The use of MMF as part of non-MTX-containing regimens is recently being explored with the hope to avoid MTX related toxicities such as mucositis. With most of studies involved nonmyeloablative conditioning[28,32,33] although there were several studies with myeloablative conditioning,[28,31] MMF has been shown to provide equivalent immunosuppressive activity with regard to occurrence of acute GvHD, and a reduction in mucositis and duration of neutropenia, but a possibly increased risk of viral infections.[29,30,31]

T Cell Depletion - An Effective Non-Pharmacologic Immunosuppression

With the recognition that T lymphocytes are central players in the pathophysiology of GvHD, donor T-cell depletion (TCD) has been employed in experimental and clinical approaches to control this undesirable clinical entity. In many instances, TCD can dramatically reduce the incidence of GvHD even in the absence of post-transplantation immunosuppressive therapy. Ex vivo T cell depletion using various techniques – e.g. soybean agglutination, elutriation or, later on, positive CD34 selection of stem cells – have been reported for many years. In addition, several antibodies such as Alemtuzumab (Campath) and antithymocyte globulin (ATG) have been incorporated into transplant conditioning regimens and serve as powerful in vivo T cell depletion agents. The availability of these effective T cell depleting strategies has resulted in less severe GVHD and has broadened the application of hematopoietic transplant to patients with only a partially HLA matched donor available.

Pre –Clinical Models and Early Clinical Studies

A series of studies performed in animal models revealed that allogeneic marrow or spleen cells that were depleted of T cells rescued the recipient from lethal irradiation without causing fatal GVHD, despite disparity of MHC between the donor and host. [34, 35, 36] In the late 1970s, it became clear from murine models that even minor alloantigen differences could stimulate GVHD, and that contamination of the marrow with as few as 0.3% T lymphocytes (3×10^4 cells) could be sufficient to cause lethal GVHD.[37] Subsequent clinical observations have shown that GVHD can be effectively prevented by infusing less than 1-5 x 10^5 T cells/kg of recipient body weight. [38, 39] However, early enthusiasm for the ex vivo removal of immunocompetent T-cells from the marrow graft, as will be discussed below, was tempered by an increased risk of graft failure, delayed immune reconstitution, increased Epstein-Barr virus associated posttransplantation lymphoproliferative disorders (PTLD), and increased rate of disease relapse, revealing the new and important limitations associated with TCD BMT.

Strategies of T Cell Depletion

To address these persistent concerns in humans, a myriad of T cell depletion strategies have been developed and employed over the past three decades to minimize GVHD and maximize antitumor and anti-infective effects. (Table 1). They can be broadly classified as *ex vivo* or *in vitro* TCD. Most *ex vivo* strategies are primarily dependent on either (i) negative selection techniques by physical separation (which include differential agglutination with lectins followed by rosetting with sheep red blood cells, [6,40] counterflow centrifugal elutriation, [41,42,43] or fractionation on density gradients.[44]); (ii) antibody-based purging; or (iii) positive selection of CD34+ stem cells. In contrast, most *in vivo* TCD that has been employed clinically in the human setting involves the incorporation of either antithymocyte globulin (ATG) or monoclonal antibodies such as alemtuzumab in the pretransplant conditioning regimen. The prolonged half lives of ATG and alemtuzumab allow the active compound to persist in the circulation and therefore elimination of T cells of the infused allograft. Another new strategy that has recently been explored involves administration of high-dose cyclophosphamide after transplant induced immune tolerance, thus reducing GvHD and graft rejection. [45]

The availability of effective TCD techniques provides a pivotal platform in the development of haploidentical transplant. [46] It also leads to the enthusiastic application of TCD in allogeneic HSCT with the general anticipation that pharmacological immunosuppression in this setting is not adequate. While large bodies of clinical evidence attests to the efficacy of TCD strategies in crossing the immunological barrier and GvHD suppression, it has also revealed new and important limitations associated with TCD HSCT. These include potentially a higher incidence of graft failure, relapse, and complications associated with delayed immune reconstitution with resultant risk of infection and Epstein-Barr virus associated post transplant lymphoproliferative disorders.

Table 1. Methods of T Cell Depletion

1) Ex Vivo TCD

1.1 Negative Selection

Physical - DACS (Density adjusted cell sorting)
- Counterflow centrifugal elutriation

Immunological – Soybean lectin and erythrocyte rosette
Monoclonal antibody + rabbit/human complement
Monoclonal antibody formulated as immunotoxin
Monoclonal antibody bound to magnetic beads

Photodynamic Cell Purging

1.2 Positive Selection

CD34+ immunoadsorption column (eg: CliniMACS)

2) In Vivo TCD

Monoclonal Antibody (eg: Alemtuzumab/ Campath)
Antithymocyte Globulin (eg: Thymoglobulin)
Posttransplantation Cyclophosphamide

i. Early Development in TCD

Early efforts at TCD were thus intended to maximally purge lymphocytes without compromising hematopoietic precursors. Positive and/or negative selection of the hematopoietic stem cells are the most commonly used techniques in graft manipulation today. In the negative selection, unwanted T cells are eliminated from the allogeneic grafts. The early techniques of negative selection developed were based on combining E-rosetting and soy bean lectin aggutinination, which removes cells producing graft versus host reactions by differential agglutination with the galactose binding lectin soybean agglutinin.[36] This approach had first been attempted in animal models [36], then applied in transplantation for patients with severe combined immunodeficiency and leukemia.[6 , , 47] Investigators in Perugia made further advancements in successful T cell depletion in pioneering the 'mega-dose' CD34+ stem cell dosage. This approach utilizes G-CSF mobilized peripheral blood stem cells and bone marrow cells, both *ex vivo* depleted of T cells by soybean agglutination and E-rosetting, following an intensive total body irradiation (TBI) -based conditioning regimen. Clinical studies showed convincingly that prompt engraftment was achieved with low occurrence of GVHD. [70, 48]

Since the 1990s, several investigators have started evaluating haploidentical transplant by using partial T cell depletion combined with intensive immunosuppression. Hanslee-Downey et al [49] were among the early pioneerers in exploiting a novel sequential immunomodulation strategy pre- and post-transplant using *ex vivo* T-cell depletion with the $T_{10}B_9$ monoclonal antibody and *in vivo* T-cell lysis with immunotoxin H65-RTA, following an intensive TBI-based myeloablative conditioning. Seventy-two patients received partially mismatched related donor grafts from haploidentical family members using this treatment protocol. The engraftment rate of 88%, 16% probability of acute GVHD grade II-IV and 51 % probability of extensive chronic GVHD were encouraging. At a median follow-up of 21.5 months, the 2-year disease free survival (DFS) was 31%, with 53% probability of DFS seen among the low risk patients.

These studies highlighted the feasibility of partial T cell depletion in preventing GVHD in mismatched hematopoietic transplant and the importance of post-grafting immunosuppression in lowering the risk of graft failure, significantly broadening the array of patients who may now be offered immunotherapy from those with matched donors to those with at least a partially matched family member..

ii. Recent Advances in T Cell Depletion

While a wide range of T cell depleting techniques have been employed, three different strategies of T cell depletion have emerged to show promising results: (1) Positive CD34+ selection; (2) *ex vivo* CD3+/CD19+ T cell depletion (negative selection); (3) *in vivo* T cell depletion using alemtuzumab or ATG, and posttransplantation cyclophosphamide. While it is impossible to make a definite conclusion with regard to the best option available in the absence of propective comparative studies, some of the merits and limitations of each technique will be compared and discussed.

A wide array of monoclonal antibodies, either used alone [50, 51, 52] or in conjunction with homologous or heterologous complement, [53, 54, 55] have been employed with successful 2-4 log T cell reduction. Alemtuzumab (Campath), an anti-CD52 monoclonal antibodies, has been widely used for both *in vitro* and *ex vivo* TCD. It has been incorporated into many myeloablative and nonmyeloablative conditioning regimens with encouraging outcomes in terms of GvHD management and has also broadened the applicability of transplant using both matched and mismatched donors.[46, 93, 95, 96]

(A) Positive CD34 Selection

Using CD34+ hematopoietic stem cell selection for elimination of T-cells represents an important breakthrough in the field of HSCT, especially in the field of haploidentical transplantation. First introduced by investigators from Tuebingen, CD34+ selection was primarily developed to enrich for hematopoietic progenitor cells and passive depletion of tumour or lymphoma cell contamination in autologous apheresis product.[56,57 58] The first system available for large clinical-scale CD34+ selection was based on an immunoaffinity device using an avidin-coated column and biotinylated anti-CD34 antibody (Ceprate SC).[59] During subsequent years new methodologies based on immunomagnetic enrichment with ferromagnetic particles (Isolex 300) have been developed, which allowed for better recovery of CD34+ cells and purities between ≥95%. [58,60] The technology of immunomagnetic CD34+ selection has now been optimized towards a closed system which allows each site to adhere to the principles of good manufacturing practice, leading to approval for clinical use in Europe and the Unite States. Importantly, the availability of the $CD34^+$-enrichment technique using the CliniMACS system (Miltenyi Biotec Gmbh, Bergish Gladbach, Germany) has provided a reproducible T-cell depletion of >4.5 logs in several studies, [58] This technology, initially intended to prepare stem cell grafts for autologous transplantation was later extended to allogeneic transplantation settings. Moreover, positive stem cell selection techniques can be followed by antibody-based negative selection to further deplete specific T cell populations. Several studies have shown the feasibility of transplanting allogeneic CD34+ selected PBSC from matched related donors,[61,62,63,64,65,66] haploidentical related donors,[67,68,69,70,71,72,73, 74]unrelated donors.[75,76,77] In contrast to the time-consuming and 'difficult-to-standardize' TCD techniques by the older physical separation methods discussed above, the availability of CD34+ selection has allowed effective, reproducible TCD to be performed in a relatively simple and automated manner.

(B) CD3+/CD19+ Depletion

The delayed immune reconstitution in CD34+ selected cells is partly attributed to the absence of NK cells, monocytes or granulocytes. A negative T-and B-cells depletion strategy was thus developed to overcome this limitation. Using anti-CD3- and anti-CD19-coated microbeads on a CliniMACS device, this negative T-and B-cells (CD3/CD19) depletion strategy resulted in grafts with up to a 4 log reduction in T-cells. The CD34+ dose was approximately half of that collected from the CD34+ selection strategies reported above.[78] This approach preserves a high content of NK cells and other non-CD34+ cells in the graft, which may contribute to the important engraftment-facilitating function and graft-vs.-tumor effects after transplantation, especially in the setting of killer inhibitory receptor (KIR) mismatch situations. Further, the cellular preparations depleted of B cells also minimize development of Epstein–Barr-virus-associated lymphoproliferative diseases. This CD3/CD19-depletion approach has been tested in a pilot study of 10 patients with advanced hematological malignancies receiving transplant from mismatched donors. Using a reduced intensity conditioning regimen, the study showed that stable engraftment could be achieved in all patients with a low incidence of GVHD.[78] Treatment-related mortality was still 30% though and overall survival was 50% with 4 patients alive and in complete remission at a median follow of > 1 year. Importantly, favorable immune reconstitution with fast reconstitution of NK cells was noted with this approach, resulting in few infectious complications. In their most recent published updated report which included another 19 patients, engraftment occurred in all except 1 patient. Grade ≥2 and ≥ 3 acute GVHD occurred in 48% and 14% of patients, respectively. However, the first 100 day TRM was 20% and the event free and overall survival at 12 month were both 35%. [79] The fast engraftment seen in this CD3/CD19 group with CD34 doses as low as 5.2×10^6 $CD34^+$ cells/kg demonstrates that successful haploidentical transplant may be feasible even without mega-doses of $CD34^+$ stem cells. This may have logistic implications as mobilization and/or harvesting and processing of megadoses of CD34+ cells can be labor intensive, expensive, and place considerable demand on both the donors and the pheresis service.

(C) In vivo T Cell Depletion Using Alemtuzumab or ATG

Another method of immunosuppression commonly used to reduce graft failure and GVHD in unrelated or mismatched/haploidentical transplant is the simultaneous depletion of host and donor immune cells using ATG or alemtuzumab at the time of transplantation. Significant in vivo depletion of donor T cells from the graft can be achieved with alemtuzumab and ATG persisting in the patient's circulation for weeks after the allograft, thereby allowing a prolonged donor T cell depletion and reduction in the risk of GVHD. Several investigators have incorporated antithymocyte globulin (ATG)[80,81,82,83,84] with some confirming that the addition of ATG pretransplant reducing the risk of severe aGVHD, the incidence of extensive cGVHD, and of nonrelapse mortality (NRM)[83,84,85] This has led to the results of matched unrelated donor transplant approaching those of matched sibling donor transplants in some series.[86,87,88] However, there are also disadvantages to this approach because there is evidence for delayed immune reconstitution and a higher risk of infectious complications and of disease relapse.[89] At least one phase three study is underway in the MUD population to assess the outcomes with and without ATG in the preparative regimen.

Alemtuzumab (Campath-1H), a humanized rat monoclonal anti-CD52 antibody, targets the CD52 antigen, which is expressed by all lymphocytes, monocytes, and dendritic cells, but not by adult hematopoietic stem cells.[90] The long half-life of alemtuzumab also results in the depletion of donor $CD52^+$ cells including circulating antigen-presenting dendritic cells.[91, 92] This humanized antibody is uniquely suited to managing both graft rejection and GVHD because of its ability to deplete T cells as well as B cells from both host and recipient.[93] Furthermore, recent evidence has suggested that alemtuzumab may be selective in the T cells that it targets for elimination, thus allowing it to limit GVHD while promoting engraftment and maintaining the allogeneic antitumor effect. The preferential targeting of CD52 expressing monocyte-derived dendritic cells, and sparing of Langerhans cells and dermal-interstitial dendritic cells has been speculated to facilitate immune reconstitution and in mediating the GVL effect.[94]

Alemtuzumab have been used over the last two decades in stem cell transplantation for depletion of donor and recipient T-cells to prevent graft-versus-host disease and graft rejection.[95,96] Several clinical trials evaluated the ability of alemtuzumab to prevent GVHD following conventional, [97, 98, 99 ,100] or reduced-intensity conditioning allografts,

[101,102,103,104,105,106,107] in the settings of either matched related, unrelated or mismatched/haploidentical donor transplants.[108, 109] By depleting T cells in both the donor and the recipient, alemtuzumab has been shown to prevent development of both acute and chronic GVHD, without impairing engraftment or inhibiting the benefits associated with the graft-versus-leukemia effect. In a the study performed by the Spanish and United Kingdom (UK) Collaborative Groups for Nonmyeloablative Transplantation which analyzed data from 129 patients participating in two prospective studies,[110] investigators compared the effectiveness of alemtuzumab or methotrexate (MTX) in reducing GVHD for patients receiving the same nonmyeloablative-conditioning regimen consisting of fludarabine and melphalan. The study showed that, as compared to MTX, patients receiving alemtuzumab had significantly lower incidence of acute GVHD (21.7% versus 45.1%, $P = .006$) and chronic GVHD (5% versus 66.7%, $P < .001$), a trend toward a lower mortality rate (10% *v* 20%; $P=$ .12;), less death related to GvHD (5% *v* 33.4%). No significant differences were observed in event-free or overall survival between the two groups. However, among alemtuzumab-treated patients, there was a higher incidence of CMV reactivation (85% *v* 24%, $P< .001$), suggesting more immunosuppression.

In the context of haploidentical transplant, the use of alemtuzumab or ATG for *in vitro* TCD without any *ex vivo* graft manipulation has resulted in a low incidence of grade II-IV and III-IV acute GVHD ranging between 16-40% and 8-16%, respectively in several series.[111,108, 109]This approach, while allowing the omission of *ex vivo* graft manipulation without compromising its efficacy in risk of GVHD reduction and facilitating engraftment, also confers the advantage of simplifying the transplant procedure and lowering costs. Moreover, this technique provides the additional advantage of allowing T cell depletion to be performed in the absence of a cell-processing facility.[46,108]

(D) Posttransplantation Cyclophosphamide

Preclinical and clinical studies demonstrated that administration of high-dose cyclophosphamide after transplant induced immune tolerance, thus reducing GvHD and graft rejection [112,113, 114, 115]. Recently, Johns Hopkins University and Fred Hutchison Cancer Research Center reported a jointed phase I/II trial in 68 patients who received nonmyeloablative, unmanipulated haploidentical marrow transplant, followed by 50mg/kg per day of cyclophosphamide administered at day 3 or days 3 and 4 after transplant [116]. Graft rejection occurred in 9/66 (13%) evaluable patients. Nonrelapse mortality and relapse at 1 year were 15 and 51%, respectively. The incidence of extensive chronic GvHD at 1 year was 5%in patients who received two doses of posttransplant cyclophosphamide. These outcomes are very encouraging, although further studies with more patients and a longer follow-up are needed to confirm the feasibility of this approach.

(E) Ex-Vivo Induction of T cell Anergy

At the Dana Farber Cancer Institute, Guinan et al [117] investigated the use of costimulatory blockade to induce tolerance and thereby prevention of GVHD development. To induce anergy, donor marrow was harvested and co-cultured with irradiated mononuclear cells from the recipient in the presence of soluble CTLA-4-Ig. After myeloablative conditioning, 12 patients, almost all in advanced stages of a hematological malignancy, received marrow containing a median of 2.8 x 10^7/kg of CD3+ T cells from a mismatched/ haploidentical family member that had been treated to induce anergy. Evaluable patients engrafted at a median of 20 days (range, 14–23), with full donor chimerism observed in 8 of 10 patients in whom engraftment occurred. Of the 12 patients, 7 died of infections, multiorgan failure, hemorrhage, or relapse and 5 were alive and in remission 132 to 863 days after transplantation. Only 3 patients developed acute GVHD, confined to the gastrointestinal tract, and no deaths were attributable to GVHD. When the results were recently updated to include another 12 patients,[118] graft failure occurred in 4.2%, aGVHD grade II–III in 35% and cGVHD in 4.2%, suggesting that this strategy has not meet its stated goal of improving outcomes by inducing tolerance.

Merits and Problems with TCD

1. Acute Graft versus Host Disease

Different studies have tried to identify a threshold of T lymphocyte numbers necessary to mediate GVHD in the context of transplantation from HLA-matched related sibling donors. Reduction below 10^5 T lymphocytes per kg bodyweight of the recipient was effective in preventing acute GVHD in recipients of matched related sibling donor transplantation. [119] Most of the commonly employed *ex vivo* TCD depletion methods dependent on negative selection techniques by physical separation or antibody-based purging have consistently resulted in reduction in the incidence of grade II-IV acute GVHD to less than 20-25% after matched related transplantation, [6, 8, 41, 120, 121, 122, 123, 124,125,126] 20-50% after matched unrelated donor transplantation.[127, 128, 129, 130, 131]

Studies on transplantation using $CD34^+$ selection, on the other hand, have reported great variation in acute GVHD incidence from 8% to 100% in matched sibling donor transplant,[61,62,63,64,65,66] 9% to 50% in unrelated donor transplant, [76,77,77] and 0% to 13% in haploidentical donor transplant.[68,69,70,71,72,73,74] This variability in GVHD incidence was likely influenced by factors such as the number of $CD3^+$ cells infused, conditioning regimen, immunosuppressive agents given after transplantation, and type of $CD34^+$ selection device used.

2. Chronic Graft versus Host Disease

Whereas it has been clear that *ex vivo* TCD reduced incidences of acute GVHD after HSCT, the effect on chronic GVHD has been less well lineated. Single center studies using T-cell depleting regimens producing 2 to 4 log depletions report a low incidence of chronic GVHD[132, 133] but other studies using antibodies with narrower specificity have reported higher incidences. [134] In the recently published first large prospective randomised trial of T cell depletion in unrelated marrow transplantation,[131] 410 patients were randomized to receive TCD with either counterflow elutriation or incubation of marrow cells with T10B9 monoclonal antibody, or immunesuppression with cyclosporine/methotrexate. The study showed that TCD resulted in lower acute GVHD (grade II-IV acute GVHD 39% vs 63%) and lower early toxicity, but no reduction in the incidence of chronic GVHD. There was no statistically significant difference in survival between the recipients of TCD and unmanipulated marrow. The main caveat of the study lies in the degree of TCD with counterflow elutriation or T10B9 monoclonal antibody incubation. With only one log depletion of T cell, the conclusion of this study cannot be extrapolated to other TCD regimens. Further, with the higher incidence of fatal viral complications and also leukemia relapse observed among CML patients in the TCD arm, the study reinforces several important points: (i) For a TCD regimen to be successful it must do more than just protect against GVHD; (ii) It must also preserve graft-versus-leukemia (GVL) activity and engraftment potential and spare patients from excessive transplant-related toxicity.

3. Graft Failure

One of the main concerns with profound T cell depletion relates to the higher incidence of graft failure. Several published series between late 80s and early 90s on T-cell depleted HLA identical transplant in leukemia patients have documented significant rate of graft failure ranging between 10-30%,[135, 136, 137,138, 139, 140], with some exceeding 50%. [141, 142] In an analysis from the IBMTR of more than 3000 patients who received TCD or non-TCD BMT for leukemia, TCD was associated with a 9-fold increased risk for graft failure compared to unmanipulated marrow transplantation.[7] The mechanism of graft failure was attributed to an immune rejection mediated by anti-donor cytotoxic T-lymphocyte precursors (CTL-p) in the host [143, 144] or to competition for 'niches' from residual host stem cells,[145] either of which having survived the conditioning. In unmanipulated grafts, the presence of donor T cells usually suppresses residual host immunity, facilitating engraftment, but such suppression is abolished by profound T-cell depletion of the graft. Several other risk factors associated with higher incidence of graft failure have also been identifed and these include HLA disparity, donor-patient gender disparity, lower dose of TBI in the conditioning, donor age over 25 years, and absence of posttransplantation immunosuppression. [7, 141, 146] It was originally believed that this barrier to engraftment could be overcome by a global increase in the intensity of the conditioning regimen,[147, 148] or giving extra whole body[142] or total lymphoid irradiation.[149] However, such intensive regimens have led to unacceptable toxicity, particularly in heavily pretreated patients with advanced disease. The inclusion of total lymphoid irradiation (TLI) in the conditioning regimen, despite having lower incidence of graft failure in the setting of mismatched transplant,[149] also raised the concern of long-term side effects of irradiation, particularly among pediatric patients.

More recently, focus has been shifted towards further depletion of host immune cells with concurrent use of immunosuppressive agents such as fludarabine,[70] antithymocyte globulin (ATG)[70,111 ,150] alemtuzumab[98,100,108,109]and other anti-T cell antibodies.[151] in which several clinical studies have demonstrated similar immunosuppressive effect to allow prompt and robust engraftment without excessive toxicity. Such approach have successfully reduced incidence of graft rejection of TCD transplant using both HLA matched related sibling donor,[98,110,152], matched unrelated donor,[100,153] mismatched/haploidentical donor following both ablative and nonmyeloablative conditioning.[46]

Probably the most important development in preventing rejection has been the concept that escalation of the stem cell dose directly contributes to the likelihood of establishing donor type chimerism. Increasing the donor stem cell dose may facilitate competition with residual host stem cells for available niches. Additionally, it was realized that cells within the $CD34^+$ compartment possessed potent veto activity, which neutralize host alloreactive CTL, and the greater the number of $CD34^+$ cells, the greater the induction of tolerance.[154, 155] Aversa et al from University of Perugia, Italy, pioneered a strategy in which a 'mega-dose' of vigorously T-cell depleted, GCSF-mobilized PBSCs from haploidentical donors was transplanted following a TBI/thiotepa/fludarabine/antithymocyte globulin based conditioning regimen. With this approach, traditional barriers such as graft failure and GVHD could be overcome, but the incidence of TRM (mainly resulting from infection) was 40%. [70, 74]This group further tried to refine this approach for large-scale clinical studies by using automated devices for $CD34^+$ cell purification and has published the outcome in104 patients with high-risk acute leukemias. Notable features of this study were reliable and reproducible $CD34^+$ cell purification, high engraftment rates (Engraftment was achieved in 100 of 101 evaluable patients.), and prevention of GVHD despite the use of haploidentical donors.[74]

4. Relapse

Numerous clinical studies involving T-cell replete marrow have demontrated the inversion relationship between leukemia relapse and GVHD,[5,156, 157] suggesting the important role of antileukemic effect exerted by the allograft. Such graft-versus-leukemia(GVL) effect may be further abrogated by extensive T-cell depletion. Several retrospective studies have documented higher leukemic relapse after TCD BMT, especially for CML.[5,7, 158,159,160]

In an attempt to further improve on engraftment and overcome the major drawback of TCD BMT, investigators from Memorial Sloan Kettering and Perugia modified the conditoning protocol by adding antithymocyte globulin and thiotepa to the conditioning regimen to prevents rejection of extensively T-cell–depleted bone marrow by soybean agglutination and E-rosetting technique.[161,162] In a small cohort of patients with acute leukemia, the two group have shown low relapse rate of <20% in patients and favorable 5 year disease free survival exceeding 70% among patients with AML in remission. Importantly, there was no graft rejection seen, suggesting that robust engraftment without GVHD can be attained in patients of TCD HLA identical transplant without adverse effects on relapse rate.

In contrast to results obtained with TCD in acute leukemia, the outcome of TCD transplant in CML patients was clearly associated with markedly enhanced relapse rate. Therefore, for almost 10 years beginning in the mid 1980s since this problem was recognised, there was very little enthuasism using TCD in the transplant for patients with CML. However, the increase in CML relapse is not as apparent after TCD transplantation using matched unrelated marrow. [163,164] Several studies showed encouragingly low probability of relapse despite the use of TCD graft, suggesting that patients receiving unrelated TCD marrow grafts for CML can achieve durable engraftment with a low incidence of severe GVHD and apparent preservation of GVL reactivity. In contrast to these encouraging results from the retrospective analysis, the prospective randomized trial of TCD in unrelated donor transplant yielded a slightly different result with less favorable outcome for CML patients. Wagner et al reported a higher relapse of was observed after TCD only in patients with CML, but not in patients with AML in the large prospective randomised trial of T cell depletion in unrelated marrow transplantation.[131] Nevertheless, the risk of relapse after TCD in patients with CML in chronic phase remains lower in unrelated donor transplant than that reported after TCD with sibling donors.[159,160]

The success of DLI in salvaging CML patients after BMT[165] has led many researchers to investigate the potential of using delayed T-cell add-back to eliminate residual disease after TCD BMT. However, the high risk of GVHD associated with this approach has tempered the enthusiasm in exploring this option.

Paradoxically, clinical reports of patients with advanced acute myeloid leukaemia (AML) undergoing haploidentical SCT, suggest a relatively low incidence of GVHD and a low relapse rate.[70,166] Extensive elegant work by the investigators in Perugia suggested that donor NK alloreactivity, a biological phenomenon which is unique to mismatched transplants, may play a significant role in this GVL effect in mismatched transplants.[167,168]. The encouraging results seen in the mismatched donor transplant using alemtuzumab-containing conditioing regimen may, in part, be derived from the known benefits of alemtuzumab sparing $CD56^+$ natural killer and cytotoxic T cells, while depleting $CD8^+$ and $CD4^+$ cells.[108]This realization that NK cells from HLA-mismatched donor can exert an anti-leukemia effect against the patients' blasts in the absence of HLA-antigenic engaging killer-inhibitory receptors (KIR) has provided the important framework for the haploidentical transplant, as will be discussed in the following section.

5. Delayed Immune Reconstitution

A major problem limiting the efficacy of TCD HSCT is the issue of delayed immune reconstitution resulting in high TRM and relapse, and also higher probability of reactivation for viruses such as CMV,[169,170,171] and EBV, leading to EBV-associated B-cell lymphoprolifcrative disorders (EBV-LPDs) (as discussed in the following section). Apart from the cytoreductive conditioning and extensive T-cell depletion, functional status of thymus of patient also contributes to post-transplant immune recovery. In adult patients, the capacity for thymic-derived T cell production is greatly diminished as a result of age-related thymic involution,[172] and tissue damage to the thymic epithelial cells caused by cytoreductive conditioning.[173, 174] A slow recovery in $CD4^+$ T cell repertoire is associated with an increased risk of post transplant opportunistic infections, and is the most important cause of mortality in adults undergoing haploidentical transplant, reaching as high as 40% in some studies.[70] Multiple strategies of graft engineering involving depletion of T-cells from the graft have reduced the incidence of GVHD but have not resulted in significant improvements in survival outcomes due to higher rates of infection and relapse. The recent introduction of nonmyeloablative conditioning in haploidentical transplant has resulted in high rate of engraftment and acceptable transplant-related toxicities. However, problems related to delayed immune reconstitution and relapse continues to be impediment.[108] Clearly, expediting immune reconstitution during the early post-transplant period, thereby protecting the host from infection and perhaps generating a graft-versus-tumor effect against disease relapse, remains a critical research objective.

In allogeneic HSCT using mismatched donor, the pattern of immune reconstitution is influenced by, among many factors, age of the patients and type of conditioning (both of which affects thymic function), HLA disparity, the degree of T depletion, $CD34^+$ cell dose infused, *in vitro* T depleting effect of agents such as ATG or alemtuzumab, and whether GVHD occurs post transplant. Waller et al [175] analyzed the kinetics of immune reconstitution and incidence of GVHD in 28 adult patients (median age 31 years, range 21-56 years) with very high-risk hematological malignancies who received ATG conditioning and lymphocyte-depleted, CD34+ cell-enriched HPC grafts from partially HLA-matched related donors. The study showed that normal numbers of blood NK cells and B-cells recovered within 1–2 months of transplant, but blood T-cell counts were below normal for more than 1 year with slower recovery seen in older in older patients as compared to the younger patients The low numbers of circulating T-cells contributed to death due to infections or EBV lymphoproliferative disorders in 21/28 patients. The results suggest that slow T-cell recovery was not due to effects of residual active ATG in the plasma posttransplant, but was rather a result of ex vivo T-cell depletion and in vivo ATG purging of donor T-cells combined with poor thymic function.

As compared to adult patients, pediatric patients receiving myeloablative haploidentical transplant showed a striking difference with more favorable profile in their immune reconstitution. In a prospective study of immune reconstitution post-CD34-selected haploidentical SCT in 20 children, Eyrich et al[176] showed that the reconstitution of functioning T-, B- and NK-cell compartments occurred within the first post-transplant year. The more rapid immune reconstitution in the pediatric setting may be attributed to the higher $CD34^+$ cell doses infused and also because of the presence of intact thymic function. $CD34^+$ cell with a megadoses of >20 × 10^6/kg appear to enhance the recovery of CD3 and CD4 lymphocyte populations.[68] The more favorable immune recovery seen in the pediatric cohort resulted a slightly lower incidence of fatal infectious complications (18%) as compared to the group with predominance of adults as reported by Aversa et al, [74] which had a higher incidence (25%) of early lethal infections. Similarly, in another pediatric series using reduced conditioning that was devoid of TBI and ATG, rapid recovery of $CD3^+$ T-cells, T-cell receptor (TCR) excision circle counts, TCRβ repertoire diversity and natural killer (NK)-cells was observed during the first 4 months post-transplantation. [177] The results compared favorably to a group of patients who received myeloablative conditioning regimen and also patients described in other haploidentical studies,[178] suggesting that reduced intensity conditioning allows more rapid immune reconstitution.

6. Epstein–Barr-Virus-Associated Post-transplant Lymphoproliferative Disease (EBV-PTLD)

T-cell depletion using both i*n vivo* and *in vitro* technique, has been identified as an important predisposing factors for Epstein–Barr-virus-associated posttransplant lymphoproliferative disease (PTLD).[179, 180, 181, 182, 183, 184, 185] In a survey of 235 transplant centers,[179] the risk factors for PTLD in the first year after transplant included: (1) unrelated or HLA-mismatched donors (relative risk (RR)=4.1), (2) T-cell depletion (RR=12.7) and (3) the use of antithymocyte globulin (ATG) (RR=6.4) or anti-CD3 monoclonal antibodies (RR=43.2) for the prophylaxis or treatment of graft rejection and/or graft-versus-host disease (GVHD). PTLD occurred in 8% of HSCT recipients with two risk factors and 22% of recipients with three risk factors. Consistent with the essential role of T cells in controlling the proliferation of latent EBV-infected B-cells, each of these risk factors is associated with prolonged and severe T-cell immunodeficiency. In fact, methods of T-cell depletion that selectively target T cell or T- and NK-cell populations confer a significantly higher risk of PTLD than methods that deplete both T- and B cells.[179, 186, 187] For example, in a study of over 2500 allogeneic transplants, the use of alemtuzumab (that deplete both T- and B cells) for *in vitro* or *in vivo* T-cell depletion was associated with PTLD in only 1.3% of recipients,[96] which is not much different from the rate in patients transplanted with unmodified marrow.[188] This risk reduction was believed to be due to the depletion of both T and B cells by alemtuzumab, thereby removing donor B cells that are potentially infected with EBV from the donor marrow. In addition, other TCD approach employing the CD34+ positive selection strategy [74] for indirect depletion of T and B lymphocytes from PBSC, and the negative T-and B-cells (CD3/CD19) depletion strategy[78] has also resulted in grafts depleted of B cells, thereby avoiding the development of EBV-PTLD.

The use of IFN-α, intravenous γ-globulin, reduction of immunosuppression reduction and high-dose acyclovir are some of the representative strategies employed in the treatment against EBV-LPDs. The response rates with these approaches have been disappointing. [189,190] While reduction in immunosuppression is the most established therapy for PTLD, there are significant risks with this treatment resulting in increased risk for GVHD with significant risk for morbidity and mortality.

Cellular or adoptive immunotherapy, given therapeutically or prophylatically, remains one of the most established strategies for treatment of PTLD. The observation that unselected donor leukocytes can be efficacious in reconstituting the recipient's immune system has prompted the use of donor leukocyte infusions in treating and preventing PTLD.[191] Administration of unselected bulk of DLI [192, 193]has been proven to be effective treatment of many cases of PTL, but was associated with the risk of GVHD. A strategy to limit the risk of GVHD is the administration of EBV-specific CTLs cultivated in vitro from donor lymphocytes.[194, 195, 196] While this strategy is effective, the significant resources and logistics associated with the creation of patient-specific EBV-specific CTLs limits the widespread use of this treatment. The alternative strategy that is more feasible and widely applicable include the use of the anti-CD20 monoclonal antibody rituximab,[197,198,199] which has been shown to be effective in several case series. Despite the lack of randomized trials to support preemptive treatment based on PCR testing, the efficacy of preemptive rituximab demonstrated so far has provided argument for several centers to accept this pre-emptive approach as a standard of care.[200] More recent emphasis was in the preventive strategies for patients at high risk of developing PTLD. Frequent PCR-based quantitative monitoring may allow early detection of EBV reactivation and hence preemptive therapy by rituximab, thereby improving outcome in patients at high risk of EBV-LPD.[201]

Haploidentical Transplantation

Haploidentical hematopoietic stem cell transplantation (HSCT) provides an opportunity for nearly all patients to benefit from HSCT when a human leukocyte antigen (HLA) genotypically matched sibling is not available.[46] It presents an easier logistic and practical alternative to matched unrelated donor transplantation as well. This may be especially important when dealing with a patient suffering from a disease with a rapid tempo and also for non-Caucasian patients, in whom the chances of finding an available matched unrelated match are still low. Early attempts of haploidentical or partially matched BMT with T-cell replete marrow graft following a myeloablative conditioning has been disappointing, with high transplant-related mortality from GVHD, graft failure, delayed immune reconstitution, vulnerability to life threatening infections and relapse. [202,203] Recent advances with effective T-cell depletion, the use of 'megadose' of stem cells, earlier detection of severe infections combined with better antimicrobial therapy and reduced intensity conditioning has significantly decreased the early transplant related mortality and GVHD, while enabling prompt engraftment, hence advancing the therapeutic benefit of haploidentical transplantation. However, the cardinal problems related to delayed immune reconstitution allowing post-transplant infectious complications and relapse remain, limiting the efficacy of haploidentical HSCT.

In single institution studies, grade II to IV GVHD incidence ranging between 8% to 40% has been reported in recipients of HLA-mismatched myeloablative HSCT after ex vivo ± in vivo TCD using monoclonal antibody or immunomagnetic CD34 selection [49, 71,74,111, 204, 205],

The most encouraging results have come from Perugia, where the investigators pioneered the 'mega-dose' approach by infusing G-CSF mobilized peripheral blood and bone marrow stem cells, both ex vivo depleted of T cells by soybean agglutination and E-rosetting, [206]following an intensive TBI-based conditioning regimen. Although engraftment was prompt with low occurrence of GVHD, subsequent follow-up showed difficulty with both late rejection and/or graft failure. These events resulted in increased transplant-related mortality in excess of 60%, leading to subsequent modification of treatment protocols, [70] which included: (i) substituting cyclophosphamide with fludarabine; (ii) The use of GCSF-mobilized peripheral blood progenitor cells instead of bone marrow grafts; (iii) lower dose of TBI; (iv) Positive immunoselection of peripheral blood $CD34^+$ cells using the Clinimacs device (Miltenyi Biotec) instead of the soybean agglutination and E rosetting. These modifications have resulted in favorable outcome in a large series of high-risk acute leukemia, with sustained full donor type engraftment in over 95%, rapid hematopoietic recovery and a very low incidence of acute GVHD grade II–IV without the need for any post-transplant immune suppression as prophylaxis.[74,207] In their more recently published report,[74] 104 patients with high risk leukemia (67 AML and 37 ALL) were transplanted between 1999 and 2004 following the modified transplant protocol of the Perugia group. Engraftment was achieved in 100 of 101 evaluable patients. Acute and chronic GVHD developed in 8% and 7% of evaluable patients, respectively. Patients in any remission had a remarkable event-free survival of 47 ± 6%. The cumulative incidence of relapse in patients transplanted in remission from natural killer alloreactive donors was 14%, whereas it was 28% in the non-alloreactive donors. For patients transplanted in relapse, the corresponding relapse rates were 33% and 45%, respectively, emphasizing the importance of pre-transplant disease control and presence of NK alloreactivity.

High transplant-related mortality in the range of 35-40%, contributed mainly by post-transplant infectious complications and relapse, remain important barriers to overcome.[74,208] This has important implication as the high TRM associated with this procedure will limit its use only in otherwise healthy, younger patients. To extend allogeneic HSCT to older patients with comorbidities, reduced-intensity or nonmyeloablative conditioning lacking significant regimen related toxicities has been developed. The clinical outcome of patients undergoing haploidentical/mismatched transplant using the reduced-intensity preparative regimens have been published by several groups.[46, 78,79, 108,109,209,210, 211] Most of these studies include patients of poor prognostic group with either relapsed chemoresistant or primary refractory hematological diseases. The results showed that this reduced intensity conditioning regimen is associated with less immediate regimen-related toxicities. Importantly, despite the less ablative conditioning regimen and the use of mismatched donors, graft failure rate is low, ranging between 0% and 17%. This is attributed to a combination of factors including the use of immunosuppressive regimens and the effective ex vivo ± in vivo TCD strategies employed. The incidence of grade III-IV acute GVHD is lower than 20% and the non-relapse mortality is in the range between 10-30%. While these reduced-intensity preparative regimens have decreased immediate procedural mortality and GVHD, cardinal problems related to delayed immune reconstitution causing post-transplant infectious complications and relapse remain. It remains to be seen if these barriers can all be safely overcome to result in long-term improvements in survival. As will be discussed in the following section, new directions in the use of adoptive cellular immunity appear promising.[212] Preliminary data has demonstrated the great potential of selective allodepletion in rapidly reconstituting immunity without GVHD.[213, 214] It appears that in some T cell-depleted haploidentical transplants, the benefit of NK alloreactivity is expected to encourage the greater use of haploidentical transplants for a larger number of leukemia patients without matched donors.[215] In addition, there are emerging data to suggest the use of NIMA-mismatched donors in providing an especially attractive strategy for patients to further minimize the risk of GVHD.[216, 217, 218, 219]

Strategies to Improve Outcome of Patients with T Cell Depletion

1. Selective Depletion

In an effort to diminish the problems of engraftment failure and relapse probability risk of ex vivo TCD, recent investigations have focused on the depletion of selective T cell subsets. One of the promising approaches is to selectively remove the T cells responsible for mediating GVHD, while conserving GvL and anti-microbial immune responses. This can be accomplished by deleting T cells that become activated in response to recipient APC. This approach has the advantage that alloreactive T cells are permanently eliminated and cannot influence the function of the remaining T cells. In several murine transplant models, GVHD can be reduced or prevented by removal or inactivation of alloreactive donor T cells using anti-CD25, [220, 221] anti-CD69[222] anti-CD95[223] or photodepletion.[224] This promising approach has been tested by a number of clinical trials involving both HLA matched-sibling donor and haploidentical donor transplantations, and the results suggest that the concept is feasible. [213,214,220,225] In a recently published report, Solomon *et al.*[213] performed transplantations on 16 older patients (median age, 65 years) with selective allodepletion allografts following reduced-intensity conditioning and compared their results with a historical cohort of older transplant recipients receiving unmanipulated allografts. The results demonstrate that ex vivo selective depletion of alloreactive T cells from PBSC allografts, using an anti-CD25 immunotoxin, is feasible and safe and that GVHD severity may be diminished in patients treated by this approach. Furthermore, the severity of GVHD was found to be related to the efficiency of selective allodepletion, as measured by the helper T-lymphocyte precursor (HTLp) frequency assay. Finally, unlike other methods of T-cell depletion, engraftment, GVL, and immune recovery were not adversely affected in these patients. More recently, Amrolia *et al.* [214] reported the results from a dose-escalation study using allodepleted T cells following haploidentical transplantation in 16 patients with a median age of nine years (range, 2–58), treated mostly for high-risk hematologic malignancies. Each patient was scheduled to receive three infusions of allodepleted donor T cells on days 30, 60 and 90 after HSCT. Eight patients received dose level 1 (10^4 cells/kg/dose) and eight patients received dose levels 10^5 cells/kg/dose. Only two patients developed significant acute GVHD, followed by extensive, chronic GVHD, with death in one of those patients from liver failure associated with GVHD and adenovirus. Patients at dose level 1 had T-cell reconstitution consistent with other patients undergoing haploidentical HSCT without allodepleted T-cell add back. However, patients at dose level 2 (10^5 cells/kg/dose) showed significantly improved T-cell recovery time, particularly at 3–5 months after HSCT, which is most often the time period in which patients die of infection following haploidentical HSCT.

While this selective allo-depletion approach represents an important step toward the goal of engineering stem cell transplants to rapidly reconstitute immunity without causing GVHD, several concerns and limitations remain to be addressed before it can be more widely applied: (1) Firstly, selective depletion techniques are cumbersome and expensive in time and materials. Improved and simpler techniques will be needed before the approach is universally applicable in routine transplant centers. (2) Secondly, the best technique to eliminate alloreactive T cells remains to be determined. There is a continuous need to tailor the selective depletion technique for different transplant situations, in particular whether the transplant is between HLA-matched related donor-recipient pairs or between unrelated or mismatched pairs, and whether the transplant is for malignant or non-malignant disease. (3) Thirdly, there is currently no generally accepted technique to determine whether a selective allo-depleted product will be free of significant GVHD risk. The correlation between the clinical results (predicting the risk of GVHD) and the *in vitro* tests available such as MLR and HTLp need to be validated with more clinical studies. (4) The optimal number of T cells, including the allowable number of residual allo-reactive T cells, to include in the graft remains unknown and may vary among donor-recipient pairs. (5) Lastly, it is important to note that not all data obtained in murine or other animal models can be extrapolated to the clinic. The preliminary clinical reported so far requires further validation in a large patient cohort to better define the optimal strategies for each situation.

2. Cotransplantation of Mesenchymal Stem Cell

In addition to HSCs, bone marrow contains a second type of stem cells—the mesenchymal stem cells (MSCs) capable of giving rise to multiple mesenchymal lineages [226, 227] Convincing evidence shows that mesenchymal stem cells (MSCs) possess immunomodulatory properties, which may play a role in the maintenance of peripheral tolerance, the induction of transplantation tolerance and control of autoimmunity.[228] In allogeneic stem cell transplant, MSCs may be used to enhance engraftment of white blood cells and platelets, modulare the immune system system, as prophylaxis to prevent GVHD, and treatment of established GVHD. The first experience with the use of MSC was reported in two patients for the prevention and treatment of acute GVHD after HLA-matched or mismatched HCT. [229, 230] Following the encouraging results of these anecdotal case reports, the immunosuppressive capacities of MSC to prevent GVHD has been evaluated in several clinical studies. In an open-label multicenter clinical trial involving adult patients undergoing transplantation from an HLA-identical sibling, MSC infusion has been shown by Lazarus et al to be safe and possibly to accelerate hematopoietic recovery, as well as to reduce the incidence of both acute and chronic GvHD. [231] Ball et al recently reported the results of a phase I–II study in children undergoing haploidentical HSC transplantation. The co-transplantation of MSC from the same HSC donor was associated with a significant reduction of graft failure rate as compared to historic controls.[232] Although very encouraging, the long-term outcome of both anecdotal and full series is not yet available. More recently, Ning et al from Beijing published the results of the first randomised trial addressing benefits and disadvantages of MSC infusions in the context of HSC allografting. [233] The study showed that while cotransplantation successfully prevents GVHD, it is not without its drawback as the prevention of GVHD is associated with a higher incidence of leukemia relapse. Further large-scale randomized studies are needed to evaluate the potential benefits and hazards of MSC-cotransplantation in malignant hematopoietic diseases.

3. Suicide Gene Insertion

One means of modifying GVHD reactions in vivo that has attracted continuing interest is to insert a specific marker gene that would allow T cells to be selectively depleted should GVHD occur. The best characterized method involves transducing donor lymphocytes with herpes simplex virus thymidine kinase (HSV-tk) gene. Transduced cells are then selected and infused into patients, either as part of the graft or as a donor lymphocytes infusion. If GVHD should occur and require therapeutic intervention, ganciclovir is given to eliminate transfected cells. Such approach has been used in several clinical trials without significant acute toxicity. This approach, pioneered by Claudio Bordignon in Milan[234] and recently reviewed by his group,[234] represents the widest clinical application of T cell–targeted gene therapy to date. More than 100 patients have been treated worldwide to date in several phase 1 and 2 studies. Plans are underway for a phase 3 study with industry support.[234] This approach seeks to preserve the graft-versus-infection and graft-versus-leukemia potential of donor lymphocytes while providing a safety valve for abrogating graft-versus-host disease (GVHD) if it occurs and proves clinically problematic. In the earliest study, the investigators from Milan[235] used an HSV–TK-modified DLI to treat EBV–LPD or relapsed leukemia after allogeneic T-cell-depleted HSCT in a small population of patients and showed the modified cells had antitumor efficacy, persisted in the circulation and could be eliminated by the administration of ganciclovir. Tiberghien et al.[236] administered HSV–TK-positive T cells in conjunction with a T-cell-depleted graft to 12 HSCT recipients and also confirmed the persistence of HSV–TK cells; however, results in subsequent studies in which HSV–TK donor T cells administered following non-T-cell-depleted grafts have not shown the persistence of the gene-modified cells in most patients. Bonini et al, in a dose-finding clinical protocol, explored the strategy of TK^{+}-cell add-back to prevent disease relapse and promoting immune reconstitution after haploidentical transplant.[237] In their study enrolling 8 patients with high risk hematologic malignancies who underwent haploidentical transplant were enrolled, TK^{+}-cell add-back at a dose of 1×10^{7}/kg was identified as an effective dose for preventing disease relapse and promoting immune reconstitution after haplo-HCT. Patients who received the highest dose of TK^{+} cells, circulating T cells were rapidly detected. *Ex vivo* analyses showed that engrafted T cells were fully functional memory Thl/Tcl T cells, with a wide TCR repertoire, able to proliferate and lyse viral and allogeneic targets. Immune reconstitution significantly reduced the incidence of viral infections in all patients and prevented leukemic relapse in 2/3 patients. Technical difficulties include the problem of ensuring that all transplanted T cells are properly transduced, so as to prevent escape of nontransduced cells from ganciclovir treatment, and the difficulty of conserving a broad T-cell repertoire during in vitro expansion to incorporate the gene. Whether this technology can be fully expoited in HSCT will depend upon the ability to define and comply with rigorous conditions for scaling up production of suicide gene modified cells under the norms of good manufacturing practices, and to provide appropriate clinical validation to these technologies.

4. Prophylatic/Pre-emptive DLI Infusion

Despite significant reduction in transplantation-related mortality over the past few years using the TCD graft, there has been no clear reduction in disease relapse, which still surpasses 50% among the high-risk patients in some series. [49,74] Apart from the inclusion of high proportion of high risk patients or patients with refractory diseases at the time of transplant, the high relapse rate is attributable to the delayed immune recovery and abrogated GvL effect with the use of TCD graft. Intensification of conditioning regimens is unlikely to compensate for the loss of T-cell-related GvL effect, as the benefit usually is offset with the increase the regimen-related toxicity. Additional post transplant strategies such as donor lymphocyte infusion are potential therapeutic option for relapse prevention.

Donor lymphocyte infusions (DLI) provides direct and potent GvL activity to treat relapse in patients who have undergone HLA-matched, related or unrelated HSCT,[238, 239, 240, 241, 242] nonmyeloablative HSCT[243, 244] and also haploidentical HSCT.[245, 246, 247, 248, 249] Despite the undeniable efficacy of donor lymphocytes, their extensive exploitation is limited by the risk of severe and potentially life-threatening GvHD, which occurs in 30-60% of patients receiving DLI. [240,241,242]

In studies in which TCD strategy was employed, the higher relapse rate inherent to the protocol prompted the need to frequently use DLI [250,152] to promote graft-vs-malignancy activity, thereby rendering patients to the undesired risk of GVHD toxicity. In an attempt to induce a GVM effect, which may be compromised by the T-cell depletion procedure, several groups have looked into the feasibility of prophylatic DLI to eliminate residual disease after TCD HSCT. The observation that graft vs malignancy response can be achieved in patients in whom GVHD did not develop has led investigators to explore approached that could limit GVHD without compromising GVL. Based on earlier clinical and correlative laboratory studies that implicated CD8+ T cells as major contributors to GVH reactions, [251, 252] several groups have examined the effects of selective infusion of T cell subsets on GVHD.

The published phase I and phase II studies have suggested that depletion of CD8 T cells from either the allotransplant or from DLIs efficiently reduces the incidence and severity of GVHD.[251, 253, 254, 255] Importantly, CD8-depleted DLIs can induce significant disease remissions in patients with myeloma or chronic myeloid leukemia (CML) relapse.[254,255,256] Moreover, the delayed T-cell add-back strategy employed in some of these TCD clinical trials offers the theoretical advantage over early T cell infusion in that it allows attainment of early alloengraftment without GVHD, and provides T cell add back only when the patient is further removed from conditioning therapy and the associated inflammatory cytokine milieu. In this manner, it was hoped that the GVHD associated with delayed DLI is associated with a substantially lower risk of GVHD than the early T cell infusion. In fact, preliminary results suggest that this strategy is feasible, and addback can be performed without a prohibitive risk of GVHD.[257] Randomized studies confirmed that CD8-depletion of DLIs or bone marrow maintains considerable antileukemic activity while reducing GVHD.[258, 259] More recently, Meyer et al from Berlin[260] have shown that prophylactic transfer of CD8-depleted donor lymphocytes into TCD reduced-intensity HSCT patients accelerated immune reconstitution, resulting in increased circulating CD4 T-cell numbers as well as enhanced frequencies of CMV-specific CD4 and CD8 T cells in several lymphopenic patients, and was associated with a low risk of inducing severe GVHD. Despite these encouraging results, this approach is not without limitations. Despite T-cell-depleted transplantation and the use of nonmyeloablative conditioning regimen, nearly half of the patients were prevented from receiving DLI because of development of GvHD [254,256,260] Ongoing studies will define the optimal nonmyeloablative transplantation regimen to both avoid the toxicity of transplantation and provide a platform for the administration of DLI.

In haploidentical SCT, studies have been initiated in which purified donor NK cells have been used in DLI with the aim to facilitate engraftment and induce GVT effects. [261, 262] Although no firm conclusions can be made regarding the clinical efficacy of NK-cell-based DLI at this stage, the available data indicate that NK-cell infusions are safe and can generate antitumour responses and long-term remission in some patients after leukemia relapse. The development of NK-cell-based DLI presents new possibilities to treat patients with tumour relapse after haploidentical or cord-blood SCT in which T-cell-based DLIs are not feasible.

5. Immunoregulatory T Cells

The immunoregulatory T (Treg) cells, which is a subpopulation of T cells co-expressing $CD4^+$ and $CD25^+$ plays a crucial role in the control of autoimmune processes. Recent *in vitro* and *in vivo* data indicate that $CD4^+$ $CD25^+$ immunoregulatory T cells can regulate alloreactivity.[263] This renders them good candidates for innovative strategies in the field of transplantation. Inducing a state of immune tolerance with immunoregulatory T cells would alleviate the need for immunosuppression, and represents a major goal of transplantation immunology. Accumulating evidence from both humans and experimental animal models has implicated the involvement of Tregs in the development of graft-versus-host disease (GVHD). The demonstration that Tregs could separate GVHD from graft-versus-tumor (GVT) activity suggests that their immunosuppressive potential could be manipulated to reduce GVHD without detrimental consequence on GVT effect. In the murine studies, it has been shown that if $CD4^+CD25^+$ Treg cells naturally present in the transplant product are depleted before infusion into irradiated allogeneic recipient mice, GvHD is significantly accelerated. Conversely, GvHD can be prevented by the addition of freshly isolated Treg cells to the donor product; unexpectedly, these models also show that the GvL effect is spared. [264, 265, 266, 267, 268] Infusion of *ex vivo* activated and expanded Tregs significantly inhibited lethal GVHD in several murine models.[265,266 ,266,269]

In contrast to the pre-clinical models, conflicting data have been reported with regards to the role of Tregs in the development of cGVHD in humans, with some reporting significantly increased Tregs in patients with cGVHD,[270,271] while others showing no difference or decrease in Treg when quantification using expression of a different intracellular marker, forkhead transcription factor, FoxP3, was performed. [272, 273, 274] It is possible that the apparent discrepancies between these studies simply reflect the lack of specific markers for regulatory T cells, as well as the varying strategies employed to measure the Treg population including its phenotypic definition. Utilization of additional cell surface marker such as CD127 may help to resolve these contradicting results.

Several groups are now investigating the value of infusing ex-vivo expanded donor Treg cells following HSCT. Considerable efforts have been made to expand human Tregs for use in clinical setting. Large-scale expansion of $CD4^+CD25^+$ Tregs, up to 1000 times, using anti-CD3 and anti-CD28 microbeads and high doses of IL-2 has demonstrated the feasibility of bringing this new treatment modality to the bedside. [275, 276] Many obstacles to the effective implementation of this approach remain, such as inability to define the antigenic specificities of these cells the difficulty of using cell sorting to obtain a pure Treg cell population for infusion into patients, given that FoxP3, the best Treg cell marker to date, is intracellular. Also, early infusion of Tregs together with the transplant in humans, unlike animal models. might be more complicated owing to the presence of intense inflammatory responses immediately after transplant and the routine use of immunosuppressive agents for GVHD prophylaxis. Advances in understanding the molecular basis for the activation and expansion of regulatory T cells together with ongoing clinical trails will be crucial to resolve these issues and to exploit the therapeutic potential of regulatory T cells to differentially control GvHD and facilatate immune reconstitution.

On the basis of murine models showing that the inhibitory effect on GVHD by natural killer T cells and CD4+CD25+ T cells inhibit GVHD without compromising GVL effect, [264,268] Lowsky and colleagues from Stanford University designed a nonmyeloablative conditioning protocol that contains total lymphoid irradition (TLI) and ATG for GVHD prevention in HSCT. As in preclinical models of BMT, the nonmyeloablative TLI conditioning protects against GVHD by skewing host T cell subsets to favor regulatory natural killer T cells that suppress GVHD by polarizing donor T cells toward secretion of noninflammatory cytokines such as interleukin-4. The investigators from Stanford University have studied this NM conditioning regimen that consisted of pre-transplant TLI (10 doses of 80 cGy) and ATG (5 doses of 1.5 mg/kg) to reduce acute GVHD in 37 patient receiving HSCT from either matched related donors (MRD) or matched unrelated donors.[277] Following the infusion of unmanipulated G-CSF mobilized blood containing approximately $1–3 \times 10^8$ $CD3^+$ T cells/kg with approximately $3–5 \times 10^6$ $CD34^+$ cells/kg, all patients were given post-grafting immunosuppression of mycophenolate mofetil (MMF) for 1 month, and cyclosporine with tapered withdrawal at 6 months. The regimen was well tolerated and without significant regimen related toxicity. The incidence of severe acute GVHD ($\geq$ grade II) was less than 5%. Donor chimerism was evaluated in peripheral blood CD3, CD19 and CD15 compartments and sustained high levels were achieved in almost all patients in PR or CR on entry into the protocol. Relapse of leukemia and lymphoma was comparable to previous reports of similar patients using non-myeloablative conditioning. Over 100 patients have now been reported with this approach, and the incidence of severe acute GVHD is about 4%.[278]

6. Adoptive Immunotherapy and Vaccination

Dendritic cells (DCs), NK cells, and cytotoxic lymphocytes have been shown to mediate antitumor response in HSCT. [279, 280, 281, 282 , 283]Specifically, these cells have been incorporated into vaccines or expanded and direct against tumor cells. In patients with leukaemia such as AML, ALL or CLL, malignant cells can be induced to differentiate and mature into relatively mature malignant DC capable of generating an alloimmune response. Vaccination of patients in a state of minimum residual disease after allogeneic HSCT may evoke an appropriate immune response to control the disease. The malignant DC can be used to induce a leukaemia reactive T cell response from donor cells in vitro resulting in the production of large numbers of activated T cells that may be capable of controlling the disease after allogeneic HSCT.[283] Although the feasibility of this approach has been demonstrated, the logistics of generation of these T cell responses is still complex. Further clinical and preclinical investigations are needed to improve the specificity and efficacy of these in vitro immune response.

A promising method for restoring specific immunity against infections after transplants, albeit highly specialized and cumbersome, relies upon adoptive transfer of specific T cell clones. Adoptive transfer of donor-derived virus-specific $CD8^+$ T cells has been shown to be safe and effective in prophylaxis and treatment of cytomegalovirus (CMV) and Epstein-Barr virus (EBV) infection following stem cell transplantation from an HLA-identical related and unrelated donor. [284, 285, 194] Due to the high degree of mismatching between donor and patient in haploidentical transplantation, transfer of donor T cells to improve immune reconstitution in these patients is associated with a high risk of severe acute graft-versus-host disease (GVHD). But immunotherapy with highly enriched polyclonal virus-specific $CD4^+$ T cells has been reported to be safe and effective in a small cohort of patients, including one recipient of a haploidentical transplant. [286] The most recent and exciting data have come from investigators in Perugia, who have generated large numbers of donor pathogen-specific T-cell clones, screened them individually for alloreactivity against recipient cells, identified and deleted those cross-reacting against recipient alloantigens, and infused them into 35 high-risk adults with diverse advanced-stage, heavily pretreated hematologic malignancies who had undergone haploidentical hematopoietic transplantation.[212] This study has demonstrated that transfer of immunity to *Aspergillus* and CMV to recipients of a haploidentical transplant can be performed without out triggering GVHD. Interestingly, despite small number of pathogen-specific T cells was administered; specific T-cell responses could be detected in all patients in the study. All the patients in this study showed a surprisingly prompt increase in $CD4^+$ as well as $CD8^+$ T-cell responses to CMV as soon as 3 weeks after transfer, suggesting that even extensively in vitro–cultured T cells were able to rapidly expand in vivo when administered to lymphopenic patients not receiving immunosuppressive medication for GVHD prophylaxis. When compared with a control group, patients receiving CMV-directed immunotherapy had a lower risk of CMV reactivation and disease. Importantly, this is the first study that described adoptive T-cell therapy not only for viral but also for invasive fungal infection. *Aspergillus*-directed $CD4^+$ T_h1 responses were detected in all recipients as soon as 3 weeks after the transfer, and 9 of 10 treated patients showed a decrease in their galactomannan antigenemia and resolution of pulmonary infiltrates. Although not a routine laboratory procedure, the development of such adoptive therapy clearly offers promise for improving overall outcome following haploidentical SCT by reducing infectious complications without worsening GVHD.

Conclusions

GVHD can be prevented by effective T cell depletion from the graft. Recent advances with effective T-cell depletion have significantly decreased the early transplant related mortality and risk of severe GVHD, while enabling reliable engraftment, and hence provide encouraging outcomes in both matched or mismatched donor transplantation. However, while they have broadened the array of patients able to be offered immunotherapy to those without a fully matched sibling, post-transplant infections and relapse remain important barriers to overcome. Therefore, we have yet to provide clear and convincing evidence that these advancements in graft manipulation have translated into improvement in overall survival following traditional HSCT in the matched sibling setting. A key challenge is to balance the positive and negative effects of donor T cells to optimize outcome. New directions in the use of adoptive cellular immunity, immunoregulatory T cells, mesenchymal stem cell and selective allodepletion in rapidly reconstituting immunity without GVHD appear promising. The data presented to date provides an important framework for future improvements via more appropriate patient and donor selection, development of conditioning regimens that are safer yet result in reliable engraftment, and more effective strategies that eliminate the high risk of severe GVHD while preserving anti-tumor and anti-microbial immunocompetence. The full therapeutic potential of allogeneic HSCT will not be realized until approaches to separate GVH and GVL are developed.

References

[1] Storb R, Thomas ED. Allogeneic bone marrow transplantation. *Immunol Rev* 1983; 71:77.

[2] Thomas ED. Bone marrow *transplant*ation for malignant diseases. *J Clin Oncol* 1983;1: 517.

[3] Socie G, Stone JV, Wingard JR, et al. Long-term survival and late deaths after allogeneic *bone marrow transplantation.* Late Effects Working Committee of the International Bone Marrow Transplant Registry. *N Engl J Med* 1999;341:14-21.

[4] Ferrara JL , Levy R and Chao NJ. Pathophysiologic mechanisms of graft–versus–host disease. *Biol Blood Marrow Transplant* 1999; 5:347–356.

[5] Horowitz MM, Gale RP , Sondel PM, et al. Graft-versus-leukemia reactions after *bone marrow transplant*ation. *Blood* 1990;75: 555–562.

[6] Reisner Y, Kapoor N, Kirkpatrick D, et al. Transplantation for severe combined immunodeficiency with HLA-A, B, D, DR incompatibility parental marrow cells fractionated by soybean agglutinin and sheep red blood cells. *Blood.* 1983;61:341-348.
[7] Marmont AM, Horowitz MM, Gale RP, et al. T-cell depletion of HLA-identical transplants in leukemia. *Blood* 1991;78: 2120–2130.
[8] Maraninchi D, Gluckman E, Blaise D, et al. Impact of T-cell depletion on outcome of allogeneic *bone marrow transplant*ation for standard-risk leukaemias. *Lancet* 1987;2: 175–178.
[9] Keever CA, Small TN, Flomenberg N, et al. Immune reconstitution following bone marrow *transplant*ation: comparison of recipients of T-cell depleted marrow with recipients of conventional marrow grafts. *Blood* 1989;73:1340–1350.
[10] Storb R, Deeg HJ, Pepe M, et al. Methotrexate and cyclosporine versus cyclosporine alone for prophylaxis of graft-versus-host disease in patients given HLA-identical marrow grafts for leukemia: long-term follow-up of a controlled trial. *Blood.* 1989; 73:1729-1734.
[11] Storb R, Deeg HJ, Pepe M, et al. Graft-versus-host disease prevention by methotrexate combined with cyclosporin compared to methotrexate alone in patients given marrow grafts for severe aplastic anaemia: long-term follow-up of a controlled trial. *Br J Haematol.* 1989;72:567-572.
[12] Storb R, Deeg HJ, Whitehead J, et al. Methotrexate and cyclosporine compared with cyclosporine alone for prophylaxis of acute graft versus host disease after marrow transplantation for leukemia. *N Engl J Med.* 1986 20;314:729-735.
[13] Sorror ML, Leisenring W, Deeg HJ, et al. Twenty-year follow-up of a controlled trial comparing a combination of methotrexate plus cyclosporine with cyclosporine alone for prophylaxis of graft-versus-host disease in patients administered HLA-identical marrow grafts for leukemia. *Biol Blood Marrow Transplant.*2005;11:814-815.
[14] Locatelli F, Bruno B, Zecca M, et al. Cyclosporin A and short-term methotrexate versus cyclosporin A as graft versus host disease prophylaxis in patients with severe aplastic anemia given allogeneic *bone marrow transplant*ation from an HLA-identical sibling: results of a GITMO/EBMT randomised trial. *Blood* 2000;96:1690-1697.
[15] Chao NJ, Schmidt GM, Niland JC, et al. Cyclosporine, methotrexate, and prednisone compared with cyclosporine and prednisone for prophylaxis of acute graft-versus-host disease. *N Engl J Med.* 1993; 329: 1225–1230.
[16] Weisdorf DJ, Anasetti C, Antin JH, et al. Allogeneic *bone marrow transplant*ation for chronic myelogenous leukemia: comparative analysis of unrelated versus matched sibling donor transplantation. *Blood* 2002; 99:1971–1977.
[17] Champlin RE, Schmitz N, Horowitz MM, et al. *Blood* stem cells compared with bone marrow as a source of hematopoietic cells for allogeneic transplantation. *Blood* 2000; 95:3702–3709.
[18] Chao NJ, Snyder DS, Jain M, et al. Equivalence of 2 effective graft-versus-host disease prophylaxis regimens: results of a prospective double-blind randomized trial. *Biol Blood Marrow Transplant* 2000; 6:254–261.
[19] Loughran TP, Deeg HJ, Dahlberg S, et al. Incidence of hypertension after marrow transplantation among 112 patients randomized to either cyclosporine or methotrexate as graft-versus-host disease prophylaxis. *Br J Haematol.* 1985;59: 547–553.

[20] Cutler C, Li S, Kim HT, et al. Mucositis after allogeneic hematopoietic stem cell transplantation: a cohort study of methotrexate- and non-methotrexate-containing graft-versus-host disease prophylaxis regimens. *Biol Blood Marrow Transplant* 2005; 11:383–388.

[21] Ho VT, Weller E, Lee SJ, et al. Prognostic factors for early severe pulmonary complications after hematopoietic stem cell transplantation. *Biol Blood Marrow Transplant* 2001; 7:223–229.

[22] Nash RA, Antin JH, Karanes C, et al. Phase 3 study comparing methotrexate and tacrolimus with methotrexate and cyclosporine for prophylaxis of acute graft-versus-host disease after marrow transplantation from unrelated donors. *Blood.* 2000; 96: 2062-2068.

[23] Ratanatharathorn V, Nash RA, Przepiorka D, et al. Phase III study comparing methotrexate and tacrolimus (prograf, FK506) with methotrexate and cyclosporine for graft-versus-host disease prophylaxis after HLA-identical sibling *bone marrow transplant*ation. *Blood* 1998; 92:2303–2314.

[24] Yanada M, Emi N, Naoe T, et al. Tacrolimus instead of cyclosporine used for prophylaxis against graft-versus-host disease improves outcome after hematopoietic stem cell transplantation from unrelated donors, but not from HLA-identical sibling donors: a nationwide survey conducted in Japan. *Bone Marrow Transplant* 2004; 34:331–337.

[25] Antin JH, Kim HT, Cutler C, et al. Sirolimus, tacrolimus, and low-dose methotrexate for graft-versus-host disease prophylaxis in mismatched related donor or unrelated donor transplantation. *Blood* 2003;102:1601-1605.

[26] Benito AI, Furlong T, Martin PJ, et al. Sirolimus (rapamycin) for the treatment of steroid-refractory acute graft-versus-host disease. Transplantation 2001;72:1924-29.

[27] Cutler C, Kim HT, Hochberg E, et al. Sirolimus and tacrolimus without methotrexate as graft-versus-host disease prophylaxis after matched related donor peripheral *blood* stem cell *transplantation. Biol Blood Marrow Transplant.*2004;10:328-336.

[28] Nash RA, Johnston L and Parker P, et al. A phase I/II study of mycophenolate mofetil in combination with cyclosporine for prophylaxis of acute graft-versus-host disease after myeloablative conditioning and allogeneic hematopoietic cell transplantation. *Biol of Blood Marrow Transplant* 2005; 11: 495–505.

[29] Neumann F, Graef T, Tapprich C, et al. Cyclosporine A and mycophenolate mofetil vs cyclosporine A and methotrexate for graft-versus-host disease prophylaxis after stem cell transplantation from HLA-identical siblings. *Bone Marrow Transplant* 2005; 35 :1089–1093.

[30] Mohty M, de Lavallade H, Faucher C, et al. Mycophenolate mofetil and cyclosporine for graft-versus-host disease prophylaxis following reduced intensity conditioning allogeneic stem cell transplantation. *Bone Marrow Transplant* 2004; 34: 527–530.

[31] Bolwell B, Sobecks R, Pohlman B, et al. A prospective randomized trial comparing cyclosporine and short course methotrexate with cyclosporine and mycophenolate mofetil for GVHD prophylaxis in myeloablative allogeneic bone marrow transplantation. *Bone Marrow Transplant* 2004; 34:621–625.

[32] Basara N, Blau WI, Kiehl MG, et al. Mycophenolate mofetil for the prophylaxis of acute GVHD in HLA-mismatched bone marrow transplant patients. *Clin Transplant.* 2000;14;121–126.
[33] Vogelsang GB, Arai A. Mycophenolate mofetil for the prevention and treatment of graft-versus-host disease following stem cell transplantation: preliminary findings. *Bone Marrow Transplant* 2001;27:1255–1262.
[34] Dicke KA, van Hoot JIM, van Bekkum DW. The selective elimination of immunologically competent cells from bone marrow and lymphatic cell mixtures; II: mouse spleen cell fractionation on a discontinuous albumin gradient. *Transplantation.* 1968;6:562-570.
[35] Müller-Ruchholtz W, Wottge HU, Müller-Hermelink HK. *Bone marrow transplant*ation in rats across strong histocompatibility barriers by selective elimination of lymphoid cells in donor marrow. *Transplant Proc.* 1976;8:537-41.
[36] Reisner Y, Itzicovitch L, Meshorer A, Sharon N. Hemopoietic stem cell transplantation using mouse bone marrow and spleen cells fractionated by lectins. *Proc Natl Acad Sci U S A*. 1978;75:2933-6.
[37] Korngold R, Sprent J. Lethal graft-versus-host disease after *bone marrow transplant*ation across minor histocompatibility barriers in mice: prevention by removing mature T cells from marrow. *J Exp Med*. 1978;148:1687-1698.
[38] Verdonck LF, de Gast GC, van Heugten HG, Dekker AW. A fixed low number of T cells in HLA-identical allogeneic bone marrow transplantation. *Blood.* 1990;75:776-80.
[39] Verdonck LF, Dekker AW, de Gast GC, van Kempen ML, Lokhorst HM, Nieuwenhuis HK. Allogeneic bone marrow transplantation with a fixed low number of T cells in the marrow graft. *Blood.* 1994;83:3090-6.
[40] Reisner Y, Kapoor N, Kirkpatrick D, et al. Transplantation for acute leukemia with HLA-A and B nonidentical parental marrow cells fractionated with soybean agglutinin and sheep red blood cells. *Lancet.* 1981;2:327-331.
[41] De Witte T, Hoogenhout J, de Pauw B, et al. Depletion of donor lymphocytes by counterflow centrifugation successfully prevents acute graft-versus-host disease in matched allogeneic marrow transplantation. *Blood.* 1986;67:1302-1308.
[42] Noga SJ, Donnenberg AD, Schwartz CL, Strauss LC, Civin CI, Santos GB. Development of a simplified counterflow centrifugation elutriation procedure for depletion of lymphocytes from human bone marrow. *Transplantation.* 1986;41:220-228.
[43] Wagner JE, Donnenberg AD, Noga SJ, et al. Lymphocyte depletion of donor bone marrow by counterflow centrifugal elutriation: results of a phase I clinical trial. *Blood.* 1988;72:1168-1176.
[44] Lowenberg B, Wagemaker E, van Bekkum DW, et al. Graft-versus-host disease following transplantation of "one log" versus "two log" T-lymphocyte depleted bone marrow from HLA-identical donors. *Bone Marrow Transplant*. 1986;1:133-140.
[45] Luznik L, O'Donnell PV, Symons HJ, et al. HLA-haploidentical bone marrow transplantation for hematologic malignancies using nonmyeloablative conditioning and high-dose, posttransplantation cyclophosphamide. Biol Blood Marrow Transplant. 2008; 14:641-50.

[46] Koh LP, Rizzieri DA, Chao NJ. Allogeneic hematopoietic stem cell transplant using mismatched/haploidentical donors. *Biol Blood Marrow Transplant* 2007;13:1249-67.

[47] Buckley RH, Schiff SE, Schiff RI, et al. Hematopoietic stem-cell transplantation for the treatment of severe combined immunodeficiency. N Engl J Med. 1999 ;340 :508-16.

[48] Aversa F, Tabilio A, Terenzi A, et al. Successful engraftment of T-cell-depleted haploidentical "three-loci" incompatible transplants in leukemia patients by addition of recombinant human granulocyte colony-stimulating factor-mobilized peripheral *blood* progenitor cells to bone marrow infusion. *Blood* 1994; 84**:** 3948–3955.

[49] Henslee-Downey PJ, Abhyankar SH, et al. Use of partially mismatched related donors extends access to allogeneic marrow transplant. *Blood.* 1997;89:3864-3872.

[50] Prentice HG, Blacklock HA, Janossy G, et al. Use of anti-T-cell monoclonal antibody OKT3 to prevent acute graft versus host disease in allogeneic *bone marrow transplant*ation for acute leukemia. *Lancet.* 1982;1:700-703.

[51] Filipovich AH, McGlave PB, Ramsay NKC, et al. Pretreatment of donor bone marrow with monoclonal antibody OKT3 for prevention of acute graft versus host disease in allogeneic histocompatible bone marrow transplantation. *Lancet.* 1982;1:1266-1269.

[52] Martin PJ, Hansen JA, Thomas ED. Preincubation of donor bone marrow cells with a combination of murine monoclonal anti-T-cell antibodies without complement does not prevent graft-versus-host disease after allogeneic marrow *transplantation.* J Clin Immunol. 1984;4:18-22.

[53] Waldmann HG, Hale G, Cividalli G, et al. Elimination of graft-versus-host disease by in vitro depletion of alloreactive lymphocytes with a monoclonal rat anti-human lymphocyte antibody (Campath-1). *Lancet.* 1984;2:483-486.

[54] Mitsuyasu RT, Champlin RE, Gale RP, et al. Treatment of donor bone marrow with monoclonal anti-T-cell antibody and complement for the prevention of graft versus host disease. *Ann Intern Med.* 1986;105:20-26.

[55] Soiffer RJ, Murray C, Mauch P, et al. Prevention of graft-versus-host disease by selective depletion of CD6-positive T lymphocytes from donor bone marrow. *J Clin Oncol.* 1992;10:1191-2000.

[56] Handgretinger R, Lang P, Ihm K et al. Isolation and transplantation of highly purified autologous peripheral CD34(+) progenitor cells: purging efficacy, hematopoietic reconstitution and long-term outcome in children with high-risk neuroblastoma. *Bone Marrow Transplant.* 2002; **29:**731–736.

[57] Lang P, Schumm M, Taylor G et al. Clinical scale isolation of highly purified peripheral CD34+ progenitors for autologous and allogeneic transplantation in children. *Bone Marrow Transplant.* 1999;**24:** 583–589.

[58] Schumm P, Lang P, Taylor G et al. Isolation of highly purified autologous and allogeneic peripheral CD34+ cells using the CliniMACS device. *J. Hematother.*1999;**8**: 209–218.

[59] Heimfeld S, Fogarty B, McGuire K, Williams S, Berenson RJ. Peripheral blood stem cell mobilization after stem cell factor or G-CSF treatment: rapid enrichment for stem and progenitor cells using the CEPRATE immunoaffinity separation system. *Transplant Proc.* 1992 ;24:2818.

[60] Rowley SD, Loken M, Radich J, et al. Isolation of CD34+ cells from blood stem cell components using the Baxter Isolex system. *Bone Marrow Transplant.* 1998 ;21:1253-62.

[61] Elmaagacli AH, Peceny R, Steckel N, et al. Outcome of transplantation of highly purified peripheral *blood* CD34+ cells with T-cell add-back compared with unmanipulated bone marrow or peripheral blood stem cells from HLA-identical sibling donors in patients with first chronic phase chronic myeloid leukemia. *Blood.* 2003;101:446-53.

[62] Finke J, Brugger W, Bertz H, et al. Allogeneic transplantation of positively selected peripheral *blood* CD34+ progenitor cells from matched related donors. *Bone Marrow Transplant.* 1996 ;18:1081-6.

[63] Bensinger WI, Buckner CD, Shannon-Dorcy K, et al. Transplantation of allogeneic CD34+ peripheral *blood* stem cells in patients with advanced hematologic malignancy. *Blood.* 1996;88:4132-4138.

[64] Link H, Arseniev L, Bahre O, Kadar JG, Diedrich H, Poliwoda H. Transplantation of allogeneic CD34+ blood cells. *Blood.* 1996;87:4903-4909.

[65] Urbano-Ispizua A, Solano C, Brunet S, et al. Allogeneic transplantation of selected CD34+ cells from peripheral blood: experience of 62 cases using immunoadsorption or immunomagnetic technique. Spanish Group of Allo-PBT. *Bone Marrow Transplant.* 1998;22:519-525.

[66] Vij R, Brown R, Shenoy S, et al. Allogeneic peripheral blood stem cell transplantation following CD34+ enrichment by density gradient separation. *Bone Marrow Transplant.* 2000;25:1223-1228.

[67] Handgretinger, M. Schumm, P. Lang et al. Transplantation of megadoses of purified haploidentical stem cells. *Ann. NY. Acad. Sci.* 1999;872:351–361.

[68] Handgretinger, T. Klingebiel, P. Lang et al. Megadose transplantation of purified peripheral *blood* CD34(+) progenitor cells from HLA-mismatched parental donors in children. *Bone Marrow Transplant.* 2001;27: 777–783.

[69] Klingebiel T, Handgretinger R, Lang P, et al. Haploidentical transplantation for acute lymphoblastic leukemia in childhood. *Blood Rev.* 2004;18:181-192.

[70] Aversa F, Tabilio A, Velardi A, et al. Treatment of high-risk acute leukemia with T-cell-depleted stem cells from related donors with one fully mismatched HLA haplotype. *N Engl J Med.* 1998; 339:1186-93.

[71] Lang P, Greil J, Bader P, et al. Long-term outcome after haploidentical stem cell transplantation in children. *Blood Cells Mol Dis.* 2004;33:281-287.

[72] Kato S, Yabe H, Yasui M, et al. Allogeneic hematopoietic transplantation of CD34+ selected cells from an HLA haplo-identical related donor. A long-term follow-up of 135 patients and a comparison of stem cell source between the bone marrow and the peripheral blood. *Bone Marrow Transplant.* 2000; 26: 1281-1290.

[73] Walker I, Shehata N, Cantin G, et al. Canadian multicenter pilot trial of haploidentical donor transplantation. *Blood Cells Mol Dis*. 2004;33:222–226.

[74] Aversa F, Terenzi A, Tabilio A, et al. Full haplotype-mismatched hematopoietic stem-cell transplantation: a phase II study in patients with acute leukemia at high risk of relapse. *J Clin Oncol.* 2005 ; 23:3447-3454.

[75] Bornhäuser M, Platzbecker U, Theuser C, et al. CD34+-enriched peripheral *blood* progenitor cells from unrelated donors for allografting of adult patients: high risk of graft failure, infection and relapse despite donor lymphocyte add-back. *Br J Haematol.* 2002; 118:1095-103.

[76] Lang P, Handgretinger R, Niethammer D, et al. Transplantation of highly purified CD34+ progenitor cells from unrelated donors in pediatric leukemia. *Blood.* 2003;101:1630-6.

[77] Bunjes D, Buchmann I, Duncker C, et al. Rhenium 188-labeled anti-CD66 (a, b, c, e) monoclonal antibody to intensify the conditioning regimen prior to stem cell transplantation for patients with high-risk acute myeloid leukemia or myelodysplastic syndrome: results of a phase I-II study. *Blood* 2001; 98: 565-572.

[78] Bethge WA, Haegele M, Faul C, et al. Haploidentical allogeneic hematopoietic cell transplantation in adults with reduced-intensity conditioning and CD3/CD19 depletion: fast engraftment and low toxicity. *Exp Hematol.* 2006;34:1746-1752.

[79] Bethge WA, Faul C, Bornhäuser M, et al. Haploidentical allogeneic hematopoietic cell transplantation in adults using CD3/CD19 depletion and reduced intensity conditioning: an update. *Blood Cells Mol Dis*. 2008;40:13-9.

[80] Marsh J, Schrezenmeier H, Marin P, et al. Prospective randomized multicenter study comparing cyclosporin alone versus the combination of antithymocyte globulin and cyclosporin for treatment of patients with nonsevere aplastic anemia: a report from the European *Blood* and Marrow Transplant (EBMT) Severe Aplastic Anaemia Working Party. *Blood* 1999;93: 2191–2195.

[81] Byrne JL, Stainer C, Cull G, et al. The effect of the serotherapy regimen used and the marrow cell dose received on rejection, graft-versus-host disease and outcome following unrelated donor *bone marrow transplant*ation for leukaemia. *Bone Marrow Transplant* 2000; 25: 411–417.

[82] Finke J, Schmoor C, Lang H et al. Matched and mismatched allogeneic stem-cell transplantation from unrelated donors using combined graft-versus-host disease prophylaxis including rabbit anti-T lymphocyte globulin. *J Clin Oncol* 2003; 21: 506–513.

[83] Bacigalupo A, Lamparelli T, Bruzzi P, et al. Antithymocyte globulin for graft-versus-host disease prophylaxis in transplants from unrelated donors: 2 randomized studies from Gruppo Italiano Trapianti Midollo Osseo (GITMO). *Blood* 2001; 98: 2942–2947.

[84] Basara N, Baurmann H, Kolbe K, et al. Antithymocyte globulin for the prevention of graft-versus-host disease after unrelated hematopoietic stem cell transplantation for acute myeloid leukemia: results from the multicenter German cooperative study group, *Bone Marrow Transplant* 2005;35: 1011–1018.

[85] Remberger M, Storer B, Ringden O, et al. Association between pretransplant thymoglobulin and reduced non-relapse mortality rate after marrow transplantation from unrelated donors. *Bone Marrow Transplant* 2002 ;29:391–397.

[86] Kalhs P, Brugger S, Reiter E, et al. Low transplant-related mortality in patients receiving unrelated donor marrow grafts for leukemia. *Bone Marrow Transplant* 1999;23: 753–758.

[87] Duggan P, Booth K, Chaudhry A, et al. Unrelated donor BMT recipients given pretransplant low-dose antithymocyte globulin have outcomes equivalent to matched sibling BMT: a matched pair analysis. *Bone Marrow Transplant* 2002; 30:681–686.
[88] Finke J, Bertz H, Schmoor C, et al. Allogeneic *bone marrow transplant*ation from unrelated donors using in vivo anti-T-cell globulin. *Br J Haematol* 2000:111:303–313.
[89] Bacigalupo A. Antilymphocyte/thymocyte globulin for graft versus host disease prophylaxis: efficacy and side effects. *Bone Marrow Transplant* 2005; 35: 225–231.
[90] Hale G, Rebello P, Brettman LR. Blood concentrations of alemtuzumab and antiglobulin responses in patients with chronic lymphocytic leukemia following intravenous or subcutaneous routes of administration. *Blood* 2004;104:948-955.
[91] Klangsinsirikul P, Carter GI, Byrne JL, Hale G, Russell NH. Campath-1G causes rapid depletion of circulating host dendritic cells (DCs) before allogeneic transplantation but does not delay donor DC reconstitution. *Blood.* 2002;99: 2586-2591.
[92] Buggins AGS, Mufti GJ, Salisbury J, et al. Peripheral *blood* but not tissue dendritic cells express CD52 and are depleted by treatment with alemtuzumab. *Blood.* 2002;100: 1715-1720.
[93] Hale G, Slavin S, Goldman JM. Alemtuzumab (Campath-1H) for treatment of lymphoid malignancies in the age of nonmyeloablative conditioning? *Bone Marrow Transplant* 2002;30:797-804.
[94] Ratzinger G, Reagan JL, Heller G. Differential CD52 expression by distinct myeloid dendritic cell subsets: Implications for alemtuzumab activity at the level of antigen presentation in allogeneic graft-host interactions in transplantation. *Blood* 2003;101:1422-1429.
[95] Chakrabarti S, Hale G, Waldmann H. Alemtuzumab (Campath-1H) in allogeneic stem cell transplantation: where do we go from here? *Transplant Proc.* 2004 ;36:1225-7.
[96] Hale G. Alemtuzumab in stem cell *transplantation.* Med Oncol. 2002;19 Suppl:S33-47.
[97] Barge RM, Brouwer RE, Beersma MF, et al. Comparison of allogeneic T cell-depleted peripheral *blood* stem cell and *bone marrow transplant*ation: effect of stem cell source on short- and long-term outcome. *Bone Marrow Transplant*. 2001;27:1053-8.
[98] Hale G, Waldmann H. Control of graft-versus-host disease and graft rejection by T cell depletion of donor and recipient with Campath-1 antibodies: results of matched sibling transplants for malignant diseases. *Bone Marrow Transplantation.* 1994;13:597-611.
[99] Das-Gupta EP, Russell NH, Shaw BE, et al. Long-term outcome of unrelated donor transplantation for AML using myeloablative conditioning incorporating pretransplant Alemtuzumab. *Biol Blood Marrow Transplant*. 2007;13:724-33.
[100] von dem Borne PA, Beaumont F, Starrenburg CW, et al. Outcomes after myeloablative unrelated donor stem cell transplantation using both in vitro and in vivo T-cell depletion with alemtuzumab. *Haematologica*. 2006 ;91:1559-62.
[101] Chakraverty R, Peggs K, Chopra R, et al. Limiting transplantation-related mortality following unrelated donor stem cell transplantation by using a nonmyeloablative conditioning regimen. *Blood.* 2002;99: 1071-1078.
[102] Ho AY, Pagliuca A, Kenyon M, et al. Reduced-intensity allogeneic hematopoietic stem cell transplantation for myelodysplastic syndrome and acute myeloid leukemia with multilineage dysplasia using fludarabine, busulphan, and alemtuzumab (FBC) conditioning. *Blood.* 2004;104:1616-23.

[103] Kottaridis PD, Milligan DW, Chopra R, et al. In vivo CAMPATH-1H prevents graft-versus-host disease following nonmyeloablative stem cell transplantation. *Blood.* 2000 ;96:2419-25.

[104] Morris E, Thomson K, Craddock C, et al. Outcomes after alemtuzumab-containing reduced-intensity allogeneic transplantation regimen for relapsed and refractory non-Hodgkin lymphoma. *Blood.* 2004 ;104:3865-71.

[105] Faulkner RD, Craddock C, Byrne JL, et al. BEAM-alemtuzumab reduced-intensity allogeneic stem cell transplantation for lymphoproliferative diseases: GVHD, toxicity, and survival in 65 patients. *Blood.* 2004 ;103:428-34.

[106] Peggs KS, Hunter A, Chopra R, et al. Clinical evidence of a graft-versus-Hodgkin's-lymphoma effect after reduced-intensity allogeneic transplantation. *Lancet.* 2005 ;365:1934-41.

[107] Hale G, Jacobs P, Wood L, et al. CD52 antibodies for prevention of graft-versus-host disease and graft rejection following transplantation of allogeneic peripheral blood stem cells. *Bone Marrow Transplant*. 2000;26:69-76.

[108] Rizzieri DA, Koh LP, Long GD, et al. Partially matched, nonmyeloablative allogeneic transplantation: clinical outcomes and immune reconstitution. *J Clin Oncol.* 2007;25: 690-697.

[109] Kanda Y, Oshima K, Asano-Mori Y, et al. In vivo alemtuzumab enables haploidentical human leukocyte antigen-mismatched hematopoietic stem-cell transplantation without ex vivo graft manipulation. *Transplantation* 2005;79:1351-1357.

[110] Perez-Simon JA, Kottaridis PD, Martino R. Nonmyeloablative transplantation with or without alemtuzumab: Comparison between 2 prospective studies in patients with lymphoproliferative disorders. *Blood* 2002;100:3121-3127.

[111] Lu DP, Dong L, Wu T, et al. Conditioning including antithymocyte globulin followed by unmanipulated HLA-mismatched/haploidentical *blood* and marrow transplantation can achieve comparable outcomes with HLA-identical sibling transplantation. *Blood.* 2006;107:3065-3073.

[112] Luznik L, Jalla S, Engstrom LW, Iannone R, Fuchs EJ. Durable engraftment of major histocompatibility complex-incompatible cells after nonmyeloablative conditioning with fludarabine, low dose total body irradiation, and posttransplantation cyclophosphamide. *Blood.* 2001;98:3456-3464.

[113]Mayumi H, Umesue M, Nomoto K. Cyclophosphamide induced immunological tolerance: an overview. *Immunobiology*. 1996;195:129-139.

[114]Mayumi H, Himeno K, Tanaka K, Tokuda N, Fan JL, Nomoto K. Drug-induced tolerance to allografts in mice. XII. The relationships between tolerance, chimerism, and graft versus-host disease. *Transplantation*. 1987;44:286-290.

[115]Luznik L, Engstrom LW, Iannone R, Fuchs EJ. Posttransplantation cyclophosphamide facilitates engraftment of major histocompatibility complex-identical allogeneic marrow in mice conditioned with low-dose total body irradiation. *Biol Blood Marrow Transplant*. 2002;8:131-138.

[116] Luznik L, O'Donnell PV, Symons HJ, et al. HLA-haploidentical bone marrow transplantation for hematologic malignancies using nonmyeloablative conditioning and high-dose, posttransplantation cyclophosphamide. *Biol Blood Marrow Transplant.* 2008; 14:641-50.

[117] Guinan EC, Boussiotis VA, Neuberg D, et al. Transplantation of anergic histoincompatible bone marrow allografts. *N Engl J Med.* 1999;340:1704-1714.
[118] Guinan EC. Costimulatory blockade *ex vivo*: results of 2 pilot clinical trials. *Blood* Cell Mol Dis 2004; 33: 204–205.
[119] Kernan NA, Collins NH, Barrett A, et al. Clonable T lymphocytes in T-cell depleted bone marrow transplants correlate with development of graft versus host disease. *Blood* 1986;68:770-73.
[120] Filipovich AH, McGlave PB, Ramsay NKC, et al. Pretreatment of donor bone marrow with monoclonal antibody OKT3 for prevention of acute graft versus host disease in allogeneic histocompatible bone marrow transplantation. *Lancet.* 1982;1:1266-1269.
[121] Mitsuyasu RT, Champlin RE, Gale RP, et al. Treatment of donor bone marrow with monoclonal anti-T-cell antibody and complement for the prevention of graft versus host disease. *Ann Intern Med.* 1986;105:20-26.
[122] Soiffer RJ, Murray C, Mauch P, et al. Prevention of graft-versus-host disease by selective depletion of CD6-positive T lymphocytes from donor bone marrow. *J Clin Oncol.* 1992;10:1191-2000.
[123] Antin JH, Bierer BE, Smith BR, et al. Selective depletion of bone marrow T lymphocytes with anti-CD5 monoclonal antibodies: effective prophylaxis for graft-versus-host disease in patients with hematologic malignancies. *Blood.* 1991;78:2139-49.
[124] Hale G, Cobbold S, Waldmann H. T cell depletion with CAMPATH-1 in allogeneic bone marrow transplantation. *Transplantation.* 1988;45:753-9.
[125] Martin PJ, Hansen JA, Buckner CD, et al. Effects of in vitro depletion of T cells in HLA-identical allogeneic marrow grafts. *Blood.* 1985; 66:664-72.
[126] Champlin R, Ho W, Gajewski J, et al. Selective depletion of CD8+ T lymphocytes for prevention of graft-versus-host disease after allogeneic bone marrow transplantation. *Blood.* 1990;76:418-23.
[127] Champlin RE, Passweg JR, Zhang MJ, et al. T-cell depletion of *bone marrow transplants* for leukemia from donors other than HLA-identical siblings: advantage of T-cell antibodies with narrow specificities. *Blood.* 2000;95:3996-4003.
[128] Soiffer RJ, Weller E, Alyea EP, et al. CD6+ donor marrow T-cell depletion as the sole form of graft-versus-host disease prophylaxis in patients undergoing allogeneic *bone marrow transplant* from unrelated donors. *J Clin Oncol.* 2001;19:1152-1159.
[129] Drobyski WR, Ash RC, Casper JT, et al. Effect of T-cell depletion as graft-versus-host disease prophylaxis on engraftment, relapse, and disease-free survival in unrelated marrow transplantation for chronic myelogenous leukemia. *Blood.* 1994;83:1980-1987.
[130] Marks DI, Bird JM, Vettenranta K, et al. T cell-depleted unrelated donor *bone marrow transplant*ation for acute myeloid leukemia. *Biol Blood Marrow Transplant.* 2000;6:646-653.
[131] Wagner JE, Thompson JS, Carter SL, et al. Effects of graft-versus-host disease prophylaxis on 3 year disease-free survival in recipients of unrelated donor bone marrow (T-cell Depletion Trial): a multicenter, randomised phase II-III trial. *Lancet* 2005;366:733-41.
[132] Papadopoulos EB, Carabasi MH, Castro-Malaspina H et al. T-cell depleted allogeneic *bone marrow transplant*ation as post remission therapy for acute myelogeneous

leukemia: freedom from relapse in the absence of graft-versus-host disease. *Blood* 1998;91:1083-1090.

[133] Hongeng S, Krance RA, Bowman LC, et al. Outcomes of transplantation with matched-sibling and unrelated-donor bone marrow in children with leukemia. *Lancet* 1997;350:767-770.

[134] Ho VT, Kim HT, Li S, et al. Partial CD8+ T-cell depletion of allogeneic peripheral *blood* stem cell transplantation is insufficient to prevent graft-versus-host disease. *Bone Marrow Transplant* 2004;34:987-994.

[135] Delain M, Cahn JY, Racadot E, et al. Graft failure after T cell depleted HLA identical allogeneic bone marrow transplantation: risk factors in leukemic patients. *Leuk Lymphoma*. 1993;11:359-368.

[136] Bordignon C, Keever CA, Small TN, et al. Graft failure after T-cell-depleted human leukocyte antigen identical marrow transplants for leukemia: II. In vitro analyses of host effector mechanisms. *Blood.* 1989 ;74:2237-43.

[137] Hale G, Cobbold S, Waldmann H. T cell depletion with CAMPATH-1 in allogeneic bone marrow transplantation. *Transplantation.* 1988;45:753-9.

[138] Mitsuyasu RT, Champlin RE, Gale RP, et al. Treatment of donor bone marrow with monoclonal anti-T-cell antibody and complement for the prevention of graft-versus-host disease. A prospective, randomized, double-blind trial. *Ann Intern Med.* 1986 ;105:20-6.

[139] Filipovich AH, Vallera DA, Youle RJ, et al. Graft-versus-host disease prevention in allogeneic bone marrow transplantation from histocompatible siblings. A pilot study using immunotoxins for T cell depletion of donor bone marrow. *Transplantation.* 1987; 44:62-9.

[140] Martin PJ, Hansen JA, Buckner CD, et al. Effects of in vitro depletion of T cells in HLA-identical allogeneic marrow grafts. *Blood.* 1985; 66:664-72.

[141] Martin PJ, Hansen JA, Torok-Storb B, et al. Graft failure in patients receiving T cell-depleted HLA-identical allogeneic marrow transplants. *Bone Marrow Transplant.* 1988;3:445-456.

[142] Patterson J, Prentice HG, Brenner MK, et al. Graft rejection following HLA matched T-lymphocyte depleted bone marrow transplantation. *Br J Haematol.* 1986;63:221-230.

[143] Reisner Y, Ben-Bassat I., Douer D., Kaploon A, et al. Demonstration of clonable alloreactive host T cells in a primate model for bone marrow transplantation. *Proc Natl Acad Sci U S A*.1986;83: 4012–4015.

[144] Kernan NA, Flomenberg N, Dupont B, O'Reilly RJ. Graft rejection in recipients of T-cell-depleted HLA-nonidentical marrow transplants for leukemia. Identification of host-derived antidonor allocytotoxic T lymphocytes. *Transplantation.* 1987;43:842-7.

[145] Lapidot T, Terenzi A, Singer TS, et al. Enhancement by dimenthyl myleran of donor type chimerism in murine recipients of bone marrow allografts. *Blood* 1989; 73: 2025–2032.

[146] Kernan NA, Bordignon C, Heller G, et al. Graft failure after T-cell-depleted leukocyte antigen identical marrow transplants for leukemia; I: analysis of risk factors and results of secondary transplants. *Blood.* 1989;74:2227-2236.

[147] Bozdech MJ, Sondel PM, Trigg ME, et al. Transplantation of HLA-haploidentical T-cell-depleted marrow for leukemia: addition of cytosine arabinoside to the pretransplant conditioning prevents rejection. *Exp Hematol.* 1985;13:1201-10.

[148] Champlin RE, Ho WG, Mitsuyasu R, et al. Graft failure and leukemia relapse following T lymphocyte-depleted *bone marrow transplants*: effect of intensification of immunosuppressive conditioning. *Transplant Proc.* 1987 ;19:2616-9.

[149] Soiffer RJ, Mauch P, Tarbell NJ, et al. Total lymphoid irradiation to prevent graft rejection in recipients of HLA non-identical T cell-depleted allogeneic marrow. *Bone Marrow Transplant.* 1991;7:23-33.

[150] Malilay GP, Sevenich EA, Condie RM, et al. Prevention of graft rejection in allogeneic *bone marrow transplant*ation: I. Preclinical studies with antithymocyte globulins. *Bone Marrow Transplant* 1989; 4: 107-112.

[151] Henslee-Downey PJ, Parrish RS, MacDonald JS, et al. Combined in vitro and in vivo T lymphocyte depletion for the control of graft-versus-host disease following haploidentical marrow transplant. *Transplantation.* 1996;61:738-745.

[152] Peggs KS, Sureda A, Qian W, et al. Reduced-intensity conditioning for allogeneic haematopoietic stem cell transplantation in relapsed and refractory Hodgkin lymphoma: impact of alemtuzumab and donor lymphocyte infusions on long-term outcomes. *Br J Haematol.* 2007 ;139:70-80.

[153] Das-Gupta EP, Russell NH, Shaw BE, et al. Long-term outcome of unrelated donor transplantation for AML using myeloablative conditioning incorporating pretransplant Alemtuzumab. *Biol Blood Marrow Transplant.* 2007;13:724-33.

[154] Bachar-Lustig E, Rachamim N, Li HW, et al. Megadose of T cell-depleted bone marrow overcomes MHC barriers in sublethally irradiated mice. *Nat Med.* 1995;1:1268-7123.

[155] Reisner Y, Martelli MF. Bone marrow transplantation across HLA barriers by increasing the number of transplanted cells. *Immunol Today.* 1995;16:437-440.

[156] Weiden PL, Flournoy N, Thomas ED, Prentice R, Buckner CD, Storb R. Antileukemic effect of graft-versus-host disease in recipients of allogeneic-marrow grafts. *N Engl J Med.* 1979;300:1068-1073.

[157] Sullivan KM, Weiden PL, Storb R, et al. Influence of acute and chronic graft-versus-host disease on relapse and survival after bone marrow transplantation from HLA-identical siblings as treatment of acute and chronic leukemia. *Blood.* 1989;73:1720-1728.

[158] Apperley JF, Mauro FR, Goldman JM, et al. Bone marrow transplantation for chronic myeloid leukaemia in first chronic phase: importance of a graft-versus-leukaemia effect. *Br J Haematol.* 1988;69:239-245.

[159] Goldman JM, Gale RP, Horowitz MM, et al. Bone marrow transplantation for chronic myelogenous leukemia in chronic phase: increased risk for relapse associated with T-cell depletion. *Ann Intern Med.* 1988;108:806-814.

[160] Wagner JE, Zahurak M, Piantadosi S, et al. Bone marrow transplantation of chronic myelogenous leukemia in chronic phase: evaluation of risks and benefits. *J Clin Oncol.* 1992;10:779-789.

[161] Papadopoulos EB, Carabasi MH, Castro-Malaspina H, et al. T-cell-depleted allogeneic bone marrow transplantation as postremission therapy for acute myelogenous leukemia:

freedom from relapse in the absence of graft-versus-host disease. *Blood.* 1998;91:1083-1090.

[162] Aversa F, Terenzi A, Carotti A, et al. Improved outcome with T-cell-depleted *bone marrow transplant*ation for acute leukemia. *J Clin Oncol.* 1999;17:1545-1550.

[163] Drobyski WR, Ash RC, Casper JT, et al. Effect of T-cell depletion as graft-versus-host disease prophylaxis on engraftment, relapse, and disease-free survival in unrelated marrow transplantation for chronic myelogenous leukemia. *Blood.* 1994;83:1980-1987.

[164] Hessner MJ, Endean DJ, Casper JT, et al. Use of unrelated marrow grafts compensates for reduced graft-versus-leukemia reactivity after T-cell-depleted allogeneic marrow transplantation for chronic myelogenous leukemia. *Blood.* 1995;86:3987-3996.

[165] Mackinnon S, Papadapoulos EB, Carabasi MH, et al. Adoptive immunotherapy evaluating escalating doses of donor leukocytes for relapse of chronic myeloid leukemia after *bone marrow transplant*ation: separation of graft-versus-leukemia responses from graft-versus-host disease. *Blood.* 1995;86:1261-1268.

[166] Ruggeri L, Capanni M, Urbani E, et al. Effectiveness of donor natural killer cell alloreactivity in mismatched hematopoietic transplants. *Science*. 2002;295:2097-2100.

[167] Ruggeri L, Capanni M, Casucci M, et al. Role of natural killer cell alloreactivity in HLA-mismatched hematopoietic stem cell *transplantation. Blood.* 1999;94:333-9.

[168] Ruggeri L, Mancusi A, Capanni M, et al. Donor natural killer cell allorecognition of missing self in haploidentical hematopoietic transplantation for acute myeloid leukemia: challenging its predictive value. *Blood.* 2007; 110:433-40.

[169] Couriel D, Canosa J, Engler H, Collins A, Dunbar C, Barrett AJ. Early reactivation of cytomegalovirus and high risk of interstitial pneumonitis following T-depleted BMT for adults with hematological malignancies. *Bone Marrow Transplant.* 1996;18:347-353.

[170] Engelhard D, Or R, Strauss N, et al. Cytomegalovirus infection and disease after T cell depleted allogeneic *bone marrow transplant*ation for malignant hematologic diseases. *Transplant Proc.* 1989;21:3101-3102.

[171] Maltezou H, Whimbey E, Abi-Said D, et al. Cytomegalovirus disease in adult marrow transplant recipients receiving ganciclovir prophylaxis: a retrospective study. *Bone Marrow Transplant.* 1999;24:665-669.

[172] Douek DC, McFarland RD, Keiser PH, et al. Changes in thymic function with age and during the treatment of HIV infection. *Nature* 1998; 396:690–695.

[173] Mackall CL, Fleisher TA, Brown MR, et al. Age, thymopoiesis, and CD4 T-lymphocyte regeneration after intensive chemotherapy. *N. Engl. J. Med.* 1995;332:143–149.

[174] Mackall CL, Fleisher TA, Brown MR, et al. Distinctions between CD8 and CD4 T-cell regenerative pathways result in prolonged T-cell subset imbalance after intensive chemotherapy. *Blood* 1997; 89:3700–3707.

[175] Waller EK, Langston AA, Lonial S, et al. Pharmacokinetics and pharmacodynamics of anti-thymocyte globulin in recipients of partially HLA-matched *blood* hematopoietic progenitor cell transplantation. *Biol. Blood Marrow Transplant.* 2003;**9:** 460–471.

[176] Eyrich M, Lang P, Lal S, et al. A prospective analysis of the pattern of immune reconstitution in a paediatric cohort following transplantation of positively selected human leucocyte antigen-disparate haematopoietic stem cells from parental donors. *Br J Haematol.* 2001;114:422-432.

[177] Chen X, Hale GA, Barfield R, et al. Rapid immune reconstitution after a reduced-intensity conditioning regimen and a CD3-depleted haploidentical stem cell graft for paediatric refractory haematological malignancies. *Br J Haematol.* 2006;135:524-532.

[178] Ball LM, Lankester AC, Bredius RGM, et al. Graft dysfunction and delayed immune reconstitution following haploidentical peripheral *blood* hematopoietic stem cell *transplantation. Bone Marrow Transplantation* 2005; 35: 35–38.

[179] Curtis RE, Travis LB, Rowlings PA, et al. Risk of lymphoproliferative disorders after bone marrow transplantation: a multi-institutional study. *Blood* 1999; 94: 2208–2216.

[180] Ash RC, Casper JT, Chitambar CR, et al. Successful allogeneic transplantation of T-cell-depleted bone marrow from closely HLA-matched unrelated donors. *N Engl J Med.* 1990;322:485-494.

[181] Bhatia S, Ramsay NK, Steinbuch M, et al. Malignant neoplasms following bone marrow transplantation. *Blood* 1996; 87: 3633–3639.

[182] van Esser JW, van der Holt B, Meijer E, *et al.* Epstein–Barr virus (EBV) reactivation is a frequent event after allogeneic stem cell transplantation (SCT) and quantitatively predicts EBV-lymphoproliferative disease following T-cell-depleted SCT. *Blood* 2001; 98: 972–978.

[183] Zutter MM, Martin PJ, Sale GE, et al. Epstein-Barr virus lymphoproliferation after bone marrow transplantation. *Blood.* 1988;72:520-529.

[184] Martin P, Shulman H, Schubach W, et al. Fatal Epstein-Barr virus associated proliferation of donor B-cells after treatment of acute graft-versus-host disease with a murine anti-T-cell antibody. *Ann Intern Med.* 1984;101:310-315.

[185] Shapiro RS, McClain K, Frizzera G, et al. Epstein–Barr virus associated B cell lymphoproliferative disorders following bone marrow transplantation. *Blood* 1988; 71: 1234–1243.

[186] Hale G, Waldmann H. Risks of developing Epstein–Barr virus-related lymphoproliferative disorders after T-cell-depleted marrow transplants. CAMPATH users. *Blood* 1998; 91: 3079–3083.

[187] Cohen J, Gandhi M, Naik P, , et al. Increased incidence of EBV-related disease following paediatric stem cell transplantation with reduced-intensity conditioning. *Br J Haematol* 2005; 129: 229–239.

[188] Hale G, Waldmann H. Risks of developing Epstein-Barr virus-related lymphoproliferative disorders after T-cell-depleted marrow transplants. CAMPATH Users. *Blood.* 1998;91:3079-83.

[189] Shapiro RS, McClain K, Frizzera G, et al. Epstein-Barr virus associated B cell lymphoproliferative disorders following bone marrow transplantation. *Blood.* 1988;71:1234-1243.

[190] Wagner HJ, Rooney CM, Heslop HE. Diagnosis and treatment of posttransplantation lymphoproliferative disease after hematopoietic stem cell transplantation. *Biol Blood Marrow Transplant.* 2002;8:1-8.

[191] Small TN, Papadopoulos EB, Boulad F, et al. Comparison of immune reconstitution after unrelated and related T-cell- depleted bone marrow transplantation: effect of patient age and donor leukocyte infusions. *Blood* 1999; 93: 467–480.

[192] Porter DL, Orloff GJ, Antin JH. Donor mononuclear cell infusions as therapy for B-cell lymphoproliferative disorder following allogeneic bone marrow transplant. *Transplant Sci* 1994; 4: 12–14.

[193] Papadopoulos EB, Ladanyi M, Emanuel D, et al. Infusions of donor leukocytes to treat Epstein–Barr virus-associated lymphoproliferative disorders after allogeneic bone marrow transplantation. *New Engl J Med* 1994; 330: 1185–1191.

[194] Rooney CM, Smith CA, Ng CY, et al. Use of gene-modified virus-specific T lymphocytes to control Epstein–Barr-virus-related lymphoproliferation. *Lancet* 1995; 345: 9–13.

[195] Rooney CM, Smith CA, Ng CY, et al. Infusion of cytotoxic T cells for the prevention and treatment of Epstein–Barr virus-induced lymphoma in allogeneic transplant recipients. *Blood* 1998; 92: 1549–1555.

[196] Gustafsson A, Levitsky V, Zou JZ, et al. Epstein–Barr virus (EBV) load in bone marrow transplant recipients at risk to develop posttransplant lymphoproliferative disease: prophylactic infusion of EBV-specific cytotoxic T cells. *Blood* 2000; 95: 807–814.

[197] McGuirk JP, Seropian S, Howe G, et al. Use of rituximab and irradiated donor-derived lymphocytes to control Epstein-Barr virus-associated lymphoproliferation in patients undergoing related haplo-identical stem cell transplantation. *Bone Marrow Transplant.* 1999;24:1253-1258.

[198] Kuehnle I, Huls MH, Liu Z, et al. CD20 monoclonal antibody (rituximab) for therapy of Epstein-Barr virus lymphoma after hemopoietic stem-cell transplantation. *Blood.* 2000; 95:1502-1505.

[199] Faye A, Quartier P, Reguerre Y, et al. Chimaeric anti-CD20 monoclonal antibody (rituximab) in post-transplant B-lymphoproliferative disorder following stem cell transplantation in children. *Br J Haematol.* 2001;115:112-118.

[200] Weinstock DM, Ambrossi GG, Brennan C, Kiehn TE, Jakubowski A. Preemptive diagnosis and treatment of Epstein-Barr virus-associated post transplant lymphoproliferative disorder after hematopoietic stem cell transplant: an approach in development. Bone Marrow Transplant. 2006 ;37:539-46.

[201] van Esser JW, Niesters HG, van der Holt B, et al. Prevention of Epstein–Barr virus-lymphoproliferative disease by molecular monitoring and preemptive rituximab in high-risk patients after allogeneic stem cell transplantation. *Blood* 2002; 99: 4364–4369.

[202] Anasetti C, Beatty PG, Storb R,et al.. Effect of HLA incompatibility on graft-versus-host disease, relapse, and survival after marrow transplantation for patients with leukemia or lymphoma. *Hum Immunol.* 1990;29:79-91.

[203] Kernan NA, Flomenberg N, Dupont B, O'Reilly RJ. Graft rejection in recipients of T-cell-depleted HLA-nonidentical marrow transplants for leukemia. Identification of host-derived antidonor allocytotoxic T lymphocytes. *Transplantation.* 1987;43:842-7.

[204] Henslee-Downey PJ, Parrish RS, MacDonald JS, et al. Combined in vitro and in vivo T lymphocyte depletion for the control of graft-versus-host disease following haploidentical marrow transplant. *Transplantation.* 1996;61:738-745.

[205] Soiffer RJ, Mauch P, Fairclough D, et al. CD6+ T cell depleted allogeneic bone marrow transplantation from genotypically HLA nonidentical related donors. *Biol Blood Marrow Transplant.* 1997;3:11-17.

[206] Tabilio A, Falzetti F, Giannoni C, et al. Stem cell mobilization in normal donors. *J. Hematother.* 1997;6: 227–234.

[207] Aversa F, Velardi A, Tabilio A, et al. Haploidentical stem cell transplantation in leukemia. *Blood Rev.* 2001;15:111-119.

[208] Lang P, Greil J, Bader P, et al. Long-term outcome after haploidentical stem cell transplantation in children. *Blood Cells Mol Dis.* 2004;33:281-287.

[209] Handgretinger R, Chen X, Pfeiffer M, et al. Feasability and outcome of reduced intensity conditioning in haploidentical transplantation. *Ann N Y Acad Sci.* 2007;1106:279-289.

[210] Ogawa H, Ikegame K, Yoshihara S, et al. Unmanipulated HLA 2-3 antigen-mismatched (haploidentical) stem cell transplantation using nonmyeloablative conditioning. *Biol Blood Marrow Transplant.* 2006;12: 1073-1084.

[211] Spitzer TR, McAfee SL, Dey BR, et al. Nonmyeloablative haploidentical stem-cell transplantation using anti-CD2 monoclonal antibody (MEDI-507)-based conditioning for refractory hematologic malignancies. *Transplantation.* 2003;75:1448–1751.

[212] Perruccio K, Tosti A, Burchielli E, et al. Transferring functional immune responses to pathogens after haploidentical hematopoietic transplantation. *Blood.* 2005;106: 4397-4406.

[213] Solomon SR, Mielke S, Savani BN, et al. Selective depletion of alloreactive donor lymphocytes: a novel method to reduce the severity of graft-versus-host disease in older patients undergoing matched sibling donor stem cell transplantation. *Blood.* 2005;106:1123-1129.

[214] Amrolia PJ, Muccioli-Casadei G, Huls H, et al. Adoptive immunotherapy with allodepleted donor T-cells improves immune reconstitution after haploidentical stem cell transplantation. *Blood.* 2006;108:1797-808.

[215] Ruggeri L, Mancusi A, Burchielli E, et al. Natural killer cell alloreactivity in allogeneic hematopoietic *transplantation. Curr Opin Oncol.* 2007;19:142-147.

[216] Shimazaki C, Ochiai N, Uchida R, et al. Non-T-cell-depleted HLA haploidentical stem cell transplantation in advanced hematologic malignancies based on the feto-maternal michrochimerism, *Blood.* 2003;101: 3334–3336.

[217] Obama K, Utsunomiya A, Takatsuka Y, et al. Reduced-intensity non-T-cell depleted HLA-haploidentical stem cell transplantation for older patients based on the concept of feto-maternal tolerance. *Bone Marrow Transplant.* 2004;34:897-899.

[218] Shimazaki C, Fuchida S, Ochiai N, et al. Non-T-cell-depleted HLA-haploidentical stem cell transplantation after reduced-intensity conditioning in advanced haematological malignancies based on feto-maternal microchimerism, *Br J Haematol.* 2004;127: 474–475.

[219] Tamaki S, Ichinohe T, Matsuo K, et al. Superior survival of *blood* and marrow stem cell transplants given maternal grafts over recipients given paternal grafts. *Bone Marrow Transplant.* 2001;28:375-380.

[220] Cavazzana-Calvo M., Fromont C, Le DF et al. Specific elimination of alloreactive T cells by an anti-interleukin-2 receptor B chain-specific immunotoxin. *Transplantation* 1990;50 : 1–7.

[221] Harris DT, Sakiestewa D, Lyons C, et al. Prevention of graft-versus-host disease (GVHD) by elimination of recipient-reactive donor T cells with recombinant toxins that target the interleukin 2 (IL-2) receptor. *Bone Marrow Transplant* 1999;23 :137–144.
[222] Koh MB, Prentice HG and Corbo M, et al. Alloantigen-specific T-cell depletion in a major histocompatibility complex fully mismatched murine model provides effective graft-versus-host disease prophylaxis in the presence of lymphoid engraftment. *Br J Haematol* 2002; 118:108–116.
[223] Hartwig UF, Robbers M., Wickenhauser C, et al. Murine acute graft-versus-host disease can be prevented by depletion of alloreactive T lymphocytes using activation-induced cell death. *Blood* 2002; 99: 3041–3049.
[224] Chen BJ, Cui X, Liu C, Chao NJ. Prevention of graft-versus-host disease while preserving graft-versus-leukemia effect after selective depletion of host-reactive T cells by photodynamic cell purging process. *Blood* 2002; 99 : 3083–3088.
[225] Andre-Schmutz I, Le DF, Hacein-Bey-Abina S, et al. Immune reconstitution without graft-versus-host disease after haemopoietic stem-cell transplantation: a phase 1/2 study. *Lancet.* 2002;360: 130-137.
[226] Pittenger MF, Mackay AM, Beck SC, et al. Multilineage potential of adult human mesenchymal stem cells. *Science* 1999; 284: 143–147.
[227] Horwitz EM, Le Blanc K, Dominici M, et al. Clarification of the nomenclature for MSC: the international society for cellular therapy position statement. *Cytotherapy* 2005; 7: 393–395
[228] Le Blanc K, Ringdén O. Immunobiology of human mesenchymal stem cells and future use in hematopoietic stem cell transplantation. *Biol Blood Marrow Transplant*. 2005; 11:321-34.
[229] Lee ST, Jang JH, Cheong JW, et al. Treatment of high-risk acute myelogenous leukaemia by myeloablative chemoradiotherapy followed by co-infusion of T cell-depleted haematopoietic stem cells and culture-expanded marrow mesenchymal stem cells from a related donor with one fully mismatched human leucocyte antigen haplotype. *Br J Haematol* 2002; 118: 1128–1131.
[230] Le Blanc K, Rasmusson I, Sundberg B, et al. Treatment of severe acute graft-versus-host disease with third party haploidentical mesenchymal stem cells. *Lancet* 2004; 363: 1439–1441.
[231] Lazarus HM, Koc ON, Devine SM, et al. Co-transplantation of HLA-identical sibling culture-expanded mesenchymal stem cells and hematopoietic stem cells in hematologic malignancy patients. *Biol Blood Marrow Transplant* 2005; 11:389–398.
[232] Ball LM, Bernardo ME, Roelofs H, et al. Cotransplantation of *ex vivo* expanded mesenchymal stem cells accelerates lymphocyte recovery and may reduce the risk of graft failure in haploidentical hematopoietic stem-cell transplantation. *Blood* 2007; 110: 2764–2767.
[233] Ning H, Yang F, Jiang M, et al. The correlation between cotransplantation of mesenchymal stem cells and higher recurrence rate in hematologic Malignancy patients: outcome of a pilot clinical study. *Leukemia* 2008; 22: 593–599.
[234] Bonini C, Bondanza A, Perna SK, et al. The suicide gene therapy challenge: how to improve a successful gene therapy approach. *Mol Ther*. 2007;15:1248–1252.

[235] Bonini C, Ferrari G, Verzeletti S, et al. HSV-TK gene transfer into donor lymphocytes for control of allogeneic graft-versus-leukemia. *Science* 1997; 276: 1719–1724.
[236] Tiberghien P, Ferrand C, Lioure B, et al. Administration of herpes simplex-thymidine kinase-expressing donor T cells with a T cell-depleted allogeneic marrow graft. *Blood* 2001; 97: 63–72.
[237] Bonini C, Ciceri F, Marktel S et al. Abrogation of GvHD and early immune reconstitution after infusion of HSV-TK engineered donor lymphocytes after haplo-identical hemopoietic stem cell transplantation. *Blood* 2002; 100:(suppl 1): 425a.
[238] Dazzi F, Szydlo RM, Cross NC, et al. Durability of responses following donor lymphocytes infusions for patients who relapse after allogeneic stem cell transplantation for chronic myeloid leukemia. *Blood.* 2000; 96: 2712-2716.
[239] Porter DL, Collins RH, Hardy C, et al. Treatment of relapsed leukemia after unrelated unrelated donor marrow transplantation with unrelated donor leukocyte infusions. *Blood.* 2000; 95:1214-1221.
[240] Kolb HJ, Schattenberg A, Goldman JM, et al. Graft-versus-leukemia effect of donor lymphocyte transfusions in marrow grafted patients. *Blood.* 1995 ;86:2041-50.
[241] Collins RH Jr, Shpilberg O, Drobyski WR, et al. Donor leukocyte infusions in 140 patients with relapsed malignancy after allogeneic bone marrow transplantation. *J Clin Oncol.* 1997;15:433-44.
[242] Porter DL, Antin JH. Donor leukocyte infusions in myeloid malignancies: new strategies. *Best Pract Res Clin Haematol.* 2006;19:737-55.
[243] Peggs KS, Thomson K, Hart DP, et al. Dose-escalated donor lymphocyte infusions following reduced intensity transplantation: toxicity, chimerism, and disease responses. *Blood.* 2004;103:1548-56.
[244] Bethge WA, Hegenbart U, Stuart MJ, et al. Adoptive immunotherapy with donor lymphocyte infusions after allogeneic hematopoietic cell transplantation following nonmyeloablative conditioning. *Blood.* 2004;103:790-5.
[245] Wu BY, Guo KY, Song CY, et al. Mixed chimera converted into full donor chimera with powerful graft-versus-leukemia effects but no graft-versus-host disease after non T cell-depleted HLA-mismatched peripheral blood stem cell transplantation, *Bone Marrow Transplant.* 2000;26:691–693.
[246] Lewalle P, Triffet A, Delforge A, et al. Donor lymphocyte infusions in adult haploidentical transplant: a dose finding study. *Bone Marrow Transplant.* 2003;31:39-44.
[247] Pati AR, Godder K, Lamb L, et al. Immunotherapy with donor leukocyte infusions for patients with relapsed acute myeloid leukemia following partially mismatched related donor bone marrow transplantation. *Bone Marrow Transplant.* 1995;15:979-81.
[248] Or R, Hadar E, Bitan M, et al. Safety and efficacy of donor lymphocyte infusions following mismatched stem cell transplantation. *Biol Blood Marrow Transplant.* 2006;12:1295-1301.
[249] Huang XJ, Liu DH, Liu KY, et al. Donor lymphocyte infusion for the treatment of leukemia relapse after HLA-mismatched/haploidentical T-cell-replete hematopoietic stem cell transplantation. *Haematologica.* 2007;92:414-417.

[250] Chakraverty R, Peggs K, Chopra R, et al. Limiting transplantation-related mortality following unrelated donor stem cell transplantation by using a nonmyeloablative conditioning regimen. *Blood.* 2002 ;99:1071-8.
[251] Champlin R, Ho W, Gajewski J, et al. Selective depletion of CD8+ T lymphocytes for prevention of graft-versus-host disease after allogeneic bone marrow transplantation. *Blood.* 1990;76:418-23.
[252] Soiffer RJ, Gonin R, Murray C, et al. Prediction of graft-versus-host disease by phenotypic analysis of early immune reconstitution after CD6-depleted allogeneic *bone marrow transplantation. Blood.* 1993;82:2216-23.
[253] Baron F, Baudoux E, Frere P, et al. Nonmyeloablative stem cell transplantation with CD8-depleted or CD34-selected peripheral blood stem cells. *J Hematother Stem Cell Res* 2002; 11:301–314.
[254] Giralt S, Hester J, Huh Y, et al. CD8-depleted donor lymphocyte infusion as treatment for relapsed chronic myelogenous leukemia after allogeneic bone marrow transplantation. *Blood* 1995; 86:4337–4343.
[255] Alyea EP, Soiffer RJ, Canning C, et al. Toxicity and efficacy of defined doses of CD4(+) donor lymphocytes for treatment of relapse after allogeneic bone marrow transplant. *Blood* 1998; 91:3671–3680.
[256] Alyea E, Weller E, Schlossman R, et al. T-cell-depleted allogeneic *bone marrow transplant*ation followed by donor lymphocyte infusion in patients with multiple myeloma: induction of graft-versus-myeloma effect. *Blood* 2001; 98:934–939.
[257] Barrett AJ, Mavroudis D, Tisdale J, et al. T cell-depleted bone marrow transplantation and delayed T cell add-back to control acute GVHD and conserve a graft-versus-leukemia effect. *Bone Marrow Transplant.* 1998 ;21:543-51.
[258] Nimer SD, Giorgi J, Gajewski JL, et al. Selective depletion of CD8+ cells for prevention of graft-versus-host disease after bone marrow transplantation: a randomized controlled trial. *Transplantation* 1994; 57:82–87.
[259] Soiffer RJ, Alyea EP, Hochberg E, et al. Randomized trial of CD8+ T-cell depletion in the prevention of graft-versus-host disease associated with donor lymphocyte infusion. *Biol Blood Marrow Transplant* 2002; 8:625–632.
[260] Meyer RG, Britten CM, Wehler D, et al. Prophylactic transfer of CD8-depleted donor lymphocytes after T-cell-depleted reduced-intensity transplantation. *Blood.* 2007;109:374-82.
[261] Passweg JR, Tichelli A, Meyer-Monard S, et al. Purified donor NK-lymphocyte infusion to consolidate engraftment after haploidentical stem cell transplantation. *Leukemia.* 2004;18:1835-1838.
[262] Passweg JR, Stern M, Koehl U, et al. Use of natural killer cells in hematopoetic stem cell transplantation. *Bone Marrow Transplant.* 2005;35:637-643.
[263] Le NT, Chao N. Regulating regulatory T cells. *Bone Marrow Transplant.* 2007;39:1-9.
[264] Hoffmann P, Ermann J, Edinger M, et al. Donor-type CD4+CD25+ regulatory T cells suppress lethal acute graft-versus-host disease after allogeneic bone marrow transplantation. *J Exp Med* 2002; 196:389–399.
[265] Trenado A, Charlotte F, Fisson S, et al. Recipient-type specific CD4+CD25+ regulatory T cells favor immune reconstitution and control graft-versus-host disease while maintaining graft-versus-leukemia. *J Clin Invest* 2003; 112: 1688–1696.

[266] Taylor PA, Noelle RJ, Blazar BR. CD4(+)CD25(+) immune regulatory cells are required for induction of tolerance to alloantigen via costimulatory blockade. *J Exp Med* 2001; 193: 1311–1318.

[267] Cohen JL, Trenado A, Vasey D, Klatzmann D, Salomon BL. CD4(+)CD25(+) immunoregulatory T cells: new therapeutics for graft-versus-host disease. *J Exp Med* 2002; 196: 401–406.

[268] Edinger M, Hoffmann P, Ermann J, et al. CD4+CD25+ regulatory T cells preserve graft-versus-tumor activity while inhibiting graft-versus-host disease after bone marrow transplantation. *Nat Med* 2003; 9: 1144–1150.

[269] Jones SC, Murphy GF, Korngold R. Post-hematopoietic cell transplantation control of graft-versus-host disease by donor CD425T cells to allow an effective graft-versus-leukemia response. *Biol Blood Marrow Transplant* 2003; 9: 243–256.

[270] Sanchez J, Casano J, Alvarez MA, et al. Kinetic of regulatory CD25high and activated CD134+ (OX40) T lymphocytes during acute and chronic graft-versus-host disease after allogeneic bone marrow transplantation. *Br J Haematol* 2004; 126: 697–703.

[271] Clark FJ, Gregg R, Piper K, et al. Chronic graft-versus-host disease is associated with increased numbers of peripheral blood CD4+CD25high regulatory T cells. *Blood* 2004; 103: 2410–2416.

[272] Miura Y, Thoburn CJ, Bright EC, et al. Association of Foxp3 regulatory gene expression with graft-versus-host disease. *Blood* 2004; 104: 2187–2193.

[273] Meignin V, de Latour RP, Zuber J, et al. Numbers of Foxp3-expressing CD4+CD25high T cells do not correlate with the establishment of long-term tolerance after allogeneic stem cell transplantation. *Exp Hematol* 2005; 33: 894–900.

[274] Zorn E, Kim HT, Lee SJ, et al. Reduced frequency of FOXP3+ CD4+CD25+ regulatory T cells in patients with chronic graft-versus-host disease. *Blood* 2005; 106: 2903–2911.

[275] Godfrey WR, Ge YG, Spoden DJ, et al. *In vitro*-expanded human CD4(+)CD25(+) T-regulatory cells can markedly inhibit allogeneic dendritic cell-stimulated MLR cultures. *Blood* 2004; 104: 453–461.

[276] Karakhanova S, Munder M, Schneider M, Bonyhadi M, Ho AD, Goerner M. Highly efficient expansion of human CD4+CD25+ regulatory T cells for cellular immunotherapy in patients with graft-versus-host disease. *J Immunother* 2006; 29: 336–349.

[277] Lowsky R, Takahashi T, Liu YP, et al. Protective conditioning for acute graft-versus-host disease. *N Eng J Med* 2005; 353:1321–1331.

[278] Strober S. Protective conditioning against GVHD and graft rejection after combined organ and hematopoietic cell transplantation. *Blood Cells Mol Dis*. 2008 ;40:48-54.

[279] Ruggeri L, Mancusi A, Burchielli E, et al. Natural killer cell alloreactivity in allogeneic hematopoietic transplantation. *Curr Opin Oncol.* 2007;19:142-147.

[280] Dazzi F, Szydlo RM, Cross NC, et al. Durability of responses following donor lymphocytes infusions for patients who relapse after allogeneic stem cell transplantation for chronic myeloid leukemia. *Blood* 2000; 96: 2712-2716.

[281] Fong L & Engleman EG. Dendritic cells in cancer immunotherapy. *Annu Rev Immunol* 2000; 18: 245–273.

[282] O'Neill DW, Adams S & Bhardwaj N. Manipulating dendritic cell biology for the active immunotherapy of cancer. *Blood* 2004; 104: 2235–2246.

[283] Falkenburg JH, Wafelman AR, Joosten P, et al. Complete remission of accelerated phase chronic myeloid leukemia by treatment with leukemia-reactive cytotoxic T lymphocytes. *Blood.* 1999;94:1201-1208.

[284] Riddell SR, Watanabe KS, Goodrich JM, et al. Restoration of viral immunity in immunodeficient humans by the adoptive transfer of T cell clones. *Science.* 1992;257: 238-241.

[285] Peggs KS, Verfuerth S, Pizzey A, et al. Adoptive cellular therapy for early cytomegalovirus infection after allogeneic stem-cell transplantation with virus-specific T-cell lines. *Lancet.* 2003;362: 1375-1377.

[286] Einsele H, Roosnek E, Rufer N, et al. Infusion of cytomegalovirus (CMV)-specific T cells for the treatment of CMV infection not responding to antiviral chemotherapy. *Blood.* 2002;99: 3916-3922.

In: Immunosuppression: New Research
Editor: Charles B. Taylor, pp. 89-113
ISBN: 978-1-60692-102-9

Chapter 3

Leucocyte Intracellular Cytokines in Lung Transplant Patients- A More Physiological Indicator of Immunosuppression than Plasma Drug Levels

Greg Hodge[1,2], Sandra Hodge[1], Paul Reynolds[1], Daniel Chambers[3] and Mark Holmes[1,4]

[1]Department of Thoracic Medicine, Royal Adelaide Hospital, Adelaide;
[2]Haematology Department, Women's and Children's Hospital, North Adelaide, South Australia;
[3]Queensland Centre for Thoracic Transplantation, The Prince Charles Hospital, Brisbane;
[4]South Australian Lung Transplant Service.

Abstract

The strong allo-immune response to the transplanted lung necessitates combined pharmacological immunosuppression to prevent graft rejection. Immunosuppressants used to prevent and treat rejection involve several classes of drugs and many target the production of pro-inflammatory cytokines by T cells, monocytes and other immune cells. Although most effective transplantation immunosuppressive strategies are based on interruption of IL-2 signaling by the calcineurin inhibitors cyclosporin A and tacrolimus, intensification of immunosupressive therapies has not led to any improvement in graft survival. Treatment with these drugs is also associated with serious adverse effects including specific organ toxicities, increased risk of developing a range of malignancies and susceptibility to infections. High inter- and intra-individual pharmacokinetic variability of both drugs may mean some patients do not require the high levels of drugs and associated adverse side effects for effective therapeutics. While current assessment of therapeutic drug levels simply involves the empirical measurement of plasma drug concentrations, there is a need for more physiological assessment of combined immunosuppression strategies, particularly at the site of action. Recent research has identified measurement of inflammatory cytokines at the cellular level using novel flow cytometric techniques as a strategy to assess the physiological response to treatment. Intracellular cytokine levels in both peripheral blood and in the airways have been investigated and have highlighted important differences in responses seen at the transplant site versus systemically. While Th1 pro-inflammatory cytokines were significantly reduced in blood T cells from transplant patients, levels of these cytokines in T cells from the airways were significantly greater in transplant patients compared with healthy control subjects. Furthermore, patients undergoing infection or rejection episodes were characterised by significantly decreased or increased Th1 intracellular T cell cytokines in the airways respectively, compared with stable lung transplant patients. To overcome patient inter-individual variability of leucocyte cytokine production, longitudinal monitoring of patient cytokines may be useful in predicting adverse episodes of rejection and/or infection. These techniques may complement or ultimately replace current standard approaches to therapeutic drug monitoring and monitoring by invasive biopsy and have the potential to improve current immunosuppression protocols, optimise individual therapy and possibly provide new therapeutic options to improve the morbidity of lung transplant patients.

Introduction

Lung transplantation is the only definitive therapy for many forms of end-stage lung disease. However, five year survival after lung transplantation is only approximately 50%. This is a disappointing outcome considering the huge expenses involved in lung transplantation and post-transplant care and the acute shortage of donor organs. Acute graft failure is more common with lungs than any other solid organ resulting in poorer short term survival after lung transplant compared with recipients of other organs. In the longer term, the principle reason for graft failure is believed to be chronic allograft dysfunction. Chronic graft failure is manifested by progressive airways obstruction and worsening shortness of breath. The clinical syndrome is referred to as “bronchiolitis obliterans syndrome” (BOS). In many cases, there is a defined pathological correlate, “obliterative bronchiolitis” (OB).

Although the precise pathogenesis of chronic graft failure is unclear, there are certain strong associations such as acute rejection; with early and repeated episodes of acute rejection significantly increasing the risk of subsequent OB. This suggests that immune mechanisms may in part underly OB and have thus lead to the hypothesis that the disorder is a form of chronic rejection. However, many patients with acute rejection do not develop OB, and some patients with OB have never experienced clinically detected acute rejection. OB may also be associated with pulmonary infections including CMV infection, primary graft dysfunction and gastro-esophageal reflux disease.

Acute and Chronic Transplant Rejection

At the cellular level, acute graft rejection is associated with a marked increase in graft T-cell infiltration, alveolar macrophages, and pro-inflammatory cytokine expression including IL-2, IFN-γ and TNF-α [2]. Acute cellular rejection involves recipient T cell recognition of HLA molecules expressed on donor-derived, antigen presenting cells (direct allorecognition) or presentation of donor derived peptides by recipient antigen-presenting cells to recipient T cells (indirect allorecognition). Once the alloantigens are recognised as foreign, the activation and production of cytokines by T lymphocytes, monocytes and other immune cells lead to the amplification of the alloimmune response.

OB is also associated with a moderate increase in graft airway T-cell infiltration, alveolar macrophages, and pro-inflammatory cytokine expression [3, 4]. Airway fibrosis is also associated with OB, which may be due to the presence of pro-fibrotic chemokines/cytokines such as MCP-1, IL-4 and TGFβ [4]. The strong alloimmune response to the transplanted lung necessitates combined pharmacological immunosuppression to prevent graft rejection. Immunosuppression has improved graft survival but leaves patients susceptible to infectious complications and malignancies. Pulmonary infections are the leading cause of morbidity and mortality in this patient group. Immunosuppressants used to prevent and treat rejection involve several classes of drugs and many target the production of pro-inflammatory cytokine by T cells, monocytes and other immune cells.

Immunosuppression

Corticosteroids

Glucocorticoids were the first immunosuppressants used in transplantation. They are the least selective agents and affect multiple cell lines, including T and B cells, monocytes, macrophages and neutrophils. In lymphocytes and monocytes, glucocorticoids exert negative regulatory effects on cytokine gene expression [5], although one study showed upregulation of IL-10 production by monocytes in the presence of low concentrations of prednisolone in vitro [6].

Calcineurin Inhibitors: Cyclosporin A (CsA) and Tacrolimus (Tac)

Calcineurin inhibitors CsA and Tac have greatly decreased the incidence of allograft rejection and are the mainstay of current immunosuppression regimes. They are more T-cell selective and their use has helped preserve other cell lines by reducing the overall incidence of infection [7, 8]. Both CsA and Tac inhibit production of IL-1β, IL-2, IL-6, IL-8, IFNγ and TNFα while Tac preferentially suppresses T-helper-type-1 (Th1) cells over Th2 cells [5].

Both agents do however upregulate TGFβ, which although having several immunosuppressive properties on pro-inflammatory cytokines, promotes matrix formation and may contribute to allograft fibrosis as observed in chronic rejection.

Antimetabolites: Azathioprine and Mycophenolate Mofetil

Azathioprine and Mycophenolate Mofetil are antimetabolites that inhibit the production of purine which is required for T and B-cell activation and proliferation. Azathioprine also acts by inhibiting CD28 costimulation [9] while Mycophenolate Mofetil reduces cytokine production through inhibition of clonal expansion [9, 10].

Other agents such as sirolimus and everolimus inhibit mRNA responsible for cell cycle progression thus blocking IL-2 postreceptor signaling and preventing T-cell proliferation [10].

Anti-lymphocyte Antibodies

Polyclonal anti-lymphocyte antibodies have a long history of use for induction of immuno-suppression and in the treatment of acute rejection, targeting different cell lines such as lymphocytes, thymocytes or specific cell lines. For example, OKT3 is a murine monoclonal anti-lymphocyte antibody directed against the T-cell receptor causing T-cell opsinisation and removal by mononuclear phagocytes [8].

Anti-cytokine Receptor Antibodies

Anti-cytokine receptor monoclonal antibodies directed against the α-chains of the CD25 molecule, a key unit of the IL-2 receptor, have also been used successfully in the transplant setting [10] due to the central role of IL-2 in regulating T-cell activation.

"Triple immunosuppression" is the common form of immunosuppression used in lung transplantation and consists of a calcineurin antagonist (cyclosporin A or tacrolimus), an antimetabolite (Azathioprine and Mycophenolate Mofetil) and corticosteroids [9]. Trough plasma drug levels of either CsA A or Tac are kept within recommended therapeutic ranges (range for CsA (80-250 μg/L) and Tac (5-20 μg/L)). However, therapeutic drug plasma concentrations are broad and may vary according to the clinical situation and the choice of immunosuppressive agents being given.

Therapeutic monitoring of single drug levels has certain limitations as the combined therapeutic effect of all drugs used should be assessed for each patient. An alternative more physiological approach has recently been suggested [11].

Cytokine Measurement in Lung Transplant Patients

There are three sites from which cells or fluid can be assessed for cytokine analysis in recipients of pulmonary allografts; blood, the bronchial epithelium and the alveolar region.

Previous methodology to measure cytokine levels in transplant patients include ELISA quantification from serum and peripheral blood mononuclear cell culture [12, 13] and RTPCR of cytokine mRNA levels [14]. Measurement of soluble cytokines by ELISA and more recently by cytometric bead arrays have proven useful for diagnosis in several disease states [15, 16]. However, cytokines bind to proteoglycan components of the cell surface or extracellular matrix [17] and have a very limited availability within the blood, effectively limiting the prognostic value of assay of soluble cytokines. Standard techniques such as ELISA are time consuming and expensive if several cytokines are quantified and give no indication of cytokine-producing cell types. Cell purification techniques lead to loss of specific cell subsets [18] and increased apoptosis of cells [19]. While RTPCR is a sensitive technique, results depend on purification of cells from heterogeneous cell populations and are subject to technical error.

The production of cytokines by cells can be assessed using a range of techniques. Several of these assays require cell activation prior to analysis. In the case of T cells this is accomplished by polyclonal stimulation with mitogens active on the cell surface or within the cell or by antigenic stimulation. Multiparameter flow cytometry offers a powerful tool to analyse multiple pro- and anti-inflammatory intracellular cytokines following polyclonal stimulation in thousands of cells by individual cell types. This technique provides information regarding not only the phenotype but also the activation state of each individual immune effector cell.

Assessment of the activation state of T-cells by measurement of cell-specific cytokine production has also been used to investigate differences in unstimulated cells in several clinical situations such as between cord and adult blood in the context of graft versus host disease [20] and effects of other therapeutics [21]. Recently, this technique has been used in preliminary studies in lung transplant patients.

Effect of Immunosuppression Protocols on Intracellular Cytokines in Blood T Cells

Until very recently it was unknown if levels of immunosuppressive drugs correlate with pro-inflammatory cytokine expression in peripheral blood T cells. As lymphocytes traffic from the blood stream to the lung and later rejoin the peripheral circulation [22], measurement of blood T cell cytokines may be reflective of graft infiltrating T-cell cytokine profiles.

The immunomodulatory effects of currently used immunosuppressive regimes on T cell cytokine production from a group of stable, non-infected lung transplant patients and control volunteers was recently assessed using the technique of intracellular cytokine analysis and multiparameter flow cytometry [11]. This study provided evidence that current immunosuppression protocols have a significant immunosuppressive effect on pro-inflammatory cytokine production by peripheral blood CD4+ T cells consistent with therapeutic intention. However, a limited effect on peripheral blood CD8+ T-cells was noted, particularly IFNγ inflammatory cytokine production in lung transplant patients (Figure 1).

All transplant patients in this study had plasma levels of CsA or Tac within their therapeutic ranges suggesting that analysis of intracellular T cell cytokine production may provide a more accurate assessment of immunosuppression than drug levels.

This study showed that immunosuppression protocols are adequate for CD8- (CD4+) but not CD8+ T-cell inflammatory cytokines, particularly IFNγ. Results from this study also showed that current immunosuppression agents increased anti-inflammatory cytokine production of IL-4 and TGFβ by T cells from lung transplant patients compared to controls (Table 1).

IL-4 negatively regulates IFNγ and IL-2 [23], pro-inflammatory cytokines that have been reportedly increased during acute rejection episodes [14]. TGFβ has also been shown to inhibit IL-2 and IFNγ production by T cells [24] and may partially explain the significantly reduced levels of IFNγ and IL-2 in peripheral blood T cells noted in this study. TGFβ has been shown to inhibit CD4+ Th1 responses compared to CD8+ T cells [25] which may help explain the observation of increased inhibition of these cytokines in CD4+ cells compared to CD8+ T cells.

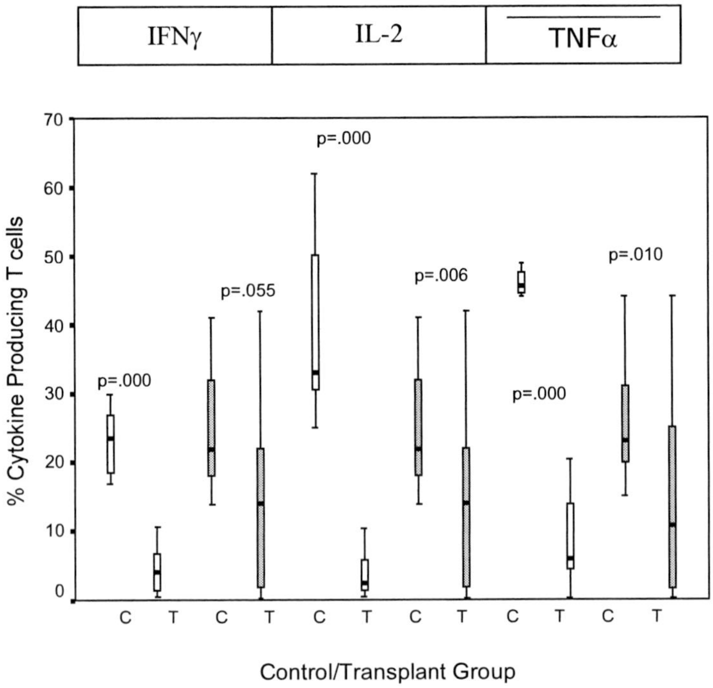

Figure 1. Box plot graphs showing the production of pro-inflammatory cytokines by CD4+ ☐ and CD8+ ▩ T-cells from the blood of lung transplant (T) and control (C) subjects following *in vitro* stimulation (mean ± SD and range). The percentage of CD4+ and CD8+ T-cells producing IL-2 and TNFα was significantly reduced from lung transplant patients compared to control. The percentage of CD4+ T-cells producing IFNγ was also significantly reduced from lung transplant patients but not the percentage of CD8+ T cells producing IFNγ. Note the marked inhibition of inflammatory T-cell cytokines in CD4+ cells compared with CD8+ cells in transplant patients compared to control group.

Table 1. The percentage of T cell subsets producing anti-inflammatory cytokines, IL-4 and TGFβ from 9 lung transplant patients (T) compared with 15 control subjects (C) (mean ± SD). There was a significant increase in IL-4 by both T-cell subsets and TGFβ by CD8+ T-cell subsets by transplant patients compared with control subjects (bold).

	IL-4		TGFβ	
	CD4	CD8	CD4	CD8
C	0.4±0.3	0.0±0.0	5.3±3.2	3.0±2.6
T	1.0±0.8	1.4±0.0	4.9±3.1	4.6±2.4
P	.019	.010	.890	.017

Increased absolute numbers of CD8+ T cells were also noted in transplant patients which is consistent with a previous report [11]. TGFβ has been shown to be co-stimulatory for CD8+ T cells but not CD4+ T cells [26]. IL-4 enhances the proliferation of precursors of cytotoxic lymphocytes and their differentiation into active cytotoxic CD8+ T cells [28]. In CsA or Tac treated mice, T-cell proliferation was shown to be suppressed in CD4+ but not CD8+ subsets [28]. These findings of increased TGFβ by CD8+T cells and increased IL-4 production by both CD4+ and CD8+ T-cell subsets may therefore be causative factors in the significant increase in cytotoxic T cells in these patients.

In contrast to acute rejection, chronic graft failure is associated with increased fibrosis in the lung. Both IL-4 [29] and TGFβ [30] have been shown to promote fibroblast proliferation in the lung. Therefore, although TGFβ and IL4 are anti-inflammatory cytokines, their increased production by cytotoxic lymphocytes that migrate to the lung may contribute to increased fibrosis noted in chronic graft rejection, hence predisposing patients receiving current immunosuppression protocols to BOS.

In an attempt to minimise the significant toxic side effects of current immunosuppression protocols [31], a number of low toxicity protocols have been developed [32]. One could hypothesise that if a transplant patient was showing signs of drug toxicity and levels of intracellular T-cell inflammatory cytokines were markedly reduced compared to control (eg., Patient B in Figure 2), the dose of drug could be reduced and therapeutic effects monitored or tailored to suit the individual patient. Alternately, if intracellular T-cell inflammatory cytokines were not reduced (eg., CD8 T cells in Patient A, Figure 2), other immunosuppressive drugs should be considered.

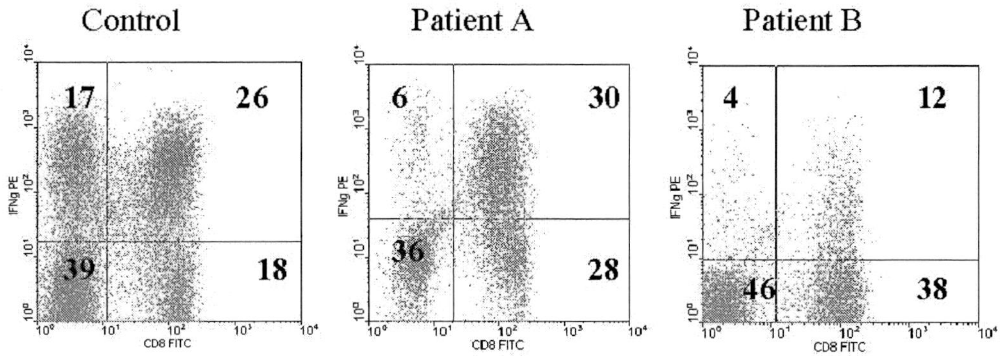

Figure 2. Representative dot plots showing the effect of immunosuppression therapy on IFNγ production by CD8+ and CD8- (CD4+) T cells from the blood of 2 lung transplant patients and control. T cells were identified by CD3 PC5 versus side scatter characteristics. Patient A shows immunosuppression of IFNγ in CD8- (CD4+) T cells but not CD8+ T cells. Patient B shows immunosuppression of IFNγ in both T-cell subsets. Note the reduced percentage of CD4 T cells and increased CD8 T cells in transplant patients compared to control.

This study showed that current immunosuppression protocols have limited effect on peripheral blood IFNγ production by CD8+ T-cells but do upregulate T-cell anti-inflammatory cytokines, TGFβ and IL4. Current protocols for reducing graft rejection in these patients may include drugs that effectively reduce IFNγ production by CD8+ T cells. Intracellular cytokine analysis using flow cytometry may be a more appropriate indicator of immunosuppression of all therapeutic drugs used than measurement of plasma CsA or Tac levels in these patients.

Effect of Immunosuppression Protocols on Blood Monocyte Cytokine and Chemokine Production

Blood monocytes that migrate to the lung form alveolar macrophages which are a major source of inflammatory cytokines/chemokines involved in the pathogenesis of lung transplant rejection. Chemokines are inflammatory mediators that specifically stimulate the directional migration of T cells and monocytes and play an important role in immune cell recruitment into sites of antigenic challenge [33] such as in the pulmonary allograft. Chemokines such as IL-8 and MCP-1 have been reportedly increased in BAL of transplant patients undergoing rejection [34]. MCP-1 induces monocyte migration and differentiation to macrophages and plays a pivotal role in BOS [35]. A recent report investigated monocyte production of cytokine/chemokine mediators in peripheral blood of lung transplant patients [36]. Intracellular cytokine/chemokine production by peripheral blood monocytes following stimulation with LPS from a group of stable lung transplant patients and control volunteers was investigated. There was a significant increase in the percentage of monocytes producing chemokines MCP-1, MCP-3 and IL-8 and anti-inflammatory cytokine IL-10, but no change in the percentage of monocytes producing IL-6, TNFα, IL-1α, IL-12, MIP-1α, MIP-1β and TGFβ (Table 2). Representative histograms showing the increase in the percentage of monocytes producing chemokines MCP-1, MCP-3 from a transplant patient is shown in figure 3.

Table 2. Monocyte cytokine/chemokine production in 9 lung transplant and 15 control subjects (% positive cells) following LPS stimulation. The percentage of blood monocytes producing IL-8, IL-10 and MCP-1 and MCP-3 was significantly increased in lung transplant patients (bold) but levels of IL-6, TNFα, IL-1α, IL-12, MIP-1α, MIP-1β and TGFβ were unchanged.

		IL-8	IL-6	TNFα	IL-10	IL-1α	IL-12	MCP-1	MCP-3	MIP1α	MIP1β	TGFβ
Controls	Mean	82.4	72.9	82.7	4.3	79.5	24.7	11.4	5.5	13.6	71.6	6.2
	SD	7.6	20.2	7.2	1.5	13.1	9.3	5.7	3.1	11.4	15.9	3.1
Patients	Mean	92.3	65.1	82.1	8.8	73.9	20.1	28.8	18.9	13.9	72.2	5.5
	SD	6.6	21.8	8.2	3.7	16.6	12.3	16.9	16.3	9.1	23.1	2.6
	P =	.039	.731	.612	.042	.714	.542	.006	.010	.875	.788	.468

Current immunosuppression protocols were shown to have limited effect on peripheral blood monocyte inflammatory cytokine production and were inadequate at suppressing monocyte chemokine production in lung transplant patients. This was the first report of increased MCP-3 in lung transplant patients. MCP-3 has been shown to be a mediator in the activation of extracellular matrix gene expression in addition to promoting leucocyte trafficking in systemic sclerosis [37]. Monocytes migrating to the lung may be acting similarly in lung transplant patients. Interestingly, it has been shown that the effects of MCP-3 can be diminished by neutralising antibody to TGFβ [38]. As TGFβ has been reported to play a major role in OB, the possible role of TGFβ – MCP-3 mediated effects clearly warrants further study.

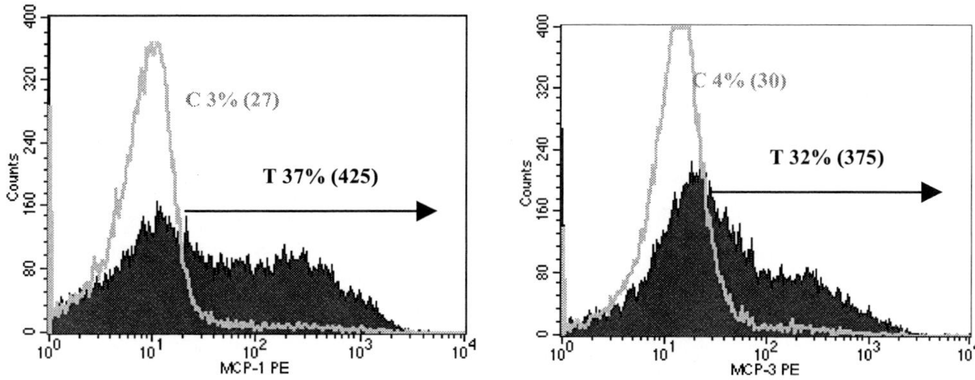

Figure 3. Representative histograms showing intracellular staining of MCP-1 and MCP-3 in peripheral blood monocytes from a transplant patient (T) and control subject (C) following LPS stimulation. The percentage of monocytes producing MCP-1 and MCP-3 was significantly increased in the lung transplant patient compared to control (marker set on negative control-not shown). The amount of MCP-1 and MCP-3 (as indicated by MFI) was also significantly increased in the lung transplant patient compared to control.

MCP-1 levels have been reported to be increased in lung allograft rejection, especially in OB [35]. Alveolar macrophages were identified as the major source of MCP-1. Blood monocytes migrating to the lung are the probable source of these high MCP-1 producers, indicating that these cells are producing MCP-1 before entering the lung. Interestingly MCP-3 has been shown to be a functional ligand for MCP-1 receptor [38]. The increased levels of monocyte MCP-3 identified in transplant patients may enhance the chemoattractant effects of MCP-1, leading to further increases in lymphocyte and monocyte recruitment in the lung.

IL-10 is a regulatory Th2 cytokine that has been shown to prevent acute rejection and OB in the animal models [39]. IL-10 and IL-4 negatively regulate Th1 cytokines IFNγ and IL-2 [23], two cytokines that are increased during acute rejection episodes [2]. MCP-1 has also been shown to upregulate IL-4 [40] and enhance Th2 polarisation [41]. Monocyte production of IL10 and MCP-1 was increased in the present study. There have been previous reports of increased T-cell production of IL-4 in lung transplant patients [11]. Taken together, these findings may explain the previous findings of significantly reduced levels of IFNγ and IL-2 in peripheral blood T cells of lung transplant patients. Increased production of IL-10 may be partially caused by treatment with immunosuppressive drugs as it has previously been shown that monocyte IL-10 production is upregulated in the presence of methylprednisolone [6]. IL-12, a Th1 cytokine that has been shown to be downregulated in the presence of methylprednisolone [6], was unchanged in monocytes from transplant patients compared with control. IL-12 synthesis has been shown to be unaltered in the presence of CsA [42]. As IL-12 is a potent inducer of cell-mediated immunity and IFNγ in T cells [23], drugs that help reduce this important regulatory cytokine may be of benefit for transplant patients. Upregulation of MCP-1 and IL-8 in BAL has recently been shown to be a predictive marker of post-transplant airway obliteration [34] which is consistent with these findings.

As described for T cells, detection of intracellular cytokines in blood monocytes may help to provide a more accurate assessment of immunosuppression than systemic therapeutic drug levels as all patients had drug plasma trough levels within their therapeutic range. The technique is relatively rapid, easy to perform and provides a detailed analysis of cytokine/chemokine levels in specific leucocyte subtypes in individual patients. The relatively large standard deviation for chemokines MCP-1 and MCP-3 in the transplant patients indicate these patients are a heterogeneous group. It would thus be of interest to serially monitor intracellular cytokines/chemokines from transplant patients with a view to detect shifts in cytokine/chemokine profiles that are indicative of transplant rejection status. These studies may reveal that patients with elevated MCP-1 and MCP-3 progress to transplant rejection earlier than patients with "normal" levels. Drugs that modulate these cytokines/chemokines may improve current protocols for reducing graft rejection in these patients.

Effect of Current Immunosuppression Protocols on Intracellular Pro- and Anti-inflammatory Cytokines in Bronchoalveolar Lavage T Cells of Stable Lung Transplant Patients

Analysis of cells and cytokines in bronchoalveolar lavage (BAL) has previously been used as an indicator of transplant rejection in humans [43, 44] and the canine model [45]. While changes in CD4/CD8 in BAL have been associated with acute and chronic rejection [43, 44], surface phenotyping gives little information regarding the activation state, as assessed by cell-specific cytokine production, of an individual cell. It has previously been shown that analysis of inflammatory cytokines in BAL and blood using ELISA may not be as reliable as analysis of intracellular cytokines using flow cytometry [46].

To overcome these problems and to investigate the immunomodulatory effects of currently used immunosuppressive regimens on BAL T-cell cytokine production, whole blood and BAL from a group of stable lung transplant patients and control volunteers was determined [47]. Results showed that there was no difference in T-cell pro-inflammatory cytokines between blood and BAL compartments in stable lung transplant patients (Table 3). In contrast, the control group showed significantly less pro-inflammatory T-cell cytokine production in BAL compared with blood (Table 4). Although there was no difference in T-cell pro-inflammatory cytokine production between blood and BAL compartments in lung transplant patients there was a significant increase in Th1 cytokines by T cells in the BAL compared to the control group (Figure 4).

Table 3. The percentage of T-cells producing intracellular cytokines in blood and BAL of the 9 stable lung transplant patients (mean ± SD). There was a significant increase in the percentage of T cells producing IL-4 and TGFβ in BAL compared to blood (bold).

	CD3		IFNγ		IL-2		IL-4		TGFβ		TNFα	
	CD4	**CD8**	**CD4**	**CD8**	**CD4**	**CD8**	**CD4**	**CD8**	**CD4**	**CD8**	**CD4**	**CD8**
Blood	55±18	44±18	7±5	17±15	6±5	5±4	1±.1	1±1	4.9±2	5±2.5	12±7	14±12
BAL	44±16	55±16	6±5	13±8	4±3	5±4	5±2	9±6	2±2	2.3±1	9±7	14±11
P	.251	.251	.965	.965	.289	.935	.001	.000	.001	.018	.479	.989

Table 4. The percentage of T-cells producing intracellular cytokines in blood and BAL of the Control group (mean ± SD). There was a significant decrease in the percentage of CD4+ and CD8+ T cells producing IFNγ, IL-2, TGFβ and TNFα and a significant increase in the percentage of CD4+ and CD8+ T cells producing IL-4 in BAL compared to blood (bold).

	CD3		IFNγ		IL-2		IL-4		TGFβ		TNFα	
	CD4	**CD8**	**CD4**	**CD8**	**CD4**	**CD8**	**CD4**	**CD8**	**CD4**	**CD8**	**CD4**	**CD8**
Blood	62±7	37±8	19±5	21±8	36±16	8±4	0.4±.3	.5±.3	5±3	3±2	43±11	24±11
BAL	70±15	29±15	2±2	1±.8	1±1	.5±.4	6±6	3±2.6	1±1	.8±.7	8±5	6±6
P	.141	.141	.000	.000	.000	.010	.003	.024	.008	.006	.000	.000

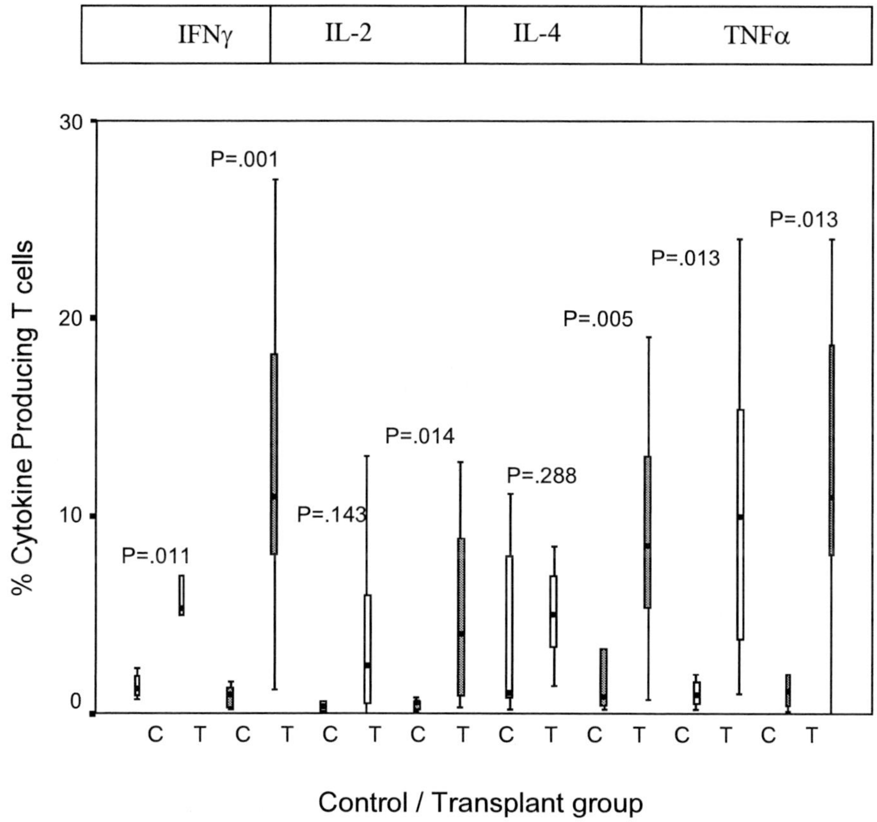

Figure 4. Box plot graphs showing the production of cytokines by BAL CD4+ □and CD8+ ■ T-cells from 9 lung transplant (T) and 10 control (C) subjects following *in vitro* stimulation (mean ± 2SD and range). The percentage of CD8+ T-cells producing IFNγ, IL-2 and IL-4 and the percentage of CD4+ cells producing IFNγ and TNFα was significantly increased in lung transplant patients. The percentage of CD4+ T-cells producing IL2 and IL4 was unchanged in lung transplant patients compared to control.

It has previously been shown that there was a good correlation between the percentage of CD8+ T cells in blood of stable lung transplant patients and IFNγ production by these cells [11]. In contrast, the present study showed that there is a poor correlation between the percentage of CD8+ T cells in BAL and IFNγ production suggesting that previous methods to quantify cytotoxic cells in BAL by immunophenotyping [44, 48] do not give accurate results of functional characteristics of these cytotoxic CD8+ T cells. There was also a significant increase in the anti-inflammatory cytokine, IL-4 in the BAL compared to blood of both the transplant and control group. Representative dot plots showing IL-4 and IFNγ production by BAL CD8+ and CD8- (CD4+) T cells from 2 lung transplant patients and controls are shown in Figure 5.

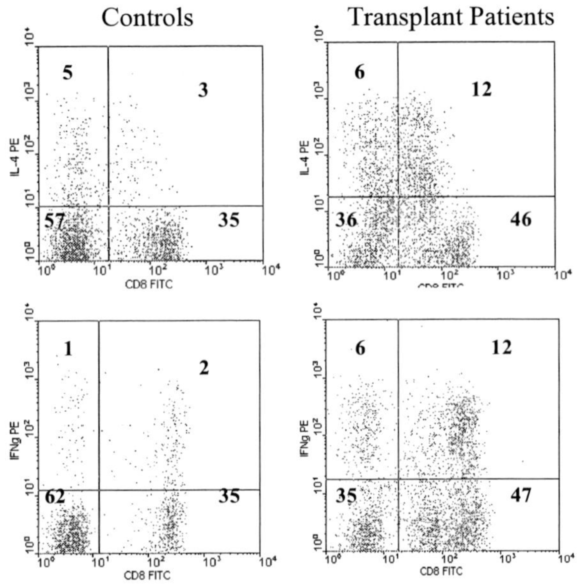

Figure 5. Representative dot plots showing IL-4 and IFNγ production by BAL CD8+ and CD8- (CD4+) T cells from 2 lung transplant patients and controls. T cells were identified by CD3 PC5 versus side scatter characteristics. Transplant patients showed an increase in IL-4 in CD8 dim but not CD8- (CD4+) T cells. Transplant patients showed an increase in IFNγ in both CD4+ and CD8 bright T cells. Note the reduced percentage of CD4+ T cells and increased CD8+ T cells in transplant patients compared to control.

IL-4 is a Th2 cytokine that provides a negative feedback on Th1 cytokine production [23], thus its reduced expression by CD8+ T cells suggests that this regulatory mechanism may be ineffective in stable transplant patients. The Th2 response may be systemic, as the same authors have recently shown increased levels of IL-10, another Th2 cytokine, by monocytes from stable lung transplant patients [36]. The anti-inflammatory cytokine, TGFβ, was also increased in CD8+ T cells in BAL of transplant patients compared with control. TGFβ has previously been shown to inhibit T-cell production of IFNγ and IL-2 [24] suggesting that the function of this regulatory mechanism is also altered in stable transplant patients. The increased sensitivity of CD4+ T cells to TGFβ in reducing Th1 responses compared to CD8+ T cells [25] may help explain the observation of increased inhibition of these cytokines in CD4+ cells compared to CD8+ T cells.

Chronic graft rejection is associated with increased fibrosis in the lung. Both IL-4 [29] and TGFβ [4] have been shown to promote fibroblast proliferation in the lung. Therefore, although TGFβ and IL4 are anti-inflammatory cytokines, their increased production by cytotoxic lymphocytes in the lung may contribute to increased fibrosis (as observed in chronic graft rejection).

This study shows that measurement of blood T-cell cytokine production in lung transplant recipients is reflective of BAL T-cell cytokine production. However, comparison of T-cell cytokine balance between the two compartments may give a more accurate indication of rejection episodes. All transplant patients in this study had plasma levels of CsA or Tac within their therapeutic range, again suggesting that analysis of cytokine production may provide a more accurate assessment of the level of immunosuppression in an individual patient This study also confirms reports that monitoring intracellular T-cell cytokine profiles may be a more appropriate indicator of patient immunosuppression and transplant status than cell phenotypes. Transplant patients were a very heterogeneous group and exhibited a broad range of inflammatory cytokines compared with controls (Figure 1). Effective reduction of T-cell pro-inflammatory cytokines in BAL through targeted use of immunosuppression may improve current protocols for prolonging graft survival in these patients. One such targeted intervention is the use of CsA in aerosolised form. Aerosolised CsA treatment has been used successfully and safely in reducing inflammatory cytokines in refractory acute rejection [49] and this therapy may be of benefit in treating lung transplant patients identified with high percentages of inflammatory cytokine producing T cells whilst minimising systemic side effects of immunosuppressive agents.

Effect of Current Immunosuppression Protocols on Intracellular pro-Inflammatory Cytokines in Bronchial intra-epithelial T Cells of Stable Lung Transplant Patients

Analysis of inflammatory cytokine profiles of intra-epithelial T cells in bronchial brushing (BB) has not previously been performed and may provide additional information to assess immune graft status in lung transplant patients.

Table 5. The percentage of T-cells producing intracellular cytokines in blood and BB of 13 lung transplant patients (mean ± SD). There was a significant decrease in the percentage of CD4+ and a significant increase in the percentage of CD8+ T cells in BB (bold). There was a significant increase in the percentage of CD8+ T cells producing IFNγ, IL-4 and TNFα, a significant decrease in the percentage of CD4+ T cells producing IL-2 and CD4+ and CD8+ T cells producing TGFβ in BB compared to blood.

	CD3		IFNγ		IL-2		IL-4		TGFβ		TNFα	
	CD4	CD8	CD4	CD8	CD4	CD8	CD4	CD8	CD4	CD8	CD4	CD8
Blood	53±11	47±11	13±7	26±15	18±13	4±4	1±.8	.9±.4	3.2±2	3±1.7	18±14	16±12
BB	37±11	63±11	17±7	40±13	8±4	3±1.6	1.2±.6	2.3±.8	2±.9	1.7±1	18±7	30±11
P	.002	.002	.085	.026	.042	.300	.179	.043	.039	.028	.738	.002

A recent study provides the first report of the use of flow cytometry to measure intracellular pro- and anti-inflammatory cytokines in BB-derived intra-epithelial T cells [50]. Results show that although there was a decrease in T-cell pro-inflammatory cytokine production in blood of transplant patients, this was not found in BAL or bronchial intra-epithelial CD8 T-cell subsets, suggesting that the same level of immunosuppression may not occur in the lung of transplant recipients (Table 5 and 6). This study also demonstrated no difference in the percentage of bronchial intra-epithelial CD8 T-cells that produce pro-inflammatory cytokines between stable lung transplant patients and control subjects (Tables 5-8) indicating that current immunosuppression protocols are ineffective at reducing pro-inflammatory T-cell cytokines in the airways of pulmonary allografts.

Table 6. The percentage of T-cells producing intracellular cytokines in BAL and BB of the 13 lung transplant patients (mean ± SD). There was a significant decrease in the percentage of CD4+ and a significant increase in the percentage of CD8+ T cells in BB (bold). There was a significant increase in the percentage of CD4 and CD8+ T cells producing IFNγ and CD8 T cells producing TNFα, and a significant decrease in the percentage of CD4+ and CD8+ T cells producing IL-4 and TGFβ in BB compared to BAL.

	CD3		IFNγ		IL-2		IL-4		TGFβ		TNFα	
	CD4	CD8	CD4	CD8	CD4	CD8	CD4	CD8	CD4	CD8	CD4	CD8
BAL	50±11	50±11	10±9	17±15	5±5	3±3	5±4	5±4	4.6±2	5±2.1	19±10	12±11
BB	37±11	63±11	17±7	40±13	8±4	3±1.6	1.2±1	2.3±2	2±.9	1.7±1	18±7	30±11
P	.006	.006	.029	.001	.100	.210	.002	.025	.035	.028	.657	.002

Table 7.The percentage of T-cells producing intracellular cytokines in blood and BB of 10 control volunteers (mean ± SD). There was a significant decrease in the percentage of CD4+ and a significant increase in the percentage of CD8+ T cells in BB (bold). There was a significant increase in the percentage of CD8+ T cells producing IFNγ and TNFα, a significant decrease in the percentage of CD4+ and CD8+ T cells producing IL-2 in BB compared to blood.

	CD3		IFNγ		IL-2		IL-4		TGFβ		TNFα	
	CD4	CD8	CD4	CD8	CD4	CD8	CD4	CD8	CD4	CD8	CD4	CD8
Blood	69±4.4	31±6.9	18±7.8	20±5	40±17	6±4	.8±.4	.5±.3	4±2	3±2	43±12	20±6
BB	36±19	64±19	15±6	45±17	10±8	3±.2	.5±.3	.9±.7	3±1	1±.3	20±6	37±17
P	.003	.003	.065	.019	.001	.038	.560	.189	.185	.064	.017	.025

Table 8. The percentage of T-cells producing intracellular cytokines in BAL and BB of 10 control volunteers (mean ± SD). There was a significant decrease in the percentage of CD4+ and a significant increase in the percentage of CD8+ T cells in BB (bold). There was a significant increase in the percentage of CD4+ and CD8+ T cells producing IFNγ and IL-2 and CD8+ T cells producing TNFα in BB. There was a significant decrease in the percentage of CD4+ and CD8+ T cells producing IL-4 in BB compared to BAL.

	CD3		IFNγ		IL-2		IL-4		TGFβ		TNFα	
	CD4	CD8	CD4	CD8	CD4	CD8	CD4	CD8	CD4	CD8	CD4	CD8
BAL	71±11	29±11	4±2.7	6±5	3±.8	.8±.7	8.5±2.4	5±2	2±2	.5±.5	14±8	7.5±6
BB	36±19	64±19	15±6	45±17	10±8	3±.2	.5±.3	.9±.7	3±1	1±.3	20±6	37±17
P	.002	.003	.041	.000	.028	.042	.001	.002	.198	.358	.530	.000

Transplant patients showed a CD4:CD8 inversion in BAL and BB consistent with a previous report [51] in contrast to control subjects who showed a CD4:CD8 inversion only in the BB compartment. The relative increase in CD8 T cells in BB may be due to an increase in proliferation of these cytotoxic cells and/or an increase in migration of these cells via specific Th1 chemokine receptors [52]. The percentage of CD8+ T cells producing IFNγ and TNFα in BB was increased compared with blood and BAL.

Representative dot plots showing IFNγ production by CD8+ and CD8- (CD4+) T cells from blood, BAL and BB in a lung transplant patient are shown in Figure 6.

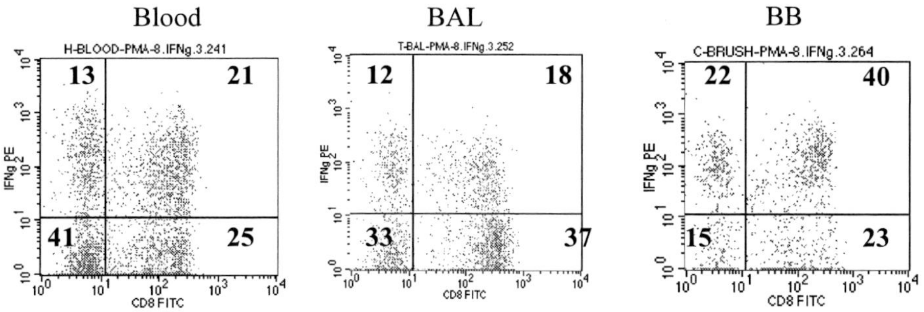

Figure 6. Representative dot plots showing IFNγ production by CD8+ and CD8- (CD4+) T cells from blood, BAL and BB in a lung transplant patient. T cells were identified by CD3 PC5 versus side scatter characteristics. Transplant patients showed an increase in the percentage of CD8+ T cells producing IFNγ in BB compared with blood. Transplant patients showed an increase in IFNγ in both CD4+ and CD8 T cells in BB compared with BAL. Note the decrease in CD4+ and increase in CD8+ T cells in BB compared with blood and BAL.

As IL-4 and TGFβ are negative regulators of Th1 inflammatory cytokines [23, 24], the findings of decreased IL-4 and TGFβ in some bronchial intra-epithelial T-cell subsets compared with blood and BAL may help explain these latter findings. Conversely, chronic rejection or OB is associated with an increase in TGF-β production [4], indicating that current immunosuppression protocols may be effective in reducing OB in lung transplant patients via this pathway.

Others have suggested that studies of intragraft immune cells may be more relevant in terms of effecting graft injury than analysis of peripheral circulating cells [53]. All transplant patients in this study had plasma levels of CsA or Tac within their therapeutic range. Our findings therefore suggest that analysis of T-cell cytokine production may provide a more accurate assessment of immunosuppression in the various compartments than systemic drug levels and show that these patients are inadequately immunosuppressed especially in the lung compartment.

A longitudinal surveillance of cell phenotypes in individuals has been suggested to identify a preclinical state of rejection [48]. Monitoring intracellular T-cell cytokine profiles may be a more appropriate indicator of patient immunosuppression and transplant status than cell phenotypes. This study demonstrates that there is compartmentalisation of pro-and anti-inflammatory CD8+ T-cell cytokine production in BB compared with blood and BAL. Drugs that effectively reduce bronchial intra-epithelial CD8+ T-cell pro-inflammatory cytokines may improve current protocols for prolonging graft survival in these patients.

Airway Infection is Associated with Increased Immunosuppression of Intracellular Th1 Cytokines in Bronchoalveolar Lavage CD8+ T Cells Compared with Stable Lung Transplant Patients

Current immunosuppression protocols to reduce lung transplant rejection include drugs to reduce pro-inflammatory Thl cytokines. However, Thl cytokine production is important in host defense against microbial infection in the lungs, particularly *Aspergillus* and *Pseudomonas spp.*, organisms shown to be leading causes of mortality in immunocompromised patients [54, 55] Excessive immunosuppression of these cytokines may leave patients susceptible to infection.

Intracellular Thl/Th2 cytokines in BAL and blood T cells from clinically stable lung transplant patients in whom potentially pathogenic organisms were isolated from BAL were compared with a culture-negative group. The predisposing pathology, cultured organism and plasma drug levels in these patients is shown in Table 9.

Table 9. Predisposing pathology and organisms isolated from "culture positive" transplant patient group

Patient	Predisposing pathology	Cultured organism	CsA / Tac levels
1	Bronchiecstasis	*Asp. Pseud.*	Tac 14.5
2	Congenital bronchial webbs	*Pseud.*	Tac 11.4
3	Cystic fibrosis	MRSA. *Pseud*	Tac 9
4	Pulmonary hypertension	*Asp. Pseud.*	CsA 276
5	Cystic Fibrosis	*Asp. Pseud.*	CsA 258
6	Emphysema	*Pseud.*	CsA 300
7	Emphysema	*Pseud.*	CsA 260
8	Emphysema	*Pseud.*	Tac 6
9	Pulmonary fibrosis	*Asp.*	CsA 349
10	Pulmonary hypertension	*E. coli*	CsA 152
11	Cystic fibrosis	*Asp.*	CsA 205
12	Emphysema	*Asp.* MRSA	CsA 235
13	Agammaglobulinaemia	*Pseud.*	CsA 185

Therapeutic range for CsA (80-250 µg/L) and Tac (5-20 µg/L).
Asp. (*Aspergillus spp.*), *Pseud.* (*Pseudomonas spp.*), MRSA (Methicillin resistant *Staphylococcus aureus*), *E. coli* (*Escherichia coli*).

Thl cytokines were significantly higher in BAL from stable, non-infected transplant recipients compared with culture-positive patients. All transplant patients in this study had plasma levels of CsA or Tac within therapeutic range (Table 9). There was no change in T cell cytokines in the blood of infected and non-infected patients (Table 10). Importantly, the majority of patients with the greatest degree of immunosuppression, as judged by intracellular Thl cytokine production in BAL, were infected with pathogenic microorganisms (Table 11).

Table 10. The percentage of T-cells producing intracellular cytokines in blood of the 13 BAL culture-negative (N) and 13 culture-positive (P) lung transplant groups (mean ± SD). There were no significant differences in intracellular cytokine production by T-cell subsets between either patient group.

	IFNγ			IL-2			IL-4			TNFα		
	CD4	CD8	CD3	CD4	CD8	CD3	CD4	CD8	CD3	CD4	CD8	CD3
N	10±6	24±17	34±12	14±12	6±5	20±9	1.4±.1	.9±.6	2±4	20±15	15±10	35±12
P	9±6	16±11	25±8	15±14	2.4±2	17±8	.9±.7	1.4±.1	2±4	15±10	18±16	33±12
P	.965	.265	.348	.935	.284	.728	.765	.785	.820	.690	.560	.889

Table 11. The percentage of T-cells producing intracellular cytokines in BAL of the 13 BAL culture-negative (N) and 13 culture-positive (P) lung transplant groups (mean ± SD). There was a significant decrease in the percentage of CD3+ T cells producing IL-2 and CD8+ T cells producing TNFα in BAL of the culture-negative compared to the culture-positive transplant group (bold).

	IFNγ			IL-2			IL-4			TNFα		
	CD4	CD8	CD3	CD4	CD8	CD3	CD4	CD8	CD3	CD4	CD8	CD3
N	9±6	22±12	31±9	5±4	5±4	10±4	6±4	11±4	17±4	12±9	15±11	27±9
P	7±6	11±8	18±8	2±2	1.7±1.1	3.7±2	6±2	6±5	12±4	12±8	8±6	20±8
P	.765	.165	.248	.218	.104	.031	.898	.157	.657	.890	.038	.200

These organisms have been shown to be the leading cause of mortality in immunocompromised patients [54, 55]. In the mouse model, lung challenge with *P. aeruginosa* resulted in significantly less severe lung pathology, bacterial loads and mortality in mice that responded with a Th1-like response [56]. Transient over-expression of IFNγ within the lungs augmented host immunity against *Aspergillus* [54]. Hence excessive suppression of Th1 cytokines may leave patients susceptible to infection. Although levels of BAL Th1 cytokines differed between patient groups, there was no difference in Th1 cytokines in blood, suggesting that reduced BAL Th1 cytokines were only associated with localised lung infection and not systemic disease.

The data shows that a cut-off value of greater than 8% CD3+ T cells producing IL-2 or 20% CD8+ T cells producing TNFα is associated with culture negative results and hence would be protective of infection in the lungs of these patients. Potent immunosuppressive drugs such as Tac and CsA cause significant toxic side effects [32]. Reducing levels of these drugs in culture-positive patients that have low Th1 cytokines would also have benefits associated with reduced organ toxicity. However, a reduction of immunosuppression due to infection must be balanced with appropriate immunosuppression of proinflammatory Th1 cytokines that have been reportedly increased in the lungs of patients undergoing graft rejection [1-3]. The degree to which transplant recipients are immunosuppressed influences their risk of infection and rejection [58]. The restoration of Th1 responses has been shown to be an important predictor of fungal infection outcome in stem cell transplantation patients [59]. Monitoring the balance of intracellular Th1 cytokines between levels associated with infection and rejection may improve morbidity in our patient group.

In conclusion, this study demonstrates that lung infection is associated with decreased intracellular Th1 cytokines in BAL T cell subsets of stable lung transplant patients. Modifying immunosuppression by monitoring intracellular Th1 cytokines in BAL T cells may improve morbidity and infection rates in this patient group.

Longitudinal Monitoring of Immunosuppression in Transplant Patients by Measurement of Intracellular T Cell Cytokines

Analysis of intracellular T cell cytokines in blood from lung transplant patients and controls showed a broad range of cells producing individual cytokines (Figure 1). To determine longitudinal changes in intracellular cytokines/chemokines in patients and controls, whole blood from several stable, non-infected lung transplant patients and control volunteers was stimulated *in vitro* and intracellular T cell cytokine production determined on several occasions over a three year period. Samples from transplant patients were collected following routine surveillance assessment and histology of bronchial biopsies showed no evidence of acute or chronic rejection. All BAL samples were negative for bacteria, fungi and viruses.

The percentage of T cell subsets producing intracellular cytokines from blood of 5 healthy control (C) volunteers on 3-8 occasions (N) (mean ± SD) are shown in Table 12. The SD of cytokines from individual subjects was significantly less compared with the overall SD of cytokines from 14 control subjects (*overall mean ± SD*), suggesting that intracellular T cell cytokines are relatively stable over time from healthy individual subjects.

The percentage of T cell subsets producing intracellular cytokines from blood of 4 stable non-infected transplant patients (P) on 3-4 occasions (mean ± SD) are shown in Table 13. The SD of cytokines from individual patients was significantly less compared with the overall SD of cytokines from 12 transplant patients (*12P*) (*overall mean ± SD*), suggesting that intracellular T cell cytokines from individual stable transplant patients are relatively stable over time.

Table 12. The percentage of T cell subsets producing intracellular cytokines from blood of 5 healthy control (C) volunteers on 3-8 occasions (N) (mean ± SD). The SD of cytokines from individual subjects was significantly less compared with the overall SD of cytokines from 14 control subjects (*overall mean ± SD*), suggesting that intracellular T cell cytokines are relatively stable over time from healthy individual subjects.

		CD3		IFNγ		IL-2		IL-4		TGFβ		TNFα	
	N	CD4	CD8	CD4	CD8	CD4	CD8	CD4	CD8	CD4	CD8	CD4	CD8
C1	8	61±2	39±2	17±2	25±2	38±3	6±1	.6±.1	.4±.1	4±.8	3±1.1	44±4	26±2
C2	4	64±3	36±2	19±2	20±2	36±3	10±1	.4±.1	.6±.1	6±1.9	2±1.2	42±4	22±3
C3	3	58±2	42±2	23±3	15±2	28±2	8±1	.3±.1	.5±.1	3±.1.1	2±1.0	36±2	24±2
C4	5	60±3	40±2	22±2	22±3	25±2	9±2	.5±.1	.3±.1	7±.1.2	4±1.4	38±3	18±2
C5	3	56±2	34±2	18±2	24±2	37±3	5±2	.4±.1	.4±.1	4±.1.4	5±1.5	50±4	29±2
14C		*62±7*	*37±8*	*19±5*	*21±8*	*36±16*	*8±4*	*0.4±.3*	*.5±.3*	*5±3*	*3±2*	*43±11*	*24±11*

Table 13. The percentage of T cell subsets producing intracellular cytokines from blood of 4 stable non-infected transplant patients (P) on 3-4 occasions (mean ± SD). The SD of cytokines from individual patients was significantly less compared with the overall SD of cytokines from 12 transplant patients (*12P*) (*overall mean ± SD*), suggesting that intracellular T cell cytokines from individual stable transplant patients are relatively stable over time.

		CD3		IFNγ		IL-2		IL-4		TGFβ		TNFα	
	N	CD4	CD8	CD4	CD8	CD4	CD8	CD4	CD8	CD4	CD8	CD4	CD8
P1	4	36±4	64±4	12±3	25±8	8±4	6±2	.6±.2	.9±.2	5±.1.5	6±1.2	9±5	9±6
P2	3	53±2	47±2	10±4	23±11	9±5	5±2	.8±.3	.6±.3	6±2.1	5±1.3	11±6	15±7
P3	3	64±3	36±3	9±1	17±5	6±3	3±1	.5±.3	.8±.1	4±.1.2	7±1.8	15±4	14±5
P4	3	48±2	42±2	7±2	16±6	25±2	7±2	.5±.1	.7±.3	7±.1.9	4±1.1	12±5	18±4
12P		*55±18*	*44±18*	*7±5*	*17±15*	*6±5*	*5±4*	*1±1*	*1±1*	*4.9±2*	*5±2.5*	*12±7*	*14±12*

Analysis of intracellular T cell cytokines in BAL and BB from lung transplant patients and controls also showed a broad range of cells producing individual cytokines (Table 3 and 4). Intracellular cytokine analyses were performed on one stable, non-infected transplant patient on three occasions and again during one occasion when the patient was undergoing acute rejection as determined by bronchial biopsy histology (A2B0). Results of the intracellular T cell cytokines from blood, BAL and BB from this patient are shown in Table 14, Figure 7 and 8 respectively.

Table 14. T cell subsets and the percentage of intracellular blood T cell cytokines from a stable transplant patient (S) on three occasions (mean ± SD) and on one occasion during an episode of acute rejection (AR). There was no significant change in CD4+ or CD8+ T cell subsets or cytokine production during the acute rejection episode.

	CD3		IFNγ		IL-2		IL-4		TNFα	
	CD4	CD8	CD4	CD8	CD4	CD8	CD4	CD8	CD4	CD8
S	53±2	47±2	12±4	23±8	9±4	3±1	.8±.3	1.1±.2	11±6	15±8
AR	60	40	10	15	2	2	.6	.9	2	2

The results from this study show that during an episode of acute rejection, there was a change in T cell subsets and intracellular cytokines in the blood of patients. There were significant increases in pro-inflammatory Th1 cytokines in BAL T cells and IL-2 production by T cells in BB. These results suggest that immunosuppression therapy may be effective in the blood compartment but not in the lungs during an episode of rejection. These data suggest that analysis of intracellular cytokines in the lung compartment, particularly in BAL T cells may be an effective, relatively non-invasive technique in the diagnosis of acute rejection episodes in lung transplant patients. Although caution must be taken when interpreting results from one patient, it will be of great interest to follow the results of these longitudinal studies on a larger cohort of lung transplant patients.

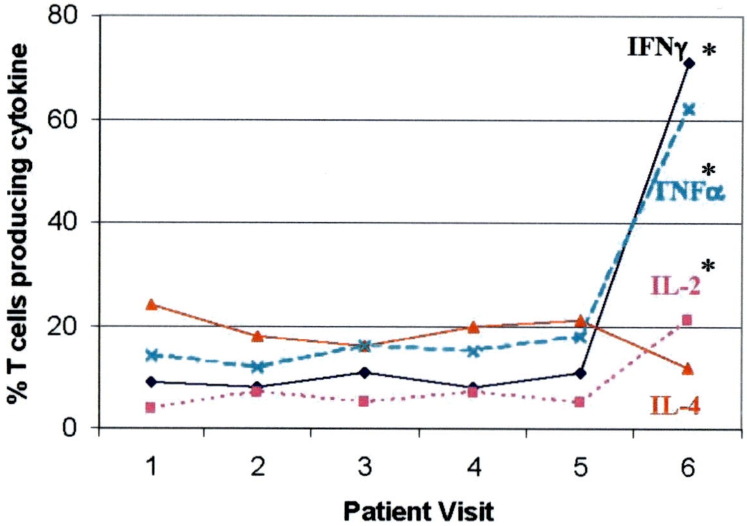

Figure 7. T cell subsets and the percentage of intracellular BAL T cell cytokines from a stable transplant patient (S) on five occasions and on one occasion during an episode of acute rejection (AR). There was a significant increase in IFNγ, IL-2 and TNFα by T cells during the acute rejection episode* (patient visit 6) but no change in IL-4 production.

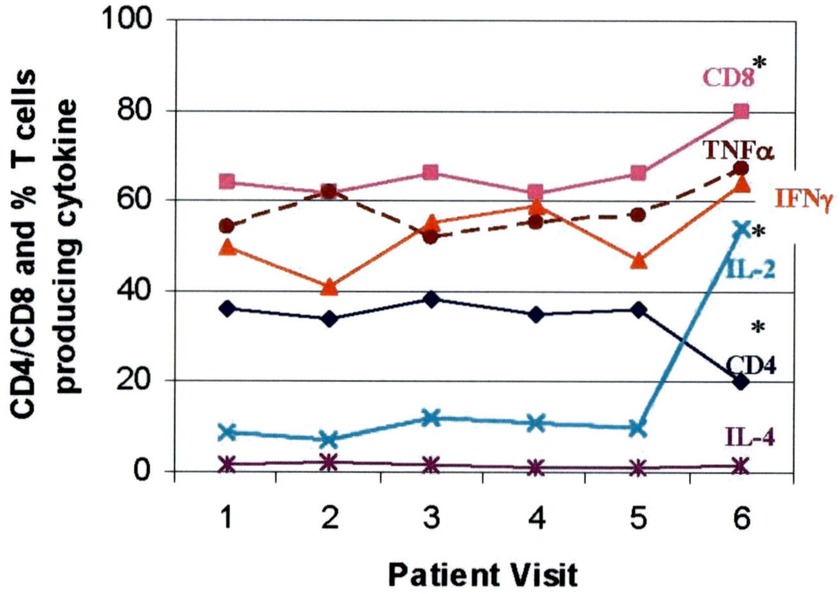

Figure 8. T cell subsets and the percentage of intracellular BB T cell cytokines from a stable transplant patient (S) on five occasions and on one occasion during an episode of acute rejection (AR). There was a significant decrease in CD4, increase in CD8 and a significant increase in IL-2 by T cells during the acute rejection episode* (patient visit 6).

Analysis of Intracellular Cytokines to Improve Therapeutic Immunosuppression Monitoring Following Lung Transplantation Now and in the Future

Assessment of immune effector cell activation state by measurement of cell-specific cytokine production across multiple immune cell subsets within the blood may provide physiological evidence of systemic levels of immunosuppression that may be more relevant than traditional therapeutic drug monitoring. Although direct examination of biopsy tissue still provides the "gold-standard" measure of allograft rejection, it is likely that analysis of intracellular cytokine expression within (assessed using bronchial brushing) or immediately adjacent to the graft (BAL) will also be of diagnostic and prognostic value. In future the clinical utility of flow cytometric evaluation of the pulmonary allograft may even extend beyond assessment of immune effector cell activation state and cell-specific cytokine production. In preliminary studies we have been able to assess protein expression by allograft epithelial cells obtained from bronchial brushings [60]. This technique may provide early information regarding impending airway fibrosis and obliteration associated with BOS. It may even be possible to adapt this technique to better assess the poorly defined entity of pulmonary allograft humoral rejection by looking for the footprint of complement activation – C4d staining [61].

Conclusion

Longitudinal monitoring of immune effector cell activation state in BAL, bronchial brushing and blood in individual patients by measuring cell-specific cytokine production may provide an early warning of impending rejection or infection. Maintaining immune effector intracellular cytokines within stable (non-infection, non-rejection) levels by regulating doses of immunosuppressant drugs may lead to reduced drug toxicity without compromising allograft function. Additionally, a considerable morbidity advantage and cost savings may be found in reduced drug costs and reduced costs associated with treatment of infection due to unnecessary immunosuppression. Although individualized monitoring of immunosuppression using intracellular cytokines as opposed to therapeutic drug monitoring is very promising, further research is required before it is likely to become of proven diagnostic utility in clinical lung transplantation.

References

[1] Boehler A and Estenne M. Post-transplant bronchiolitis obliterans. *Eur Respir Mon,* 2003, 26, 158-178.

[2] Sundaresan S, Alevy YG, Steward N, Tucker J, Trulock EP, Cooper JD, Patterson GA, Mohanakumar T. Cytokine gene transcripts for tumor necrosis factor-alpha, interleukin-2, and interferon-gamma in human pulmonary allografts. *J Heart Lung Transplant.* 1995 14(3):512-8.

[3] Neuringer IP, Walsh SP, Mannon RB, Gabriel S, Aris RM. Enhanced T cell cytokine gene expression in mouse airway obliterative bronchiolitis. *Transplantation*. 2000 69(3):399-405.

[4] El-Gamel A, Sim E, Hasleton P, Hutchinson J, Yonan N, Egan J, Campbell C,Rahman A, Sheldon S,Deiraniya A, Hutchinson RV. Transforming growth factor beta (TGF-beta) and obliterative bronchiolitis following pulmonary transplantation. *J Heart Lung Transplant*. 1999 18(9):828-37.

[5] Duncan MD, Wilkes SD. Transplant-related immunosuppression. *Proc Am Thor Soc*. 2005 2:449-455.

[6] Hodge S, Hodge G, Flower R, Han P. Methyl prednisolone upregulates monocyte IL-10 production in stimulated whole blood. *Scand J Immunol* 1999 49:548-553.

[7] Haberal M, Emiroglou R, Dalgic A, Karakayli H, Moray G, Bilgin N. The impact of cyclosporin on the development of immunosuppressive therapy. *Tranplant Proc* 2004 36:143S-147S.

[8] Levy GA. C2 monitoring strategy for optimising cyclosporin immunosuppression from the Neoral formulation. *BioDrugs* 2001 15:279-290.

[9] Norman D, Turka L. Pimer on transplantation, 2nd ed. Mt. Laurel, NJ: American Society of Transplantation 2001.

[10] Baan CC, Balk AH, van Riemsdijk IC, Vantrimpont PJ, Maat AP, Niesters HG, Zondervan PE, van Gelder T, Weimar W. Anti-CD25 monoclonal antibody therapy affects the death signals of graft-infiltrating cells after clinical heart transplantation. *Transplantation* 2003 75:1704-1710.

[11] Hodge G, Hodge S, Reynolds P, Holmes M. Intracellular cytokines in blood T cells in lung transplant patients- a more relevant indicator of immunosuppression than drug levels. *Clin and Exp Immunol*. 2005 139, 159-164.

[12] Jordan SC, Kondo T, Prehn J, Marchevsky A, Waters P. Cytokine gene activation in rat lung allografts: analysis by Northern blotting. *Transplant Proc*. 1991 23:604-606.

[13] Rondeau E, Cerrina J, Delarue F et al. Tumor necrosis alpha (TNF-alpha) production by cells of bronchiolar lavage (BAL) and peripheral blood mononuclear cells (PBMC) in cardiopulmonary transplant patients. *Transplant Proc*. 1990 22:1855-1856.

[14] Sundaresan S, Alevy YG, Steward N, Tucker J, Trulock EP, Cooper jd, Patterson GA, Mohanakumar T. Cytokine gene transcripts for tumor necrosis factor-alpha, interleukin-2, and interferon-gamma in human pulmonary allografts. *J Heart Lung Transplant*. 1995 14(3):512-8.

[15] Hodge G, Hodge S, Haslam R, McPhee A, Sepulveda H, Morgan E, Nicholson I, Zola H. Rapid detection of neonatal sepsis by simultaneous measurement of multiple cytokines using 100μL sample volumes. *Clin and Exp Immunol*. 2004 137: 402-407.

[16] Hodge G, Osborn M, Hodge S, Nairn J, Tapp H, Kirby M, Sepulveda H, Morgan E, Zola H, Revesz T. Rapid simultaneous measurement of multiple cytokines in childhood oncology patients with febrile neutropenia: increased IL-8 or IL-5 correlates with culture-positive infection. *Brit J Haem*. 2005 132, 247-248.

[17] Corti A, Poiesci C, Merli S, Cassani G. Tumour necrosis factor (TNF) alpha quantification by ELISA and bioassay: effects of TNF alpha-soluble TNF receptor (p55) complex dissociation during assay incubations. *J Immunol Methods* 1994 177:191-198.

[18] Muirhead KA, Wallace PK, Schmidt TC, Frescatore RL, Franco JA, Horan PK: Methodological considerations for implementation of lymphocyte subset analysis in a clinical reference laboratory. *Ann NY Acad Sci* 1986 468:113-127.

[19] Hodge G, Hodge S, Han P. Increased levels of apoptosis of leucocyte subsets in PBMCs compared to whole blood as shown by Annexin V binding- relevance to cytokine production. *Cytokine* 2000 12, 1763-1768.

[20] Han and G. Hodge (1999) Intracellular cytokine production and cytokine receptor interaction of cord mononuclear cells: relevance to cord blood transplantation. British *Journal of Haematology* 107, 450-457.

[21] Hodge G, Hodge S, Han, P. Allium sativum (Garlic) suppresses leucocyte inflammatory cytokine production in vitro: potential therapeutic use in the treatment of inflammatory bowel disease. *Cytometry* 2002 48, 209-215.

[22] Lehman C, Wilkening A, Lieber N, Markus R, Krug N, Pabst R, Tschernig T. Lymphocytes in the bronchiolar space reenter the lung tissue by means of the alveolar epithelium, migrate to regional lymph nodes, and subsequently rejoin the systemic immune system. *Anat Rec* 2001 264:229-236.

[23] Romagnani S. The Th1 / Th2 paradigm. *Immunology Today* 1997; 18: 263-6.

[24] Kehrl JH Transforming growth factor-β: An important mediator of immunoregulation. *Int J Cell Clon* 1991 9:438-50.

[25] Chan SY, Goodman RE, Szmuszkovicz JR, Roessler B, Eichwald EJ, Bishop DK. DNA-liposome versus adenoviral mediated gene transfer of TGF beta1 in vascularised cardiac allografts: differential sensitivity of CD4+ and CD8+ T cells to TGF beta1. *Transplantation* 2000 70:1292-301.

[26] Berthou C, Legros-Maida S, Soulie A, Wargnier A, Guillet J, Lafaurie C, Stern M, Sasportes M, Israel-Biet D. Expansion of peripheral blood perforin+ CD8+ T-cell subset in long term survival lung transplant patients. *Transplant Proc* 1996; 28(3):1964-7.

[27] Lee HM and Rich S. Differential activation of $CD8^+$ T-cells by transforming-β. *J Immunol* 1993; 151:668-677.

[28] Widmer MB and Grabstein KH. Regulation of cytolytic T-lymphocyte generation by B-cell stimulatory factor. *Nature* 1987; 326:795-98.

[29] Sempowski M, Sakiyama S, Tanida N, Fukumoto T, Monden Y, Uyama T. Interleukin-4 and interferon-gamma discordantly regulate collagen biosynthesis by functionally distinct lung fibroblast subsets. *J Cell Physiol* 1996; 167(2):290-6.

[30] El-Gamel A, Awad M, Sim E, Hasleton P, Yonan N, Egan J *et al.* Transforming growth factor beta (TGF-beta) and obliterative bronchiolitis following pulmonary transplantation. *Eur J Cardiothorac Surg* 1998; 13(4):424-30.

[31] Kuypers DR, Claes K, Evenpoel P, Maes B, Vanrenterghem Y. Clinical efficacy and toxicity profile of tacrolimus and mycophenolic acid in relation to combined long-term phermacokinetics in de novo renal allograft recipients. *Clin Pharmacol Ther* 2004, 75:434-47.

[32] Shapiro R. Low toxicity immunosuppressive protocols in renal transplantation. Keio *J Med.* 2004; 53:18-22.

[33] Taub DD, Proost P, Murphy WJ, et al. Monocoyte chemotactic protein-1 (MCP-1), -2, and –3 are chemotactic for human T lymphocytes. *J Clin Invet.* 1995; 95: 1370.

[34] Reynaud-Gaubert M, Marvin V, Thirion X, et al. Upregulation of chemokines in bronchiolar lavage fluid as a predictor of post-transplant airway obliteration. *J Heart Lung Transplant*. 2002; 21: 721.

[35] Belperio JA, Keane MP, Burdick MD, et al. Critical role for the chemokine MCP-1/CCR2 in the pathogenesis of bronchiolitis obliterans syndrome. *J Clin Invet*. 2001; 108: 547.

[36] Hodge G, Hodge S, Reynolds P, Holmes M. Upregulation of IL-8, IL-10, MCP-1 and MCP-3 in peripheral blood monocytes in stable lung transplant patients- are immunosuppression regimes working? *Transplantation* 2004 79:387-391.

[37] Ong VH, Evans LA, Shiwen X, et al. Monocyte chemoattractant protein 3 as a mediator of fibrosis: Overexpression in systemic sclerosis and the type 1 tight-skin mouse. *Arthritis Rheum*. 2003; 48:1979.

[38] Franci C, Wong LM, van Damme J, Proost P, Charo F. Monocyte chemotactic protein-3, but not monocyte chemotactic protein-2 is a functional ligand of the monocyte chemoattractant protein-1 receptor. *J Immunol*. 1995; 154: 6511.

[39] Boehler A. The role of interleukin-10 in lung transplantation. *Transpl Immunol*. 2002; 9: 121.

[40] Gonnella PA, Kondali D, Weiner HL. Induction of low dose tolerance in monocyte chemotactic protein-1 and CCR2 deficient mice. J Immunol. 2003; 170: 2316.

[41] Rose CE, Sund SS, Fu SM. Significant involvement of CCL2 (MCP-1) in inflammatory dissorders of the lung. *Microcirculation*. 2003; 10: 273.

[42] Tsiavou A, Degiannis D, Hatzigelaki E, Raptis S. Flow cytometric detection of intracellular IL-12 release: in vitro effect of widely used immunosuppressants. *Int Pharmacol*. 2002; 12: 1713.

[43] Slebos DJ, Schloma J, Boezen HM, Koeter GH, van der Bij W, Postma DS, Kauffman HF. Longitudinal profile of bronchoalveolar lavage cell characteristics in patients with good outcome after lung transplantation. *Am J Crit Care Med*. 2002 165(4):501-7.

[44] Reynard-Gaubert M, Thomas P, Gregoire R, Badier M, Cau P, Sampol J, Giudicelli R, Fuentes P. Clinical utility of bronchoalveolar lavage cell phenotype analyses in the postoperative monitoring of lung transplant recipients. *Eur J Cardiothorac Surg*. 2002 21:60-66.

[45] Chang S, Hsu H, Perng R, Shiao G, Lin C. Significance of biochemical markers in early detection of canine allograft rejection. *Transplantation* 1991 51:579-584.

[46] Tayebi H, Lienard A, Billot M, Tiberghien P, Herve P, Robinet E. Detection of intracellular cytokines in citrated whole blood or marrow samples by flow cytometry. *J Immunol Methods* 1999 229:121-30.

[47] Hodge G, Hodge S, Reynolds P, Holmes M. Increased intracellular pro- and anti-inflammatory cytokines in bronchoalveolar lavage T cells of stable lung transplant patients. *Transplantation* 2005 80:1040-1045.

[48] Slebos DJ, Schloma J, Boezen HM, Koeter GH, van der Bij W, Postma DS, Kauffman HF. Longitudinal profile of bronchoalveolar lavage cell characteristics in patients with good outcome after lung transplantation. *Am J Crit Care Med*. 2002 165(4):501-7.

[49] Keenan RJ, Zeevi A, Iacono AT, Spichty KJ, Cai JZ, Yousem SA, Ohori NP, Paradis IL, Kawai A, Griffith BP. Efficacy of inhaled cyclosporin in lung transplant recipients with refactory rejection: correlation of intragraft cytokine gene expression with pulmonary function and histologic characteristics. *Surgery* 1995 118(2):385-91.

[50] Hodge G, Hodge S, Reynolds P, Holmes M. Compartmentalisation of intracellular proinflammatory cytokines in bronchial intraepithelial T cells of stable lung transplant patients. *Clin and Exp Immunol* 2006 145:413-419.

[51] Erle DJ, Brown T, Christian D, Aris R. Lung epithelial lining fluid T cell substes defined by distinct patterns of beta 7 and beta 1 integrin expression. *Am J Respir Cell Mol Biol* 1994; 10: 237-44.

[52] Neuringer IP, Chalermskulrat W, Aris R. Obliterative bronchiolitis or chronic lung allograft rejection: a basic science review. *J Heart Lung Transplant* 2005; 24:3-19.

[53] Corris PA and Kirby JA. A role for cytokine measurement in therapeatic monitoring of immunosuppressive drugs following lung transplantation. *Cin Exp Imunnol* 2004; 139:176-178.

[54] Shao C, Qu J, He L et al. Transient expression of γ interferon promotes *Aspergillus* clearance in invasive pulmonary aspergillosis. *Clin Exp Immunol.* 2005; 142: 233.

[55] Zuercher AW, Imboden MA, Jampen S et al. Cellular immunity in healthy volunteers treated with an octavalent conjugate *Pseudomonas aeruginosa* vaccine. *Clin Exp Immunol.* 2005; 142: 381.

[56] Moser C, Johansen HK, Song Z et al. Chronic *Pseudomonas aeruginosa* lung infection is more severe in Th2 responding BALB/c mice compared to Th1 responding C3H/HeN mice. *APMIS* 1997; 105: 838.

[57] Ritchie AJ, Jansson A, Stallberg J, Nilsson P, Lysaght P, Cooley MA. The *Pseudomonas aeruginosa* quorum-swensing molecule N-3-(oxododecanoyl)-L-homoserine lactone inhibits T-cell differentiation and cytokine production by a mechanism involving an early step in T-cell activation. *Infect Immun.* 2005; 73(3):1648.

[58] Blazik M, Hutchinson P, Jose MD, et al. Leucocyte phenotype and function predicts infection risk in renal transplant recipients. *Nephrol Dial Transplant* 2005; 20(10): 2226.

[59] Safdar A, Rodriguez G, Ohmagari N, et al. The safety of interferon-gamma-1b therapy for invasive fungal infections after haemopoietic stem cell transplantation. *Cancer* 2005; 103(4): 731.

[60] Chambers DC, Holmes M, Banerjee B, et al. Epithelial to mesenchymal transition (EMT) as an indicator of airway remodeling in lung transplantation. *Am J Resp Crit Care Med*; 2008;177: A306.

[61] Magro CM, Ross P, Kelsey M, et al. Association of humoral immunity and bronchiolitis obliterans syndrome. *Am J Transplant*; 2003; 9: 1155.

In: Immunosuppression: New Research
Editor: Charles B. Taylor, pp. 115-130

ISBN: 978-1-60692-102-9

Chapter 4

Indications and Management of m-TOR Inhibitors after Liver Transplantation

Itxarone Bilbao[1,], Gonzalo Sapisochin[1], Cristina Dopazo[1], Jose Luis Lazaro[1], Leonor Pou[2], Luis Castells[3], Mireia Caralt[1], Amaia Gantxegi[1] and Ramon Charco[1]*

[1]Liver Transplantation Unit "Carlos Margarit" of the Department of General Surgery;
[2]Department of Biochemistry;
[3]Hepatology Unit of the Department of Internal Medicine; Hospital Vall Hebrón, Universidad Autónoma Barcelona, Spain
*Centro de Investigación Biomédica en Red de Enfermedades Hepáticas y Digestivas (CIBEREHD or Ciberehd) (Centre for Biomedical Research at the Hepatic and Digestive Diseases Network) Hepato-Pancreato-Biliary and Liver Transplant Service. Hospital Vall d'Hebron. Barcelona. Spain

Abstract

AIM: To assess our experience with the use and management of m-TORi after liver transplantation .
MATERIAL: From 1988 to 2007, 783 LT were performed in 725 patients. Fifty one patients (7%) received immunosuppression with m-TORi: Rapamicine 36 and Everolimus 15. Mean age was 54.8 years (r: 24-70). Indication of use, time between LT and introduction of m-TORi, efficacy, side effects and survival were analyzed.
RESULTS: Indications were: refractory rejection in the context of renal insufficiency 20 (39%), renal insufficiency 5 (10%), other CNI side effects 6 (12%), extended HCC in the explanted liver 7 (14%), HCC recurrence during follow-up 7 (14%) and de novo tumor 3 (6%). Mean time between LT and m-TORi was 18 ± 29 months with a median of 3 months (r: 10 days-122 months). Mean follow-up after conversion was 14 ± 15 months (r: 0.1-72). In

* E-mail address: ibilbao@vhebron.net. Tel: 93 2746113. Fax: 93 2746112. Address for correspondence: Itxarone Bilbao, Liver Transplant Unit, Hospital Vall d'Hebron, Paseo Vall d'Hebron, nº 119-129, 08025 – Barcelona

general, half of the patients resolved the event for which the drug was indicated. Refractory rejection was succesfully resolved in half the patients, three required re-LT and six progressed to chronic liver dysfunction with the result of five deaths due to non-resolved rejection and comorbidity. The renal insufficiency at time of conversion resolved in 11 (52%) of the 21 cases. Six out of 7 patients with recurrent HCC died at a mean follow-up of 11.5 months. Three out of 7 patients with extended HCC died at a mean follow-up of 8.2 months. The three cases of de novo tumor were coverted to m-TORi four weeks after surgery and are perfectly healthy. Half of the patients presented m-TORi-related side effects: dyslipemia in 24 (47%), infection in 9 (17.6%); diarrhea in 3 (6%), and hematologic complications in 3 (6%). Six patients (11.7%) developed acute rejection after conversion. Seventeen patients (33.3%) discontinued the drug: 6 due to inefficacy; 5 due to inter-current surgery; 3 due to resolution of the cause; and 3 due to adverse events. Patient actuarial survival was 54%, 46% and 23% at 1, 3 and 5 years post-conversion.

CONCLUSION: m-TORi are indicated in critical and irreversible situations where other immunosuppressants have failed. During the early stage, they are used for refractory rejection or as prophylaxis for recurrence of extended tumors. At any time, but specially in the late period, they are indicated in patients with serious CNI side effects, HCC recurrence, and de novo tumors.

Key Words: m-TORi, liver transplantation, indications, outcome.

Introduction

Sirolimus and Everolimus are immunosuppressive agents that inhibit the mammalian target of rapamycin (m-TOR), a proliferation signal. Both drugs inhibit growth-stimulated cell proliferation, through the formation of a complex with FK506–binding protein 12 (FKBP12). This complex blocks the phosphorylation of p70S6 kinase and subsequent protein synthesis and arrest the cell cycle in the late G1 phase (1,2). In addition, mTOR inhibitors (m-TORi) reduce the expression of vascular endothelial growth factor and the transforming growth factor-B, associated with tumor angiogenesis (3). The m-TOR signaling is activated in many tumor types, so it is an ideal target for anticancer agents. M-TORi have been used together with calcineurine inhibitors (CNI) as immunosuppression after liver transplantation (LT). Recently, m-TORi have also been used as an antiproliferative agent in oncology due to their antiangiogenic properties. Maintenance immunosuppression with m-TORi seems to reduce the incidence of de novo malignancies after solid organ transplantation (4). Furthermore, conversion to m-TORi after the development of de novo neoplasms has resulted in longer tumor-free survival (5).

Both Sirolimus and Everolimus have a similar chemical structure and mechanism of action, but differ in their pharmacokinetic properties. The elimination half-life of Everolimus is 24-35 hours as opposed to 60 hours with Sirolimus. It is administered twice a day, as opposed to Sirolimus once a day, and steady state is reached in 2-3 days versus 5-6 days for Sirolimus.

Although CNI are the first line immunosuppressants most commonly used in organ transplantation, we all know the adverse effects produced by their chronic intake. When the adverse events become serious, alternative regimens avoiding CNI are desperately sought. The m-TORi meet this need, because they help preserve renal function and do not cause hypertension or diabetes mellitus. However, among the most common adverse events of m-TORi are leukopenia, hypercholesterolemia and hyperlipidemia.

First reports about Sirolimus are dated around 1997 (6). The drug was intended to be used in combination with CNI or as a basic primary immunosuppressive therapy in de novo liver transplanted patients. However, the side effects, such as delayed wound healing, hepatic arterial thrombosis and dyslipemia, ticked this drug with a warning and limited its use as a drug of second choice after LT (7,8). Everolimus was introduced in clinical LT two years ago (9), but few personal experiences have been reported with this drug (10). The only clinical trial done with Everolimus combined with cyclosporine, had a high rate of withdrawal (11), so solid conclusions were impossible to stablish. Although nearly 10 years have passed since the introduction of m-TORi in LT, they still lack a definitive role.

Objectives

The objective of this retrospective study was to evaluate our experience and results with the use of m-TORi after LT, and to help define their role in clinical practice.

Material and Methods

Since October 1988 up to October 2007, 783 LT have been performed in 725 patients in our Unit. Fifty one (7%) received immunosuppression with m-TORi: Sirolimus 36 and Everolimus 15. Databases and medical records of this study group were reviewed, paying special attention to demographic characteristics of patients with m-TORi, causes of conversion, type of immunosuppression pre- and post-conversion, mean time between LT and introduction of m-TORi, management of doses and trough levels, efficacy, side effects, and mean follow-up post-conversion.

Demographic Characteristics

Mean age of study group at time of transplant was 54.8 ± 12 years (r: 24-70), with 11 patients (21.6%) over 65 years of age. Sex distribution was 38 male (74.5%) and 13 female (25.5%) patients. Main indications for LT were: postnecrotic cirrhosis in 20 (40%), hepatocellular carcinoma (HCC) and cirrhosis in 25 (50%), cholostatic cirrhosis in 4 (8%), and acute liver failure in 1 (2%). Half of the patients (26) were hepatitis C virus positive (HCV +), 5 patients (10%) hepatitis B virus positive (HBV +) and 3 patients (6%) were HCV and HIV coinfected patients. Concerning UNOS status, the majority of patients awaited transplant at home (86%), 11 % were hospitalized at time of transplant, and 2% were in ICU awaiting the graft. Concerning Child-Pugh classification, 15 patients (30%) were Child C, 19 patients (37%) were Child B, and 17 patients (33%) were Child A. Concerning concomitant diseases: 10 patients (20%) had a body mass index (BMI) > 30, 7 patients (14%) had arterial hypertension, 13 patients (25%) had diabetes mellitus, 5 patients (10%) had some kind of cardiopathy, 9 patients (17%) had serum creatinine > 1.5 mg/dl at time of transplant and 12 patients (23%) had undergone previous surgery of right superior abdominal quadrant, or hepatectomy or porto-systemic shunt. Data about donors and surgery are described in Table 1.

Table 1. Characteristics of recipients, donors, surgery and post-transplant evolution

CHARACTERISTIC		CONVERSION to m-TORi (n=51)
Recipient		
	Mean age	54.8 ± 12 r (24-70)
	Patients over 65 y	11 (21.6%)
	Male / female (%)	38 (74.5%) / 13 (25.5%)
	Diagnosis	
	Postnecrotic cirrhosis	21 (41%)
	HCC with cirrhosis	25 (49%)
	Cholostatic cirrhosis	4 (8%)
	Acute liver failure	1 (2%)
	HCV - HVB	26 (51%) – 5 (10%)
	ETOH	16 (31%)
	HIV	3 (6%)
	Child-Pugh A/B/C (%)	33 – 37 – 30
	UNOS(home/Hosp/ICU (%)	86 – 12 - 2
	Pre-LT associated disease	
	Renal insufficiency	9 (18%)
	Diabetes Mellitus	13 (25%)
	Arterial Hypertension	7 (14%)
	Cardiopathy	5 (10%)
	Previous surgery	12 (23%)
Donor	Mean age (years)	48±18
	Age > 70 years	6 (12%)
	Male / Female (%)	34 (67%) / 17 (33%)
	Graft steatosis > 20%	7 (14%)
Surgery	E-E / E-E+Kehr / C-J (%)	76% - 6% - 18%
	Previous portal thrombosis	8 (16%)
	Mean RBC units	4 ± 4
	Cold ischemia time (min)	420 ± 80
Time (Event to conversion)		2.7 ± 8 months (r: 0.1-54)
Mean time (LT- conversion)		18 ± 29 months (r: 0.1-122)
Median time		3 months
Patient survival (%)	1y-3y-5y	54% - 46% - 23%
Follow-up post-conversion	Mean follow-up	12 ± 14 months (r: 0.1-72)
	Median follow-up	7 months

Notes to Table 1:

HCC: hepatocellular carcinoma; HCV: hepatitis C virus; HBV: hepatitis B virus; ETOH: cirrhosis due to alcohol; HIV: human immunodeficiency virus; UNOS: United Network for Organ Sharing classification; ICU: Intensive Care Unit; LT: Liver transplantation; E-E: end to end choledoco-choledocostomy; E-E+K: end to end choledoco-choledocostomy + kehr; C-J: choledoco-jejunostomy; RBC: red blood cells; min: Minutes; r: range.

Data Analysis

The SPSS software program was used throughout. Student's t-test or the Mann-Whitney U-test was used for quantitative data. Pearson's chi-square or Fisher's exact test was used for categorical data. Data are shown as the mean ± standard deviation, or as percentages. The Kaplan-Meier method was used for survival analysis.

Results

Conversion to m-TORi over time was performed in 51 patients (7% of the series): 36 patients were converted to Sirolimus and 15 patients to Everolimus.

Sirolimus was the first m-TORi to be used in the late nineties. It was proposed as a primary immunosuppressant as a substitution of the CNI inhibitor. In our centre, the maximum application of the drug was between 2001 and 2004 (20 cases). Afterwards, the drug was used sporadically. Everolimus was introduced into clinical use more recently, at the end of 2005. Both drugs have been used in all types of transplant patients irrespective of age, sex, indication, severity of hepatopathy or concomitant diseases (Table 1).

Table 2. Causes of conversion in the group converted to Sirolimus and to Everolimus

	Sirolimus N= 36	Everolimus N=15	Total N=51
Mean time (LT to conversion) months	**16 ± 27**	**24 ± 33**	**18 ± 29**
Median time (LT to conversion) months	2.3 (r : 0.1-108)	6.5 (r: 1.5-122)	3 (r: 0.1-122)
< 12 months / > 12 months	64% - 36%	60% - 40%	63% - 37%
Indication of conversion			
CRI	5 (14%)	-	5 (9.8%)
Refractory rejection + CRI	9 (25%)	-	9 (17.6%)
Rejection	10 (28%)	1 (7%)	11 (21.6%)
CNI Adverse events	4 (11%)	2 (13%)	6 (11.7%)
Other causes	1 (3%)	2 (13%)	3 (5.9%)
Extended HCC	3 (9%)	4 (27%)	7 (13.7%)
HCC recurrence	4 (11%)	3 (20%)	7 (13.7%)
De novo tumor	-	3 (20%)	3 (5.9%)
Mean time (Event to conversion) months	**2.9 ± 9.3** (r: 0.01-54)	**2.2 ± 1.9** (r: 0.01-7)	**2.9± 8.2** (r: 0.01-54)
Follow-up post-conversion (months)	**12 ± 16**	**12 ± 7**	**14 ± 15**
Median follow-up (months)	6.5 (r: 0.1-72)	7 (r: 1.5-25)	10 (r: 0.1-72)

Notes to Table 2: LT: Liver transplantation; CRI: Chronic renal insufficiency; CNI: Calcineurine inhibitors; HCC: Hepatocellular carcinoma; r: range.

Causes of conversion in the Sirolimus group were: refractory rejection in 10 patients (28%); chronic renal insufficiency in 14 patients (39%), 9 of whom (25%) also suffered refractory rejection; neurotoxicity attributed to CNI in 4 (11%); extended HCC in explanted liver in 3 (9%); recurrence of HCC in 4 (11%); and liver dysfunction with chronic renal insufficiency in the immediate postoperative period of a retransplanted patients in 1 (3%). Causes of conversion in the Everolimus group: extended HCC in explanted liver in 4 (27%); recurrence of HCC in 3 (20%); de novo tumor in 3 (20%); neurotoxicity due to CNI in 2

(13%); refractory rejection in 1 (7%); and other causes such as sinusoidal fibrosis in 1 (7%) and graft versus host disease in 1 (7%) (Table 2).

Concerning the clinical status of patients before conversion, and taking into account that not all of them were the cause for conversion, the following complications and comorbidity were found in the Sirolimus and Everolimus groups respectively: liver dysfunction compatible with acute rejection in 19 (53%) and 1 (7%) patient; renal insufficiency in 18 (50%) and 3 (20%) patients; arterial hypertension in 12 (33%) and 4 (27%) patients; diabetes mellitus in 7 (19%) and 4 (27%) patients and dyslipemia in 5 (14%) and 3 (20%) patients.

Pre-conversion therapy in the Sirolimus group was: Tacrolimus monotherapy in 19, Tacrolimus plus MMF in 14, and MMF monotherapy in 3. Post-conversion therapy was Tacrolimus plus Sirolimus in 33 and Sirolimus monotherapy in 3. Pre-conversion therapy in the Everolimus group was: Tacrolimus monotherapy in 7, Tacrolimus plus MMF in 7, and Neoral Cyclosporine in 1. Post-conversion therapy was Tacrolimus plus Everolimus in 10; Neoral Cyclosporine plus Everolimus in 1; and Everolimus monotherapy in 4.

The mean time between LT and conversion for Sirolimus group, was 16 ± 27 months (r: 0.1-108), with a median of 2.3 months, and for Everolimus group, was 24 ± 33 months (r: 1.5-122), with a median of 6.5 months. In both groups, two thirds of patients were converted before the first year post-transplant and one third after the first year post-transplant. The mean time between the event onset and conversion to m-TORi was 2.9 ± 9.3 months (r: 0.01-54) for Sirolimus and 2.2 ± 1.9 months (r: 0.01-7) for Everolimus (Table 2).

Efficacy

The m-TORi were used to treat refractory rejection in 20 patients (19 with Sirolimus and 1 with Everolimus). Ten patients out of 19 in the Sirolimus group, and the one in Everolimus group, resolved the event properly. The clinical course in the remaining 9 were as followed: progression of liver dysfunction requiring retransplantation in 3 (two for chronic rejection and one for refractory rejection) ; progression of liver dysfunction resulting in death in 4 (severe refractory acute rejection in 1 and chronic rejection in 3) ; progression of concomitant chronic renal insufficiency to dialysis in 1, requiring reintroduction of Tacrolimus as renal function was definitely lost ; development of severe rhabdomyolysis, ventricular fibrillation and death in 1, attributed to the concomitant intake of Sirolimus and Simvastatin due to dyslipemia. (Table 3). None of them were considered for retransplantation due to non-compliance in one, coinfection of HCV and HIV with aggressive recurrence of HCV in another, aged over 75 in two cases and comorbidity with sepsis in two.

The m-TORi were used in 14 patients with chronic renal insufficiency, only in the Sirolimus group. The six patients with early conversion (mean time from LT to conversion of 3.1 months) resolved renal dysfunction. The remaining cases (mean time from transplant to conversion of 25.3 months) were unable to improve the event, with 1 patient progressing to dialysis (Table 3). If we focus in the 7 patients suffering renal insufficiency as a comorbidity, but converted for other reasons, only 2 on Sirolimus and 2 on Everolimus, experienced improvement in renal parameters.

When m-TORi were indicated for neurotoxicity (Table 3), they were totally effective in stabilizing or reversing this side effect. The types of adverse events were : 2 cerebrovascular stroke, 1 paresthesia, 1 generalized tremor, 1 tremor plus syncope and 1 Guillen-Barré Syndrome.

Table 3. Efficacy and resolution of the cause of conversion

	Sirolimus N= 36	Everolimus N=15	Total N=51
Rejection	19	1	20
Resolution	10 (52.6%)	1 (100%)	11 (55%)
Chronic renal insufficiency	14	-	14
Resolution	6 (42.8%)	-	6 (42.8%)
Neurotoxicity	4	2	6
Resolution or stabilization	4 (100%)	2 (100%)	6 (100%)
Arterial hypertension	12	4	16
Resolution or Amelioration	6 (50%)	2 (50%)	8 (50%)
Diabetes Mellitus	7	4	11
Amelioration	4 (57%)	2 (50%)	6 (54.5%)
Hepatotoxicity	-	1	1
Resolution		1(100%)	1 (100%)
HCC recurrence	4	3	7
Stabilization	0	1 (33.3%)	1 (14.3%)
Extended Hepatocellular carcinoma	3	4	7
Recurrence prevention	1 (33.3%)	3 (75%)	4 (57%)
De novo tumor	-	3	3
Recurrence prevention post-surgery		3 (100%)	3 (100%)
Follow-up post-conversion (months)	12 ± 16	12 ± 7	14 (r: 0.1-72)
Median follow-up (months)	6.5 (r: 0.1-72)	7 (r: 1.5-25)	

Notes to Table 3: r: range.

Although m-TORi were never indicated for arterial hypertension and diabetes mellitus, 16 patients had high blood pressure at time of conversion and 11 suffered insulin dependent diabetes mellitus (Table 3). Blood pressure improved in 8 patients and glucose values improved in 6 patients. Dyslipemia was present in 5 patients in the Sirolimus group (14%) and 3 patients in the Everolimus group (20%). Dyslipemia worsened in 3 patients after the introduction of Sirolimus, remaining unchanged in all the rest.

Concerning malignancies (Table 3), the four patients in whom Sirolimus was indicated for hepatocellular recurrence during follow-up, progressed to death at a mean time of 8.25 months (3-12 months). Type of recurrences were: costal and pulmonary two years after LT in the first, pulmonary 4 years post-LT in the second, costal two years post-LT in the third, and ganglionar 1 year post-LT in the last one. All of them except one were outside the Milan criteria, with multifocality and vascular invasion in the explanted liver. In the Everolimus group, three patients were converted due to HCC recurrence, progressing to death the two who were outside the Milan criteria, at a mean time post-conversion of 18 months (14-22). Type of recurrences were : intra-abdominal 122 months post-transplant in the first; pulmonary 6 months post-transplant in the second; and bone metastasis 42 months post-transplant in the third. Another indication of m-TORi was prevention in cases of extended neoplasm outside the Milan criteria, in the pathological specimen. Three patients in the Sirolimus group were converted for this reason, but two finally relapsed at a mean time of 11.5 months (r: 5-18). Four patients in the Everolimus group were converted for the same reason, but one relapsed and progressed to death 1.5 months postconversion. Three patients in the Everolimus group were converted due to "de novo" tumor appearing between 3-4 years post-transplant: squamous carcinoma of the esophagus in the first; colon carcinoma in the second; and lung carcinoma in the third. All three patients underwent surgery and oncological treatment. As soon as the patients recovered from surgery, Everolimus was introduced. The one with lung carcinoma presented recurrence 12 months post-conversion, but the other two are disease free two years post-conversion.

One patient was converted to Everolimus due to liver dysfunction with cholostasis starting at the 7th month post-transplant and progressing to severe cholostasis three months later (Table 3). Two liver biopsies at the 8th and 10th month post-transplant revealed sinusoidal fibrosis and undetermined hepatitis. After conversion, liver function was completely restored within 1 month. Another indication was a patient who presented graft versus host disease 1 month post-transplant. Immunosuppression was changed from Tacrolimus to low dosed Everolimus to reduce any associated hypersensitivity to Tacrolimus and to counterbalance the steroid bolus administered. This patient was maintained on Everolimus monotherapy at 2-3 ng/ml and did well for two months, but finally died from sepsis due to bone marrow aplasia as progression of the graft versus host disease.

Liver Graft Function after Conversion

Table 4. Adverse events, causes of discontinuation and mortality.

	Sirolimus N= 36	Everolimus N=15	Total N=51
ADVERSE EVENTS	**22 (61%)**	**4 (26.6%)**	**26 (50.9%)**
Dyslipemia	20 (55.5%)	4 (26.6%)	24 (47%)
Diarrhea	3 (8.3%)	-	3 (5.9%)
Hematological disorders	3 (8.3%)	-	3 (5.9%)
ACUTE REJECTIONS post-conversion	**6 (16.7%)**	-	**6 (11.7%)**
INFECTIONS	**8 (22.2%)**	**1 (6.7%)**	**9 (17.6%)**
CAUSES OF DISCONTINUATION	**16 (44.4%)**	**1 (6.7%)**	**17 (33.3%)**
Intercurrent surgery	5 (13.9%)	-	5 (9.8%)
Resolution of conversion cause	3 (8.3%)	-	3 (5.9%)
Retransplantation	3 (8.3%)	-	3 (5.9%)
MOF and death	2 (5.5%)	1 (6.7%)	3 (5.9%)
Non-responding rejection	2 (5.5%)	-	2 (3.9%)
CRI progressing to dialysis	1 (2.9%)	-	1 (1.9%)
CAUSES OF MORTALITY	**19 (52.8%)**	**4 (26.7%)**	**23 (45%)**
HCC recurrence	6 (16.7%)	3 (20%)	9 (17.6%)
HCV recurrence	4 (11.1%)	-	4 (7.8%)
Non-responding rejection	3 (8.3%)	-	3 (5.9%)
Pulmonary infections	2 (5.5%)	-	2 (3.9%)
MOF and sepsis	1 (2.8%)	1 (6.7%)	2 (3.9%)
Biliary complications	1 (2.8%)	-	1 (1.9%)
Gastrointestinal hemorrhage	1 (2.8%)	-	1 (1.9%)
Rhabdomyolysis	1 (2.8%)	-	1 (1.9%)
Follow-up post-conversion (months)	**12 ± 16**	**12 ± 7**	**14 (r: 0.1-72)**
Median follow-up (months)	6.5 (r: 0.1-72)	7 (r: 1.5-25)	

Notes to Table 4: MOF: Multi-organ failure; CRI: Chronic renal insufficiency; HCC: Hepatocellular carcinoma; HCV: Hepatitis C virus; r: range.

Six patients (17%) presented acute rejection after conversion to Sirolimus (Table 4). Two were so severe, that the aggressive immunosuppression ended in fatal pneumonia and aspergillosis respectively, resulting in death. Two cases were resolved with steroid bolus and reintroducing Tacrolimus in triple therapy and two cases reintroducing Tacrolimus and stopping Sirolimus once the rejection was overcome.

Side Effects and Discontinuation

Side effects related to the use of m-TORi appeared in 22 patients (61%) in the Sirolimus group and 4 patients (26.6%) in the Everolimus group (Table 4). Diarrhea appeared in 3 patients, hematological disorders in 3 patients, and dyslipemia in 24 patients. Diarrhea and hematological disorders were managed by decreasing doses and levels. Dyslipemia was managed with the introduction of hypolipemic drugs. Nine patients (17.6%) developed infections after conversion: 5 pulmonary infections (two of them clearly related to the introduction of the drug); 1 herpes zoster; 1 disseminated varicella; 1 intestinal CMV and 1 patient presenting severe infections in the context of graft versus host disease. Microorganism involved in pulmonary infections were: TBC in 2, bacterial pneumonia in 2 and pneumocystis carinii in 1.

A total of 16 patients on Sirolimus (44%) and 1 patient on Everolimus (6.7%) discontinued treatment (Table 3). Causes of discontinuation in the Sirolimus group were: retransplantation in 3, stopping the drug the day of retransplantation; multiorgan failure with death in 2, stopping the drug some days before exitus; progression to dialysis in 1, stopping the drug to prevent other adverse events; post-conversion acute rejection in 2, requiring the reintroduction of Tacrolimus and stopping of Sirolimus once the rejection was over ; intercurrent surgery in 5, requiring discontinuation of the drug in order to avoid healing problems; and resolution of the reason for conversion in 3. In the Everolimus group, 1 patient stopped the drug in the context of graft versus host, due to sepsis progressing to death.

Pharmacokinetics

Conversion to m-TORi was managed differently according to the cause of conversion. In cases of refractory rejection, Sirolimus was administered at an initial dose of 5 mg/day followed by corresponding doses to obtain levels between 5-10 ng/ml, and Everolimus at an initial dose of 0.5 mg every twelve hours, adjusting the subsequent doses to obtain trough levels around 5 g/ml. At the same time, the CNI was maintained at high doses. When the reason for conversion was CNI-related adverse events, Sirolimus was started at an initial dose of 3 mg a day and Everolimus at 0.5 mg once or twice a day. At the same time, the CNI was decreased to half the dose or completely stopped, depending on the severity of the adverse events. When m-TORi were introduced due to malignancies (extended neoplasm in the explant, cancer recurrence in the follow-up, or de novo tumor), Sirolimus was introduced at doses of 2-3 mg/day and Everolimus at doses of 0.5 mg/day, adjusting trough levels to < 5 ng/ml and < 3 ng/ml, respectively. At the same time, the CNI was drastically decreased to half levels or completely withdrawn.

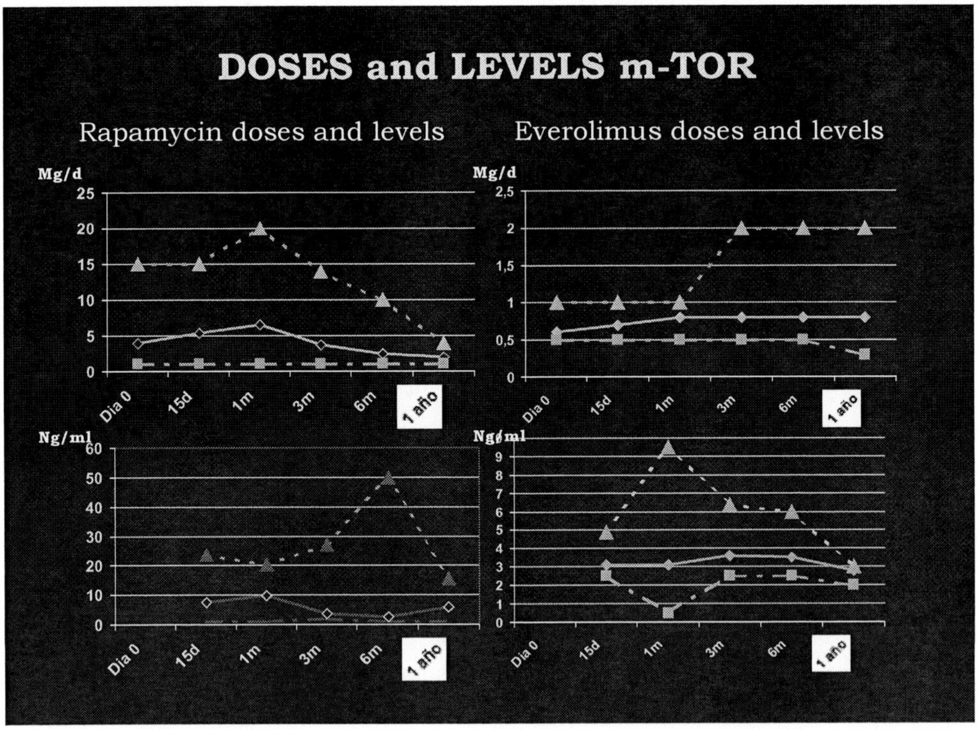

Figure 1. Doses and levels of m-TORi: Sirolimus and Everolimus.

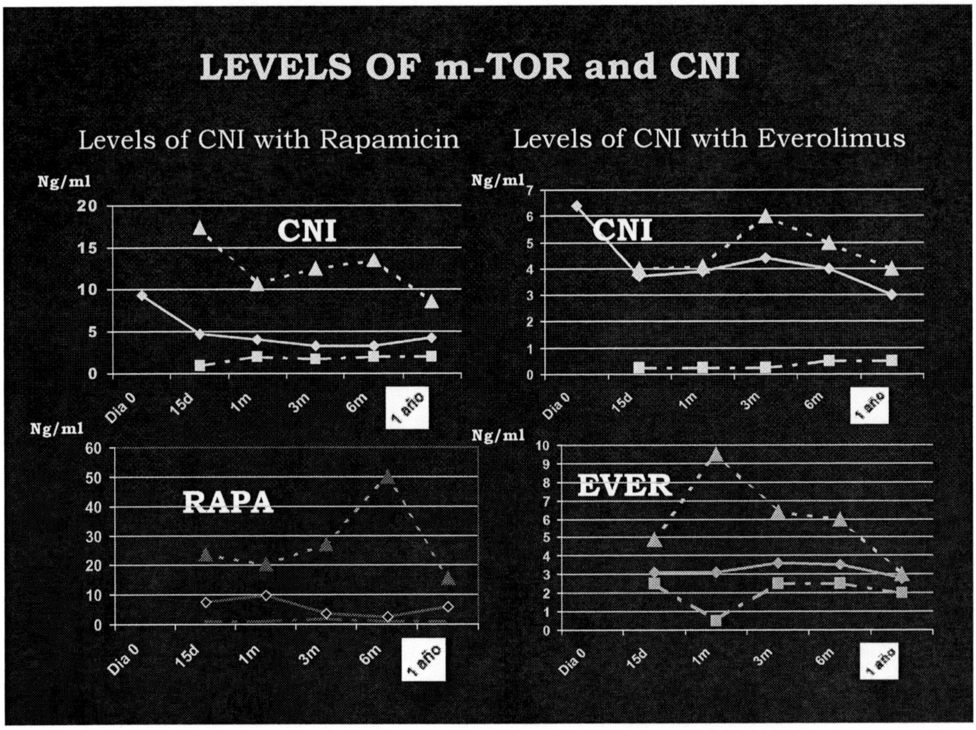

Figure 2. Levels of CNI after introduction of m-TORi.

In the follow-up after conversion, trough levels of m-TORi and CNI were regularly monitored at 15 days, 1 month, 3 months, 6 months, 9 months and 1 year post-conversion. Doses were adjusted according to trough levels, tolerability and side effects. In general, we can see that mean trough levels were in the higher recommended range for Sirolimus group, but in the lower recommended range for Everolimus group. (Figure 1 and 2).

Patient Survival and Follow-Up

All patients were followed up until death or stopping the drug. Mean follow-up in the Sirolimus group was 12 ± 16 months (r: 0.1-72 months), with a median of 6 months. Mean follow-up in the Everolimus group was 12 ± 7 months (r: 1.5-25 months), with a median of 7 months. Actuarial patient survival at 1-3-5 years after conversion was 54 %, 46 % and 23 % (Table 5). Twenty three patients were lost to follow-up (45%): 19 patients in the Sirolimus and 4 patients in the Everolimus group. Causes of death are shown in Table 4: 9 patients (18%) due to progression of HCC recurrence; 4 patients (8%) due to progression of HCV recurrence; 2 patients (4%) due to pneumonia; 2 patients (4%) due to other infections; 1 patient (2%) due to rhabdomyolysis secondary to the co-administration of Sirolimus and Simvastatin; 1 patient (2%) due to chronic biliary complications; and 1 patient (2%) from gastrointestinal hemorrhage.

Table 5. Actuarial survival table of post-conversion patients

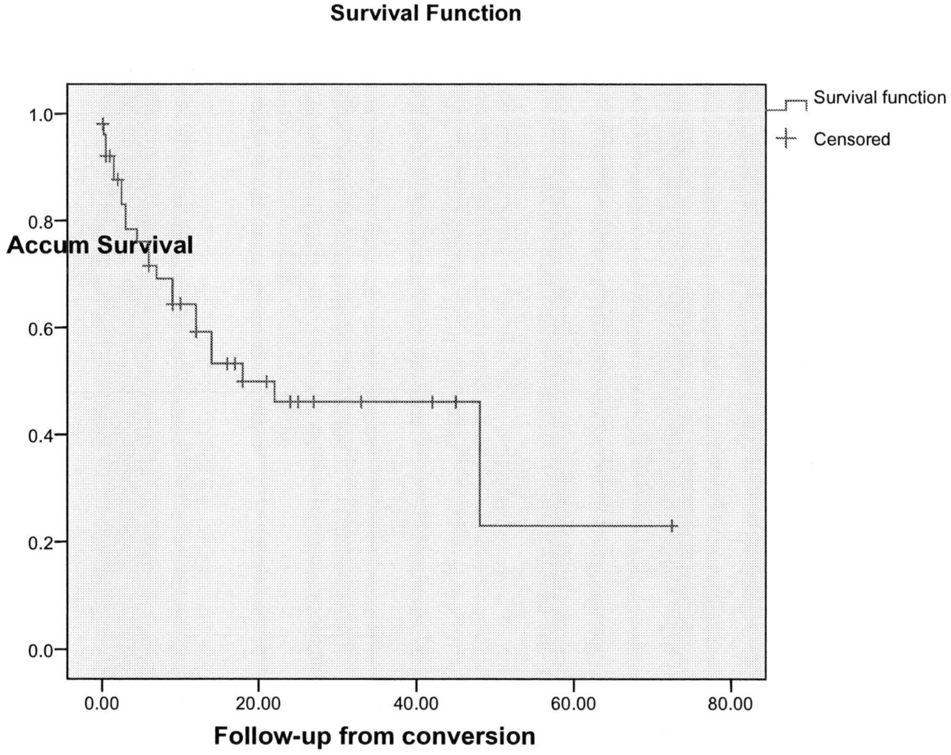

Discussion

The principal aim of this review was to study the use of m-TORi in our Unit and to help redefine the true role of these drugs in clinical practice. We present the data on Sirolimus and Everolimus separately, but we do not seek to compare the two drugs as these have been used differently, both in terms of indication and timing of use. Furthermore, with the use of Sirolimus, we learnt how to optimize the use of Everolimus, so any comparison between the two drugs would lead to totally inaccurate conclusions. This is a retrospective observational study which aims to analyze the pros and cons of the use of these drugs. The first m-TORi to be licensed as an immunosuppressant was Sirolimus. It was designed to be used as a primary immunosuppressant, to replace the widespread use of CNI. However, the first clinical trials with the drug did not take into account various common errors on launching an immunosuppressor. When a new immunosuppressant is brought out, it is first tested in kidney transplant patients and various distinctive aspects between liver and kidney transplants must be taken into account. Firstly, the liver acts as a large filter or sponge that eliminates antigens. It is therefore the least immunoreactive organ against foreign antigens. Furthermore, the liver conferes a certain level of protection to other organs when combined transplants are performed. Secondly, when the transplanted organ is the organ responsible for metabolizing the drug, starting doses should be finely adjusted to the patient's real condition, particularly in patients presenting primary graft dysfunction. This does not occur with other solid organs. Thirdly, the previous fact is further complicated with drugs with long half-lives. Excess doses take a long time to return to correct levels, while insufficient doses, due to lack of absorption, take a long time to reach the recommended steady state. All of this may lead to severe adverse effects due to over-immunosuppression or rejection due to under-immunosuppression, with early and high withdrawal rates in the clinical trials. Fourthly, the patient suffering from liver disease has a low health status as well as severe leukopenia and thrombocytopenia which complicates the use of immunosuppressor drugs with similar side effects. Fifthly, the principal end point in clinical trials with immunosuppressor drugs is often the rejection rate. This fixation in attaining a low rejection rates means that other aspects that are gaining greater importance in the long term survival of transplant patients, such as adverse effects and quality of life, are often forgotten. Sixthly, when a drug requires blood level monitoring, the procedure should be aplicable and reproductable in the majority of centers. This was not the case with Sirolimus, where only some central laboratories were capable of conducting these blood tests. Moreover, the technique was very complex and not very feasible in situations requiring urgent results. Many of these factors converged in the early clinical trials with Sirolimus. The medical community lost confidence in the drug, which was then relegated to compassionate use, in sporadic and desperate cases when other drugs have failed.

When the drug appeared in the year 2000, we started using it in all types of patients, particularly in patients presenting with rejection or CNI secondary effects in the immediate post-transplant period. The maximum number of indications was reached between 2000 and 2004. Afterwards, its use declined due to both, the self-experienced adverse events and the appearence of the warning (12-14) about the risk of arterial thrombosis. Everolimus, on the other hand, appeared much later. Our first experience was in 2005 and the principal advantage for the drug was the experience gained with Sirolimus. Furthermore, its pharmacokinetic differences, as opposed to Sirolimus, allowed 12 hourly administration and the possibility of providing much more accuracy in drug dosing, a very important fact within a scientific community which has become accustomed to this form of operating for more than two decades.

Both drugs were used in patients receiving a transplant for any cause (virus, alcohol, metabolic diseases, cholestatic diseases, tumors, acute liver failure, etc). However, HCC deserves mention as the principal indication : half the cases on Rapamycin and more than three quarters of the cases with Everolimus (Table 1). This is due to the fact that in our Unit, HCC accounts for 30% of all the LT. Moreover, the recent discovery of the m-TOR pathway in the etiopathogenic mechanisms in the development of tumor cells has conferred on it a role as an antiproliferative and anti-tumor drug. For this reason, in the past few years we have been indicating Sirolimus and more recently Everolimus in cases focusing on the oncological area, i.e. HCC. Advanced age did not constitute a contraindication for the use of m-TORi: one fifth of the indications were in patients over 65 years. M-TORi were also used in patients with concomitant diseases: co-infection with HCV and HIV viruses, diabetes mellitus, arterial hypertension, obesity, renal insufficiency, or even dyslipemia.

If we look at the timing of their use, we see that 2/3 were used within the first year post-LT and 1/3 after the first year (Table 2). Because of its initial design as a first line drug, Sirolimus was used much earlier than Everolimus. It was administered to patients as early as 10 days post-LT, with a mean of 18 months and a median of 2.3 months. In contrast, Everolimus was never used before 6 weeks post-LT, with a mean of 2 years and a median of 6.5 months. The main reasons for conversion in the case of Sirolimus were immunological (patients with unresolved rejection) and CNI adverse reactions (particularly nephrotoxicity and neurotoxicity), while in the case of Everolimus, were oncological. Because Sirolimus has been used since 2000, the follow-up of some patients in this group was much longer than in patients converted to Everolimus.

Our experience is mainly based on the Tacrolimus plus m-TORi combination. All patients, except 4, were on a Tacrolimus based regimen. Three patients were on a MMF based regimen, which was switched to Sirolimus and only 1 patient was on a Cyclosporine Neoral (CyA) regimen, maintaining a CyA and Everolimus combination. Therefore, our experience with m-TORi is as an immunosuppressant drug administered together with a CNI. We do not have much experience with m-TORi monotherapy. Only 3 patients on Sirolimus and 2 on Everolimus are on monotherapy. We do not believe that this should be its principal use, at least in the first year post-transplant, because the doses required should be excessive, causing severe adverse effects.

In terms of m-TORi doses and blood levels (Figure 1 and 2), high doses and levels were used in patients converted to Sirolimus. These doses were in the upper range of those recommended by the guidelines in the literature and previous trials. The mean starting dose was 5 mg/day, in some cases as high as 15 mg/day, with the aim of reaching initial levels of 10 ng/ml and maintaining these for the duration of follow-up. However, to prevent all the problems associated with the use of high doses of Sirolimus, patients converted to Everolimus were started on doses much lower than those recommended by Novartis SA or by preliminary studies in other organs. In our case, our mean starting dose was 0.5 mg/day and never higher than 1 mg/day. The fact that the principal reasons for conversion were patients with a high risk of tumor recurrence, warranted the use of a low dose regimen and provided evidence that despite using the minimum doses, rejections rate did not increase. This finding encouraged us to continue using these doses, in other indications such as CNI toxicity. We should also point out that despite such low starting doses, we managed to attain levels of 3 ng/ml after 15 days of administration. We always aimed not to exceed 5 ng/ml to avoid toxicity or secondary effects. In terms of the CNI doses and levels, these were reduced in almost all cases. However, there were also differences between the management of the two groups. The reduction of the Tacrolimus doses was lower when it was used in combination with Sirolimus than with Everolimus. Several conversion protocols and some clinical trials in stable patients have recommended loading doses. We have never used loading doses. We should remember that stable patients do not require high doses, as rejection is not a common problem during this period. Furthermore, in patients whose immmunosuppressant is totally converted to another, levels of the pre-conversion immunosuppressor drug are still detected for 3-5 days. Many of our patients had pre-conversion regimens based on levels less than 5 ng/ml of Tacrolimus, which indicated that they required low immunosuppression to maintain stable hepatic function. Therefore, loading doses with the accumulation of effects may even be counterproductive. In our experience, stable patients require blood levels monitoring specially sensitive to the lower drug blood ranges or even to sub-therapeutic ranges. However, the m-TORi technique does not discriminate levels under 3 or 5 ng/ml, but clinical evidence has taught us not to modify the Sirolimus or Everolimus dose despite values < 3ng/ml, provided that hepatic function remains stable.

Only half of the rejections responded to mTORi treatment (Table 3). However, the specific circumstances of the patients should be considered. In many cases, the administration of Sirolimus was started late and when other immunosuppressors had already failed, indicating an irreversible situation, more than an ineffective drug. In the cases where Sirolimus or Everolimus were started early, these were effective in resolving rejection. When the cause of conversion was CNI adverse events, these effects generally improved. It was very evident in cases of severe and life-threatening neurotoxicity which required an immediate action and less evident, in cases of well tolerated nephrotoxicity where the action taken was not immediate leading to failure of the drug in 50 % of the indications. The parallel decrease in CNI levels in patients converted to m-TORi probably led to improvements in diabetes mellitus and blood pressure in up to half of all cases. In cases in which the conversion was made due to oncological causes, our view was similar to that of other authors (15). M-TORi appear to have a good profile in preventing the recurrence or in stabilizing the disease. However, our study is an observational non-randomized non-comparative study, so we cannot make any solid conclusion. In this sense, further randomized studies are necessary to see if the time to progression is really delayed. We can only highlight that the most recent cases of conversion to m-TORi in patients outside the Milan criteria were made as early as 4-6 weeks post-transplant.

In the Sirolimus group, 17% of patients presented rejection after conversion (Table 4). Although three patients presented rejection within the first month post-LT, the other three presented it in the late post-operative period, after the third month post-LT. According to this initial experience, we have learnt that m-TORi are not suitable as a primary and single immunosuppressor agent in the immediate post-transplant period. Furthermore, rejections appearing beyond the third month post-LT, occurred when we felt confident with conversion and controls declined less often. Rejections in stable patients on m-TORi monotherapy, lasting days or weeks before attending the hospital, are difficult to resolve, because require aggressive immunosuppression prompting to the patient to succumb to pulmonary infections. Hence, in our current practice, conversion to m-TORi is not total, in other words, the patient continues for months on both drugs (m-TORi and CNI), and only after a long follow-up period with gradual decreases in the CNI, does the patient finally remain on m-TORi monotherapy.

The higher incidence of drug-related secondary effects in the Sirolimus group compared with the Everolimus group is related to the higher doses and blood levels employed and the longer follow-up with Sirolimus (Table 4). The principal adverse event was dyslipidaemia. While cholesterol and triglyceride levels can be controlled by reducing the dose and adding a statin, one of the patients with associated renal failure died due to severe rhabdomyolysis attributable to the Sirolimus and Simvastatin combination. The other adverse effect worth mentioning was pneumonia. Five patients presented pulmonary infections, two of which were clearly related with over-immunosuppression following a severe refractory rejection episode. In terms of HCV progression, we were unable to confirm any result as neither viral loads nor liver biopsies were performed after conversion.

One third of patients on m-TORi discontinued the drug during follow-up (Table 4). The higher percentage of failures with Sirolimus was due to longer follow-up and to the fact that the drug was used at a late stage and under desperate conditions when other drugs had failed. Another real problem in the long term management of m-TORi is wound complications, which would render m-TORi unadvisable in stable patients with good hepatic function who must undergo any type of intercurrent surgery. In these cases, we would recommend withdrawing the drug and then reintroducing it, if necessary, 4 weeks after the surgery.

Almost half the patients (45%) using m-TORi died during follow-up, but we should point out that drug-related deaths were in fact only 7 (13.7%). These deaths were related to: pneumonia in 2 patients, sepsis in 1 patient, rhabdomyolysis in 1 patient and refractory rejection in 3 patients (Table 4). We believe that if low doses of m-TORi are used in combination with low doses of CNI, the rates of adverse effects, discontinuations and drug-related deaths would drop considerably.

In conclusion, m-TORi have been used at excessively high doses under complex desperate situations when other immunosuppressors have failed. This has led to the failure of these drugs in terms of their indications in clinical practice. During the early post-transplant phase, they should be used in triple therapy for refractory rejection, in double therapy with CNI (both at half the normal dose) to prevent recurrence in extended tumors, and at low dose in monotherapy with steroids in cases of severe CNI adverse effects. During the later post-transplant phase, they should be used at low doses in cases with CNI adverse effects, in HCC recurrence and in the appearance of de novo tumors. Generally, m-TORi should be used with caution, not as a first line agent but as a support immunosuppressant, at low doses and prior to the appearance of severe complications. Having these premises in mind, it is responsibility of the scientific community to seek out the role that m-TORi deserve in liver transplantation so that we can regain confidence in these drugs.

References

[1] Neuhaus P, Klupp J, Langrehr JM. *M-TOR inhibitors: An overview Liver transplant* 2001; 7: 473.

[2] Dunn C and Croom K. Everolimus. A review of its use in renal and cardiac transplantation. *Drugs* 2006; 66 (4): 547-570.

[3] Luan FL, Ding R, Sharma VK, et al. Rapamycine is an effective inhibitor of human renal cancer metastasis. *Kidney Int* 2003; 63: 917.
[4] Kauffmann HM, Cherikh WS, Cheng Y, et al. Maintenance immunosuppression with Target-of-Rapamicine inhibitors is associated with a reduced incidence of de novo malignancies. *Transplantation* 2005; 80:883.
[5] Sierka D, Kumar MSA, Heifets M, et al. Successful minimization of immunosuppression (IM) and conversion to sirolimus (SLR) in kidney transplant recipients with post transplant lymphoproliferative disease (PTLD) and de novo nonskin malignancies (DNSM). *Am Jtransplant* 2004; 4 (Suppl 8): 523.
[6] Schuler W, Sedrani R, Cottens S, et al. SDZ RAD, a new rapamycin derivative: Pharmacological properties in vitro and in vivo. *Transplantation* 1997; 64: 36.
[7] Montalbano M, Neff GW, Yamashiki N, Meyer D, Bettiol M, Slapak-Green G, et al. A retrospective review of liver transplant patients treated with sirolimus from a single center: an analysis of sirolimus-related complications. *Transplantation* 2004; 78: 274-268.
[8] Kahan BD. Sirolimus: a comprehensive review. *Expert Opin Pharmacother* 2001; 78: 264-268.
[9] Chapman TM, Perry CM. Everolimus. *Drugs* 2004; 64: 861-872.
[10] Gomez-Camarero J, Salcedo M, Rincon D, Iacono O, Ripoll C, Hernando A, et al. Use of everolimus as a rescue immunosuppressive therapy in liver transplant patients with neoplasms. *Transplantation* 2007; 6 (84): 786-791.
[11] Levy G, Schmidli H, Punch J, Newhall E, Mayer D, Neuhaus P, et al. Safety, tolerability, and efficacy of everolimus in de novo liver transplant recipients: 12 and 36 month results. *Liver transplantation* 2006: 12: 1640-1648.
[12] Fortin MC, Raymond MA, Madore F, Fugère JA, Pâquet M, St-Louis G, Hébert MJ. Increased risk of thrombotic microangiopathy in patients receiving a cyclosporine-sirolimus combination. *Am J Transplant* 2004; 4 (6) : 946-52.
[13] Mac Alister VC, Peltekian KM, Malatjalian DA, Colohan S, MacDonald S, Bitter-Suermann H, et al. Orthotopic liver transplantation using low-dose tacrolimus and sirolimus. *Liver Tansplant* 2001; 7 (8): 701-708.
[14] Dunkelberg JC, Trotter JF, Wachs M, Bak T, Kugelmas M, Steinberg T, et al. Sirolimus as primary immunosuppression in liver transplantation is not associated with hepatic artery or wound complications. *Liver Transplant* 2003; 9 (5): 463-468.
[15] Zimmerman MA, Trotter JF, Wachs M, Bak T, Campsen J. Sirolimus-based immunosuppression following liver transplantation for hepatocellular carcinoma. *Liver transplantation* 2008; 14: 633-638.

In: Immunosuppression: New Research
Editor: Charles B. Taylor, pp. 131-151

ISBN: 978-1-60692-102-9

Chapter 5

Evolution of Immunosuppression in Liver Transplantation

Olga N. Tucker* and Nigel Heaton

The Liver Transplant Unit, Institute of Liver Studies, King's College Hospital, London, UK.

Abstract

We are currently entering a new era of immunosuppressive therapy in liver transplantation (LT). Since the 1980s, calcineurin inhibitors (CNI) have been the mainstay of both early and late immunosuppressive regimes following LT. The occurrence of significant adverse events with current regimes of CNI combined with tapered corticosteroids, in particular nephrotoxicity, neurotoxicity and hypertension, has been responsible for a changing view of immunosuppression with increased availability of newer potentially less toxic agents.

Combination regimes of various classes of immunosuppressive drugs, the addition of other drug types with reduction or withdrawal of CNI for treatment-related toxicity, or monotherapy with non-CNI agents are increasingly being utilised. Early corticosteroid withdrawal and steroid-free regimens have been successfully used in both children and adults. The use of induction therapy with polyclonal or monoclonal antibodies is now becoming commonplace in patients with renal dysfunction to delay CNI introduction, and to reduce acute rejection episodes. Biological induction agents have also permitted the use of steroid-free regimens and early reduction in CNI dose. Exploitation of the concept of liver tolerance with regimes to induce donor-specific systemic immunological tolerance by recipient pre-treatment, combined with low-dose post-transplant immunosuppression is an exciting and evolving field. Development of innovative immunotherapies that take advantage of natural immunoregulatory mechanisms contributing to immune privilege in the liver may challenge the need for lifelong immunosuppression in the future.

Keywords: Liver transplantation, immunosuppression

* E-mail address: olga_tucker@hotmail.com. Tel.: +353872421997; Correspondence concerning this article should be addressed to: Ms. Olga Tucker, 26 Upper Grand Canal St, Dublin 4, Ireland.

Abbreviations

ACR,	Acute cellular rejection;
ATG,	antithymocyte globulin;
AZT,	azothiaprine;
CNI,	calcineurin inhibitor;
CMV,	cytomegalovirus;
CR,	chronic rejection;
CyA,	cyclosporine;
HAT,	hepatic artery thrombosis;
HCV,	hepatitis C virus;
IL-2,	interleukin-2;
FKBP-12,	FK506-binding protein-12;
MPA,	mycophenolic acid;
MMF,	mycophenolate mofetil;
mTOR,	mammalian target of rapamycin;
LT,	liver transplantation;
POD,	postoperative day.

Introduction

Liver transplantation (LT) is the treatment of choice for patients with end stage liver disease. Improvements in immunosuppressive therapy over the last 4 decades have led to acceptable patient and graft survival rates. Current one and 5-year survival rates for liver transplant recipients are 85-90% and 70-75% respectively [1].

Immunosuppressive agents can be classified into 5 main groups: corticosteroids, calcineurin inhibitors (CNI) (cyclosporine, tacrolimus), inhibitors of purine biosynthesis (azothiaprine, mycophenolate mofetil), inhibitors of mammalian target of rapamycin (sirolimus, everolimus), and polyclonal or monoclonal antibodies (anti-thymocyte globulin, anti-lymphocyte globulin, OKT3, anti-interleukin-2 receptor antibodies (dacliximab, basiliximab), anti-CD52 antibody (campath 1-H)) [2]. Other agents include FTY720, which selectively reduces the circulating mature lymphocyte population, and FK778 which inhibits de novo lymphocyte pyrimidine synthesis and tyrosine kinase activity [3,4].

Following LT, most standard immunosuppressive regimes include a CNI with tapered corticosteroids, followed by long-term single agent CNI administration. To improve patient compliance, quality of life, and long-term graft and patient survival, efforts have been focused on developing new protocols that are less toxic and more effective [5]. Newer regimes include combination protocols of different immunosuppressive drug classes, different drug types to enable reduction or withdrawal of CNI for treatment-related toxicity, monotherapy with non-CNIs, steroid-free transplantation, the use of pre-transplant biological induction agents, and more recently, induction of immune tolerance [6-10]. In addition to attenuation of drug-related toxicity, optimization of immunosuppression may reduce the incidence of malignancy and recurrence of autoimmune hepatitis and hepatitis C. The evolution of immunosuppression in LT is discussed with emphasis on recent trials and potential future therapies.

Evolution of Immunosuppression

Following the recognition by Medawer in 1944 that organ rejection was an immunological event, the determination of the optimal level of immunosuppression to achieve long-term graft and patient survival following LT with maintenance of quality of life has been sought [11]. In the early 1960s, total body irradiation, anti-metabolites, 6-mercaptopurine and its derivative, azothiaprine (AZT), and corticosteroids were utilized with significant toxic side effects [12-15]. The combination of AZT and prednisolone was a major advance, and led to the first human liver transplant in 1963 [16].

Introduction of Cyclosporin and Tacrolimus

Improvement in post-transplant survival rates were not seen until the introduction of CNIs in the form of cyclosporine (CyA), when 1-year survival rates rose from 27% to 74% [17]. Cyclosporine, a cyclic endecapeptide, was originally isolated from the fungus Trichoderma Polysporum. It forms an active complex with cyclophilin, a cytoplasmic receptor, which binds to calcineurin resulting in inhibition of its phosphatase activity preventing activation of nuclear transcription factor which is pivotal for the upregulation of cytokine expression necessary for T cell activation. Cyclosporin is available in both oral and parenteral formulations. The standard oral formulation (Sandimmune®) is a hydrophobic compound which requires bile for absorption. A microemulsified formulation (Neoral®) was subsequently developed which demonstrated improved pharmacokinetics with better bioavailability, and reduction in the severity of episodes of acute cellular rejection (ACR) [18]. Triple therapy with CyA, AZT and prednisolone resulted in improved graft and patient survival, and was widely adopted as the standard immunosuppressive regime to prevent early allograft rejection following LT [19,20].

In 1989, tacrolimus (Prograf, FK506) was introduced. Tacrolimus is a macrolide, derived from the fungus Streptomyces Tsukubaensis that also acts by suppression of T cell activation. It binds to the intracellular protein, immunophyllin FK506-binding protein-12 (FKBP-12), which complexes with the Ca^{+2}-dependent serine-threonine phosphatase calcineurin inhibiting cytokine-induced T cell gene transcription, and therefore G_0 to G_1 transition [21]. This CNI has a 100-fold greater *in vitro* and 10-fold *in vivo* potency to inhibit T cell responses than CyA. Two large multicenter, randomized trials comparing tacrolimus with CyA as primary and maintenance immunosuppression demonstrated lower acute, steroid-resistant, and chronic rejection (CR) episodes, but higher adverse events with tacrolimus with similar patient and graft survivals at one year [22,23]. A further multicentre randomised controlled trial, the TMC trial, comparing tacrolimus and microemulsified CyA, confirmed improved early patient survival, a lower retransplantation rate and CR episodes with tacrolimus after the first year of LT [24]. A similar incidence of neurotoxicity and nephrotoxicity was seen in both, but tacrolimus was associated with a higher incidence of new-onset diabetes [24]. The recent publication of 3 year data confirmed the benefit of tacrolimus over CyA with a higher percentage of patients alive with their original graft, but no statistical difference in terms of mortality or retransplantation rate [25]. Evaluation of 5 year results of a prospective randomized trial comparing CyA microemulsion and tacrolimus for primary immunosuppression by Gonzalez-Pinto et al reported similar survival and ACR episodes, but higher rates of serious adverse events and CR episodes with CyA [26]. While longer-term follow-up studies have not consistently demonstrated a significant survival advantage with tacrolimus, significantly lower rates of graft loss and re-transplantation are reported [27-29].

Introduction of Mycoplenolate Mofetil

Mycoplenolate mofetil (MMF, CellCept(R)), a morpholinoethyl ester of mycophenolic acid (MPA), suppresses T and B cell proliferation by inhibiting inosine monophosphate dehydrogenase, a key enzyme in de novo purine synthesis [30]. Mycophenolic acid induces activated T-lymphocyte apoptosis, decreases the recruitment of lymphocytes and monocytes into sites of inflammation and graft rejection, and suppress production of inducible nitric oxide synthase by depleting tetrahydrobiopterin [30]. Mycoplenolate mofetil also downregulates IL-2 receptor expression and several adhesion receptors on T and B cells resulting in reduced T cell proliferation and immunoglobulin production respectively. The advantages of MMF are the relative absence of nephrotoxic, neurotoxic and hepatotoxic effects. Also, MPA inhibits the proliferation of human B lymphocytes transformed by the Epstein-Barr virus, and therefore may decrease the risk of lymphoma [30]. Due to its effect on both cellular and humoral mediated rejection, MMF may also attenuate the progression of CR-related intimal proliferation and arteriopathy [31].

The role of MMF as a component of primary immunosuppressive regimes after LT remains controversial. Initial reports demonstrated excellent graft and patient survival with the use of MMF combined with a tapered steroid dose, and CyA microemulsion or tacrolimus at 6 months [32]. In a randomized comparative study of MMF or AZT in combination with CyA and steroids, MMF was superior to AZT in preventing ACR in the first 6 months following LT with equivalent graft survival at one year [33]. However, in a prospective randomised trial comparing low dose corticosteroids with CyA and MMF, tacrolimus and MMF or tacrolimus after LT, no significant difference in survival was seen at 18 months, and fewer ACR episodes were documented in the tacrolimus groups. No additional benefit was observed in the tacrolimus, MMF and corticosteroids group compared to dual therapy [34]. In a subsequent study, no difference in graft or patient survival was seen at one year, however, more than 50% of the MMF group withdrew due to gastrointestinal and haematological side effects [35]. Long-term results of triple induction therapy with MMF and low-dose steroids in combination with either tacrolimus or CyA, have not demonstrated significant beneficial effects although pharmacological synergy is seen between MMF and tacrolimus [36].

Mycophenolate mofetil has been successfully employed as a secondary immunosuppressive agent in LT recipients with steroid-resistant ACR, CR, or CNI-induced toxicity. It is an effective alternative immunosuppressive agent in patients failing CNI-based therapy with an acceptable long-term safety profile [32]. Randomized studies of CNI replacement with MMF in patients with treatment-related toxicity has resulted in improvement in renal dysfunction, reduction in uric acid concentration, and blood pressure. A retrospective review of the role of MMF in the treatment of steroid-resistant ACR, CR, chronic graft dysfunction, and CNI-induced toxicity demonstrated safety and effectiveness as rescue therapy with acceptable patient and graft survival of 93% and 88% respectively, improvement in CNI-related toxicity, and acute and chronic graft dysfunction [37]. Side effects including gastrointestinal disorders or bone marrow toxicity occurred in 31% [37]. A further study of MMF as monotherapy or in combination with low-dose CNI in patients with CNI-induced renal dysfunction, demonstrated significant improvement in renal function with minimal rejection and no graft loss [38]. However, an increased risk of ACR of 4.5-29% has been observed with MMF monotherapy [39,40]. Other limiting adverse effects include nausea, vomiting, diarrhea, and dose-dependent bone marrow suppression.

Introduction of Sirolimus

Sirolimus (Rapamune®) is a potent inhibitor of antigen-induced proliferation of T cells, B cells, and antibody production [41]. Sirolimus complexes with FKBP-12 preventing the activation of cell-cycle-specific phosphatidylinositol kinases, known as mammalian target of rapamycin (mTOR) inhibitors, resulting in blockage of signals transduced by a variety of growth factor receptors to the nucleus [41]. It also inactivates 70-kDa-S6 kinase (P70S6k) resulting in selective inhibition of the synthesis of new ribosomal proteins with prolongation of cell cycle progression from G_1 to S phase. Similar to MMF, it has no reported nephrotoxic effects. Sirolimus has been used in LT as primary therapy combined with reduced CNI dose and prednisolone, or as conversion therapy in patients with CNI-related nephrotoxicity or neurotoxicity [42,43]. In two major studies on sirolimus as a primary immunosuppressive agent combined with either tacrolimus or CyA with a corticosteroid taper, the rates of acute and steroid-resistant rejection were significantly lower than in historical controls [44,45].

Because of its mode of action, sirolimus has profound effects on a variety of cell types including haematopoietic progenitor cells, lymphocytes and mesenchymal cells. The side-effect profile including dose dependent hyperlipidemia, thrombocytopenia, anaemia, leucopenia, lymphocoele, and gastrointestinal disturbances were delineated during prospective controlled trials in renal transplantation [46]. Concerns exist regarding the association of sirolimus with a higher incidence of hepatic artery thrombosis (HAT). The Wyeth Study 211 to determine the safety and efficacy of the combination of sirolimus, CyA, and tapered corticosteroids compared to tacrolimus and tapered corticosteroids as primary immunosuppression after LT demonstrated higher rates of wound complications and vascular thrombosis involving the hepatic artery, portal vein or both [47]. Further analysis by an external Data Safety Monitoring Board in conjunction with a case-by-case analysis concluded that technical and donor factors were partly responsible for the high incidence of vascular thrombosis. A subsequent phase II study, Wyeth Study 220, comparing tacrolimus and tapered corticosteroids with sirolimus, reduced dose tacrolimus, and tapered corticosteroids again noted a higher incidence of HAT in the sirolimus group [47]. These findings prompted an FDA warning against the use of sirolimus as early immunosuppressive therapy after LT. Two further reports from the University of Edmonton demonstrated one case of HAT with sirolimus use during a mean follow-up period of 23 months following LT [44,48]. Dunkleberg et al recently reviewed 170 patients transplanted between January 2000 and June 2002, who were administered sirolimus as primary immunosuppression with a CNI and a 3-day corticosteroid taper compared to historical controls administered a CNI and a 14-day corticosteroid taper, with or without MMF [43]. Multivariate analysis failed to show an association between sirolimus therapy and hepatic artery or wound complications. Hepatic artery complications occurred in 5.3% compared to 8.3% of historic controls, and the incidence of wound complications was similar between the 2 groups [43]. Hepatotoxicity has also been reported with sirolimus use [49]. In view of concerns regarding toxic effects, the minimum dosage of sirolimus necessary to achieve the appropriate immunological objective is advised [47].

Recent Advances in Immunosuppression Following Liver Transplantation

As previously discussed standard immunosuppression regimes typically include a CNI with or without corticosteroids. However, as CNIs can result in toxicity requiring reduction or withdrawal of treatment including nephropathy, neurotoxicity, hypertension, hyperlipidaemia, diabetes, hyperuricemia, hypercholesterolaemia, infection, and increased incidence of malignancy several alterations to immunosuppressive regimes have been suggested [22,23]. These include the combination of different classes of immunosuppressive agents, addition of different drug types with reduction in CNI dose, monotherapy with non-CNIs, early corticosteroid withdrawal or steroid-free regimens, and induction therapy with polyclonal or monoclonal antibodies.

Combination Immunosuppressive Regimes

Several combination immunosuppressive regimes have been reported. Animal studies have shown that sirolimus and tacrolimus act synergistically to prevent rejection [50,51]. Similar findings have been reported in both adult and paediatric recipients following LT [44,48,52,53]. When sirolimus is added to reduced-dose tacrolimus regimens low rates of ACR are seen with preservation of renal function. A primary immunosuppressive regime by McAlister et al. with sirolimus and low dose tacrolimus (target trough levels, 7 and 5 ng/mL respectively) with corticosteroid weaning by 3 months, demonstrated acceptable patient and graft survival rates. Acute cellular rejection rates of 14% were seen during a follow-up period of 23 months (range 6-35 months), and complete steroid withdrawal was achieved in 91% [44]. Importantly, near normal renal function, glucose control, and lipid metabolism were seen without additional medication in 84%. Cytomegalovirus (CMV) infection occurred in only 4 patients, however, HAT was seen in one patient [44]. In a retrospective review of paediatric patients with ACR and renal impairement following LT, tacrolimus dose reduction (target level 7.5ng/mL) and commencement of sirolimus improved hepatic and renal dysfunction [54]. Other reports confirm effective immunosuppression with lower doses of both CyA and sirolimus when co-administered, compared to the higher doses required for each when given alone.

Mycophenolate mofetil also appears to have a synergistic effect with tacrolimus. A long term prospective randomized study by Fisher et al. demonstrated acceptable patient and graft survival, and incidence of rejection and infection in regimes using MMF induction and maintenance combined with either CyA or tacrolimus and corticosteroid taper [55]. However, renal dysfunction was higher in the CyA group. Others report superior results for MMF combined with tacrolimus compared to CyA and tacrolimus for primary immunosuppression [56]. When combined with tacrolimus or CyA, MMF is effective in the treatment of steroid-resistant ACR, CR, and chronic graft dysfunction [37]. Improvements in CNI-induced toxicity have been demonstrated following CNI dose reduction with MMF addition [37]. In a small prospective study of CNI-induced renal failure, MMF addition permitted CNI-dose reduction of 70%, with early improvement in serum creatinine which was maintained for 5 years (range 3.1-6.0) without major side effects [57]. A significant reduction in serum creatinine was observed in 88%, with normalization in 41%. Based on these observations, addition of MMF within 6 months of LT was recommended in the presence of CNI-induced renal dysfunction [57].

Sirolimus has been combined effectively with MMF following CNI withdrawal for treatment-related toxicity [58]. In a small retrospective study of late conversion with mean follow-up of 137 days (range 26-258), 7 patients with CNI-related renal (n=6) and neurological (n=1) toxicity were converted to sirolimus and MMF an average of 62 months (range 37-118) following LT [59]. Patient and graft survival were 100% with no episodes of ACR or infection. Renal function improved in 83%, with resolution of neurological symptoms in the single affected patient. Hypertriglyceridaemia, hypercholesterolaemia, and exanthema occurred in 3 patients, which were reversible with dose reduction or therapy cessation in 2 [59].

Unfortunately, treatment options remain limited for patients with CR. A combination of MMF and tacrolimus is beneficial in patients with low bilirubin levels [60]. Sirolimus combined with tacrolimus (trough level 8-10ng/ml) may be beneficial in the setting of CR, but drug-related side effects are common [60].

Mycophenolate Mofetil Monotherapy

Monotherapy with MMF was first evaluated in 5 patients with CyA-induced renal impairment [61]. Significant improvements in renal function were seen without major side effects. Mild steroid-responsive ACR occurred in one patient after 3 months [61]. However, the efficacy and safety of MMF monotherapy was questioned following the publication of other trials. A randomised study assessing MMF monotherapy in 28 patients with CNI-related renal dysfunction demonstrated an improvement in renal function, blood pressure and uric acid concentration, but there was an increased risk of ACR. Three reversible episodes of ACR were seen in 14 patients, whereas none occurred in the CNI group [40]. Also, 8 of the 14 patients required continuing maintenance steroids.

A further randomised controlled trial of MMF monotherapy in CNI-related renal failure demonstrated improvement in renal function, but was prematurely terminated when 3 of 5 patients developed ACR of which 2 required retransplantation [62]. Subsequently, Fairbanks et al retrospectively examined 16 patients converted from a CNI to MMF monotherapy for renal insufficiency a median of 2,056 days (range, 606-5,893) after LT. Monotherapy with MMF was associated with a 19% significant risk of allograft rejection even among long-term transplant survivors resulting in 2 deaths and one retransplantation [63]. A longer term study over a median of 27 months evaluating 45 patients with chronic CNI-related renal dysfunction commenced on MMF demonstrated a considerable improvement in serum creatinine [38]. Sixteen of the 45 patients were commenced on MMF monotherapy while the remainder received a combination of MMF and reduced dose CNI. Over 33 months (range 7-45) only one patient experienced steroid-responsive ACR. Eleven of 29 patients treated with MMF and low dose CNI, developed refractory ACR. Of these, 5 experienced further rejection episodes at a median of one month after MMF introduction, of which 4 were treated successfully with bolus steroids and CNI dose increase [38]. It was concluded that MMF was an effective renal sparing agent particularly as monotherapy, and a history of refractory rejection may predict a poorer outcome [38]. The evidence from published trials of the impact of MMF monotherapy on ACR remains contradictory. Although the trials are limited by small numbers, caution is advised prior to commencing MMF monotherapy, and if converted, patients should be closely monitored for rejection episodes.

Sirolimus Monotherapy

Sirolimus has been shown to be an effective substitute for tacrolimus in treatment-related renal insufficiency after LT, without an increase in episodes of ACR during conversion [64]. Fairbanks et al prospectively analysed changes in renal function after conversion from a CNI to sirolimus monotherapy for treatment-related toxicity [65]. Renal function improved in 71%. Only one patient developed biopsy-proven ACR, which was successfully managed with sirolimus and MMF. Two patients discontinued sirolimus due to oral ulceration and interstitial pneumonitis [65]. A further retrospective review by Nair et al evaluated the safety of CNI therapy withdrawal after introduction of sirolimus monotherapy in chronic CNI-related renal insufficiency at least 3 years following LT [66]. A significant improvement in serum creatinine and blood urea nitrogen was observed at 6 months following conversion, with a trend to improved creatinine clearance at 6 months to one year. None developed ACR, HAT, or allograft dysfunction [66].

Steroid-Free Immunosuppressive Regimes

Steroids have traditionally been employed in primary immunosuppressive regimes, and as first-line treatment of ACR. Although steroids are potent anti-inflammatory agents their mode of action is non-specific, and their use is associated with numerous side effects including hypertension, hyperlipidaemia, infection, poor wound healing, diabetes, osteoporosis, and cushingoid habitus. To reduce morbidity several groups have withdrawn steroids soon after LT, used steroids only as induction treatment, or employed steroid-free regimens. Up to 1999, 16 published reports with a total of 901 patients were available on the role of early steroid withdrawal of which only 2 were randomized controlled trials [67]. Steroid withdrawal was achieved in approximately 85%, with no adverse effect on graft or patient survival, no significant increase in the incidence of acute or chronic rejection, and a reduced incidence of adverse events including effects on blood pressure, cholesterol levels, hyperglycaemia, and obesity [67]. Tisone at al. reported that LT for hepatitis C could be performed successfully without steroids using CyA and AZT [68]. Episodes of ACR were treated by CyA dose increase, with only 10% requiring intravenous steroids [68]. A further prospective study by Rolles et al. examined outcome following steroid-free monotherapy with tacrolimus or CyA [69]. Two-thirds of patients in both groups demonstrated biopsy proven

ACR. Pulsed steroid therapy was required to treat ACR in 60% of tacrolimus and 40% of CyA treated patients [69].

Trotter et al initiated a prednisone-free immunosuppressive regime in 2000, with a 3-day tapered dose of methylprednisolone, with either tacrolimus or CyA and sirolimus addition. In their first report, patient and graft survivals of 92% and 89% respectively were demonstrated [45]. Ten of 33 patients (30%) experienced 12 episodes of ACR compared with 70% in historical controls. Steroid resistant rejection was reduced with requirement for OKT3 in only 3% compared to 37% in historical controls [45]. A further report analyzing results over a 2 year period, demonstrated a significant reduction in CMV disease to 2% compared to 17% in historical controls [70]. In 2003, Pirenne et al reported 3 year results of a prospective study on steroid-free primary immunosuppression after LT [7]. Tacrolimus (trough level 8-10ng/ml) and AZT (1-2mg/kg) were commenced postoperatively, and steroids were given in the event of ACR, tacrolimus or AZT toxicity where dose reduction or withdrawal was required. Three year patient and graft survival were 95% and 100% respectively. Steroids were reintroduced in 10 patients (48%). Acute rejection occurred in 5 patients (23%), of whom 4 responded to a single course of intravenous steroids, with one requiring steroids and ATG. Six further patients received steroids for non-immune reasons including drug toxicity. Of the patients who received steroids, 70% were withdrawn at last follow up [7]. The authors suggested that a steroid-free regimen including an anti-lymphocyte agent such as MMF or AZT with low dose CNI provides sufficient immunosuppression, and may be safer. This prospective trial demonstrated the long term safety and feasibility of steroid-free primary immunosuppression in a single centre.

Subsequently, Reding et al. demonstrated that the combination of tacrolimus and basiliximab was a safe alternative to tacrolimus and steroids following paediatric LT [71,72]. Twenty children who received combined tacrolimus and basiliximab were compared to a matched historical control group who received tacrolimus and steroids. At one year, rejection-free survival was 75% in the tacrolimus-basiliximab group compared to 50% in the steroid group. Importantly, growth in the first year was significantly better, with a reduced need for antihypertensives in the steroid-free group [71]. Since 2001, Reding et al employ a steroid-free primary immunosuppression protocol of tacrolimus and basiliximab in their pediatric population [8,73].

The Concept of Immune Privilege and Induction of Immune Tolerance

The liver has been described as an immune-privileged organ [74]. Liver allografts have an ability to protect themselves from host adaptive immunity, and may induce systemic immunoregulatory effects that facilitate transplantation of other organs. The liver is also an excellent site for tissue allografts with recent successful implantation of islet allografts in the treatment of type I diabetes mellitus [75,76]. Also, in humans donor and recipient HLA mismatching does not appear to negatively influence outcome after LT [74]. Immune privilege is thought to be an active process with promotion of immune tolerance. A number of cellular and molecular mechanisms have been proposed including donor derived passenger leucocytes creating peripheral microchimerism, antigen presentation by hepatocytes inducing T cell apoptosis, LPS activation of innate and adaptive immunity, kupffer cell-mediated immunosuppression, T cell inactivation, and immune deviation phenomena amongst others

[74]. Manipulation of immunoregulatory mechanisms to suppress adaptive immunity and protect the transplanted allograft by enhancing immune privilege would have enormous clinical benefit.

Tolerance has been described in animal models, in patients following bone marrow transplantation, and recipients of liver grafts who have discontinued treatment after a prolonged period of good function [77,78]. To reduce morbidity from current regimens many have advocated the use of low-dose or no-dose maintenance immunosuppression through the induction of donor-specific systemic tolerance by self-limiting interactions between host and donor derived leukocytes. Operational tolerance exists when good function is maintained in the grafted organ indefinitely without maintenance immunosuppression after a short induction procedure. 'Almost' or prope tolerance occurs when graft acceptance is maintained by a low, non-toxic maintenance immunosuppressive regimen that may not be required indefinitely [6].

Profound T cell depletion in rhesus monkeys treated with a CD3 diphtheria immunotoxin results in tolerance to renal allografts [79]. Calne et al examined a similar model in humans following renal transplantation using alemtuzamab (Campath 1H, C1H) to reduce circulating peripheral blood lymphocytes. Campath 1H is a humanized anti CD52 monoclonal antibody directed against the CD25 antigen present on the surface of T cells, B cells, natural killer (NK) cells, and monocytes. It blocks the interaction of interleukin-2 (IL-2) with its receptor, resulting in rapid deletion of circulating T and B cells with intravenous administration preventing an aggressive lymphocytic immune response after transplantation. Campath 1H was administered intravenously at day 0, and day one with addition of low dose CyA monotherapy at day 3. After 24 months, 29 patients had good graft function, and 5 episodes of steroid-responsive ACR were recorded [80].

Starzl et al. advocate tolerance induction by recipient pretreatment to reduce host-versus-graft response of the organ recipient, with the lowest possible maintenance immunosuppression dose to further reduce the clonal response [81]. In a prospective trial 82 patients awaiting kidney, liver, pancreas or intestinal transplantation were pretreated with 5mg/kg of rabbit anti-thymocyte globulin (ATG) and 1-2g methylprednisolone, followed by tacrolimus monotherapy commenced an day one (target trough 10μg/ml). Thirty five of the 82 patients (43%) had an adjunct infusion of donor bone marrow cells. Patient and graft survival was 95% and 89% respectively at one year. Of the 17 patients who received a liver graft, 11 were receiving spaced tacrolimus monotherapy at 13-17 months with 3 patients on a single weekly dose [81]. Administration of donor bone marrow cells to increase the load of donor leucocytes has improved allograft survival in experimental models [82]. However, no advantage was seen in this subgroup of patients in Starzl's study. A similar study has been performed by Tzakis et al. who administered Campath 1H (n=40) followed by low dose tacrolimus aiming at a 12 hour trough level of 5-10ng/ml with dose tapering if there was no rejection, compared to a historical control group (n=50) who received tacrolimus and low dose steroids [83]. Steroids were given as premedications prior to the Campath 1H doses. Preliminary results indicated that Campath 1H and low dose tacrolimus provided effective immunosuppression with good patient and graft survival at one year, and preservation of renal function. This study was criticized for small numbers, short follow-up, and lack of randomization with comparison to historical controls [83].

Delayed introduction of maintenance immunosuppression is possible with the use of biological induction agents [84,85]. Immune activation has been associated with long-term survival in animal models [86]. In a recent study, Tector et al. used rabbit ATG (RATG) and delayed tacrolimus introduction to minimize ACR and steroid pulse use. Three doses of RATG, and methylprednisolone followed by a steroid taper were administered to 120 patients, with tacrolimus introduction on day 3/4 aiming for a target level of 8-12ng/ml for 3 months, and 5-8ng/ml thereafter. Acute rejection occurred in 4.5% within the first 2 months, with an overall incidence of 6.2% during follow-up. Five patients (4.5%) developed CMV infection.

Biological induction immunosuppression has also been utilized effectively to permit steroid-free regimens and early reduction in CNI dose. Steroids may counteract an active tolerogenic response beneficial to the graft and patient. The administration of steroids has been shown to reduce tolerance induced by donor specific blood transfusion [87]. A 2 phase prospective randomized trial by Eason et al. of 119 liver transplant recipients of a steroid-free regimen of RATG induction therapy, or methylprednisolone followed by a 3 month steroid taper with maintenance MMF and tacrolimus demonstrated excellent survival, and decreased immunosuppression-related complications [88]. In phase I, 71 patients were given maintenance tacrolimus immunosuppression to achieve a level of 10-12ng/ml by day 5, and MMF for 3 months, with prednisone taper added to the steroid group. In phase II, MMF was discontinued after 2 weeks. Patient and graft survival were similar in both groups. In phase I, the incidence of ACR was 25% in the RATG and 31% in the steroid group. The incidence of ACR was unchanged when MMF was discontinued in phase II. A significant increase in steroid-requiring rejection in the steroid group (50%) was seen compared to RATG (6.6%), while none in either group developed CR. The incidence of CMV was 5% in the RATG group compared to 23% in the steroid group. De novo diabetes was also higher in the steroid (14%) compared to the RATG group (2%).

Anti-Interleukin 2 Receptor Antibody Therapy

Basiliximab (Simulect®) and daclizumab (Zenapax®) are high affinity IL-2 receptor (IL-2R) monoclonal antibodies. Monoclonal antibodies against IL-2 receptor (IL-2Rab) offer the possibility of selective immunosuppression with inhibition of the proliferation of activated T cells. Daclizumab is a molecularly engineered human immunoglobulin G1 monoclonal antibody that binds to, and blocks the IL-2 receptor [89]. Basiliximab is a human/mouse chimeric antibody which blocks the α subunit of the IL-2 receptor [90]. According to the 2003 United States Scientific Registry of Transplant Recipients (SRTR) Annual Report the use of an induction agent in patients undergoing LT has increased to 18% of patients with the majority (13% of all patients) receiving either basiliximab or daclizumab [91].

Induction therapy with daclizumab was shown to be effective in reducing ACR in renal transplant recipients. In an early study, daclizumab was given as induction therapy to 32 patients, with enrollment of 7 in a pilot study to determine its efficacy with steroids and MMF without a CNI. The remaining patients received daclizumab, MMF, and steroids, with CNI introduction within the first week. The pilot study was halted when all patients suffered ACR compared to 36% outside the pilot study. The incidence and severity of ACR correlated with the delay in CNI therapy introduction [92]. Currently, daclizumab is used in combination with MMF, steroids and delayed introduction of CNI in patients undergoing LT with preoperative renal failure or at high risk of postoperative renal dysfunction [93]. Eckhoff et al. examined the use of daclizumab in patients at risk of renal insufficiency following LT [93]. Daclizumab

(2 mg/kg) was administered to 39 patients before organ engraftment and on POD 5 (1 mg/kg) with delayed CNI introduction when renal function recovered. This regime was compared to a control group of 58 patients who received immediate postoperative tacrolimus. Maintenance immunosuppression consisted of steroids, tacrolimus, or CyA, and MMF in selected patients. The daclizumab group had improved renal function by POD 7, and significantly less ACR episodes in the first 6 months compared to controls (18% versus 40%) with similar patient survival rates [93]. Another prospective trial compared 54 patients administered a single dose of postoperative daclizumab with delayed tacrolimus introduction at day 7, while 47 patients received immediate tacrolimus [94]. Both groups also received MMF and steroids. Again, the ACR rate was lower in the daclizumab compared to controls (26% versus 49%). Dialysis requirement was lower with daclizumab and delayed tacrolimus introduction, compared to low-dose tacrolimus [95].

Daclizumab induction has been used successfully in early withdrawal of steroid protocols with reported biopsy confirmed ACR rates of 6-9% [96,97]. Similar results are seen with basiliximab. In a phase III prospective randomized multicenter trial induction therapy of a single basiliximab dose with CyA and steroids in 188 patients lower biopsy confirmed ACR at 6 months were seen (35%) compared to a placebo group (43%) [98].

In paediatric LT recipients, basiliximab and daclizumab use are associated with significant reduction in ACR episodes [99,100]. Basiliximab is also effective as rescue therapy in steroid-resistant rejection [101]. Aw et al prospectively evaluated the safety and efficacy of basiliximab in treating biopsy-proven steroid-resistant rejection in 7 paediatric liver recipients. Primary immunosuppression consisted of CyA, AZT, and prednisolone in 4 and tacrolimus and prednisolone in 3 patients who had undergone retransplantation for CR (n=2) and hyperacute rejection (n=1). Four had received 2 cycles of high-dose steroids, and 3 a single cycle, and all were converted to tacrolimus followed by MMF addition. Five children received 2 doses of basiliximab (10 mg, 3-7 days apart), and 2 received a single dose. Five children were rejection-free at a median follow-up of 22 months (range 5-32). Biochemical abnormalities persisted in the remaining 2 recipients, and both developed CR [101].

Recurrence of Hepatitis C Virus and Immunosuppression

Hepatitis C (HCV)-related chronic liver disease is a common indication for LT, and clinically significant HCV recurrence occurs in up to 50% of recipients within one year. Hepatitis C positive recipients have a 3-fold increased risk of death if they experience an episode of ACR, which increases to 5-fold with steroid-refractory rejection [102]. The development of techniques to minimize the recurrence risk, and improve outcome is vital. Proposed methods include steroid-free regimens, induction immunosuppression, preemptive anti-viral therapy or selective use with histological diagnosis of recurrence.

Steroids have been implicated in a higher viral replication risk and recurrence of HCV after LT. Steroid boluses are associated with increased serum HCV RNA concentrations of 4-100-fold, frequency of acute hepatitis, histological severity of recurrent hepatitis, and earlier time to recurrence [103-105]. The occurrence of ACR, treatment of ACR, steroid bolus use, and the number of ACR episodes during the 1st year after LT are associated with early severe HCV recurrence within 2 years [106]. Induction therapy may reduce HCV recurrence. In patients treated with RATG the incidence of recurrent HCV was significantly reduced to 50% compared to 71% in those treated with a steroid-containing regimen [85].

The effect of CNI use on HCV recurrence remains controversial. A 4-yr follow-up of 99 consecutive LT patients randomized to receive maintenance CyA or tacrolimus with a steroid taper after MMF induction demonstrated similar patient and graft survival, similar ACR, but significantly lower rejection and lower clinically recurrent hepatitis in a subgroup with HCV receiving tacrolimus [55]. These findings have been supported by other groups [107].

The role of anti-IL2Rab therapy in HCV is controversial. In a single study, 41 patients (HCV positive n=21; HCV negative n=20) received induction therapy with daclizumab, MMF, and steroids followed by tacrolimus and a steroid taper. Hepatitis C positive patients administered daclizumab had earlier onset of hepatitis, jaundice, greater histological activity, and a more rapid progression [108]. In contrast, basiliximab, CyA, and steroids, reduced ACR with good safety and tolerability profiles. In a large double-blind randomized placebo-controlled trial, 381 HCV seropositive patients were administered basiliximab (n = 188) or placebo (n = 193) on days 0 and 4, with CyA and steroids. At 6 months, biopsy-confirmed ACR rates were 35% in the basiliximab group compared to 43% in placebo [98]. A single-arm, open-label, multicenter study involving 101 patients following LT (HCV positive n=31; HCV negative n=70) were administered basiliximab on day 0 and 4, with CyA, steroids, and AZT. At 6 months, the incidence of biopsy confirmed ACR was 23%, with more frequent episodes in HCV-positive (29%) than HCV-negative groups (20%) [109].

Pre-emptive analysis of cytokine gene polymorphisms to identify those at risk for HCV recurrence after LT are promising [110,111]. A correlation between transforming growth factor β1 (TGF-β1) gene polymorphism, and the degree of hepatic fibrosis in recipients with recurrent HCV has been demonstrated [112]. Also, HCV genotype determination may predict outcome. Genotype II (1b) and IV appear to be predictors of poor outcome, whereas genotype III is associated with a more favorable outcome [113,114].

Conclusion

Rapid advances in the field of immunosuppression over the last 4 decades have contributed to dramatic improvements in graft and patient survival following LT. Future developments will need to concentrate on tailoring treatment regimens to the individual patient, with the aim of significant dose reduction or complete withdrawal of immunosuppressive agents in the long-term. The potential to develop innovative therapies to enhance natural immunoregulatory mechanisms and create an artificial immune privileged state to protect the transplanted liver allograft holds tremendous promise for the future of transplantation.

References

[1] Busuttil RW, Lake JR: Role of tacrolimus in the evolution of liver transplantation. *Transplantation* 2004, 77:S44-S51.

[2] Furukawa H, Todo S: Evolution of immunosuppression in liver transplantation: contribution of cyclosporine. *Transplant.Proc.* 2004, 36:274S-284S.

[3] Suzuki S: FTY720: mechanisms of action and its effect on organ transplantation (review). *Transplant.Proc.* 1999, 31:2779-2782.

[4] Jin MB, Nakayama M, Ogata T, Fujita M, Mino K, Taniguchi M, Suzuki T, Shimamura T, Furukawa H, Todo S: A novel leflunomide derivative, FK778, for immunosuppression after kidney transplantation in dogs. *Surgery* 2002, 132:72-79.

[5] Galbraith CA, Hathaway D: Long-term effects of transplantation on quality of life. *Transplantation* 2004, 77:S84-S87.

[6] Calne RY: Prope tolerance: the future of organ transplantation--from the laboratory to the clinic. *Transplantation* 2004, 77:930-932.

[7] Pirenne J, Aerts R, Koshiba T, Van Gelder F, Roskams T, Schetz M, Verhaegen M, Lauwers P, Fevery J, Nevens F: Steroid-free immunosuppression during and after liver transplantation--a 3-yr follow-up report. *Clin.Transplant.* 2003, 17:177-182.

[8] Reding R, Gras J, Bourdeaux C, Wieers G, Truong QD, Latinne D, Sokal E, Janssen M, Lerut J, Otte JB, de Ville de GJ: Stepwise minimization of the immunosuppressive therapy in pediatric liver transplantation. A conceptual approach towards operational tolerance. *Acta Gastroenterol.Belg.* 2005, 68:320-322.

[9] Reding R, Gras J, Truong DQ, Wieers G, Latinne D: The immunological monitoring of alloreactive responses in liver transplant recipients: a review. *Liver Transpl.* 2006, 12:373-383.

[10] Starzl TE: Chimerism and tolerance in transplantation. *Proc.Natl.Acad.Sci.U.S.A* 2004.

[11] Medawer PB: The behavior and fate of skin autografts and skin homografts in rabbits. *J Anat* 1944, 78:176.

[12] Calne RY: The rejection of renal homografts. Inhibition in dogs by 6-mercaptopurine. *Lancet* 1960, 1:417-418.

[13] Woodruff MF, Nolan B, Wilson TI, Robson JS, Lambie AT, Clark JG: Homotransplantation of kidney in patients treated by preoperative local irradiation and postoperative administration of an antimetabolite (imuran). Report of six cases. *Lancet* 1963, 186:675-682.

[14] Billingham RE, Krohn PL, Medawer PB: Effect of cortisone on survival of skin homografts in rabbits. *Br.Med.J* 1951, 4716:1157-1163.

[15] Dempster WJ, Lennox B, Boag JW: Prolongation of survival of skin homotransplants in the rabbit by irradiation of the host. *Br.J Exp.Pathol.* 1950, 31:670-679.

[16] Starzl TE, Marchioro TL, Vonkaulla KN, Hermann G, Brittain RS, Waddell WR: Homotransplantation of the liver in humans. *Surg.Gynecol.Obstet.* 1963, 117:659-676.

[17] Starzl TE, Klintmalm GB, PORTER KA, Iwatsuki S, Schroter GP: Liver transplantation with use of cyclosporin and prednisone. *N.Engl.J Med.* 1981, 305:266-269.

[18] Graziadei IW, Wiesner RH, Marotta PJ, Porayko MK, Dahlke LJ, Wilson SM, Steers JL, Krom RA: Neoral compared to Sandimmune is associated with a decrease in histologic severity of rejection in patients undergoing primary liver transplantation. *Transplantation* 1997, 64:726-731.

[19] Gugenheim J, Samuel D, Saliba F, Castaing D, Bismuth H: Use of cyclosporine A in combination with low-dose corticosteroids and azathioprine in liver transplantation. *Transplant.Proc.* 1988, 20:366-368.

[20] Otto MG, Mayer AD, Clavien PA, Cavallari A, Gunawardena KA, Mueller EA: Randomized trial of cyclosporine microemulsion (neoral) versus conventional

cyclosporine in liver transplantation: MILTON study. Multicentre International Study in Liver Transplantation of Neoral. *Transplantation* 1998, 66:1632-1640.

[21] Lepre CA, Thomson JA, Moore JM: Solution structure of FK506 bound to FKBP-12. *FEBS Lett.* 1992, 302:89-96.

[22] A comparison of tacrolimus (FK 506) and cyclosporine for immunosuppression in liver transplantation. The U.S. Multicenter FK506 Liver Study Group. *N.Engl.J Med.* 1994, 331:1110-1115.

[23] Randomised trial comparing tacrolimus (FK506) and cyclosporin in prevention of liver allograft rejection. European FK506 Multicentre Liver Study Group. *Lancet* 1994, 344:423-428.

[24] O'Grady JG, Burroughs A, Hardy P, Elbourne D, Truesdale A: Tacrolimus versus microemulsified ciclosporin in liver transplantation: the TMC randomised controlled trial. *Lancet* 2002, 360:1119-1125.

[25] O'Grady JG, Hardy P, Burroughs AK, Elbourne D: Randomized controlled trial of tacrolimus versus microemulsified cyclosporin (TMC) in liver transplantation: poststudy surveillance to 3 years. *Am.J.Transplant.* 2007, 7:137-141.

[26] Gonzalez-Pinto IM, Rimola A, Margarit C, Cuervas-Mons V, Abradelo M, varez-Laso C, Londono MC, Bilbao I, Sanchez-Turrion V: Five-year follow-up of a trial comparing Tacrolimus and cyclosporine microemulsion in liver transplantation. *Transplant.Proc.* 2005, 37:1713-1715.

[27] Chen JW, Pehlivan M, Gunson BK, Buckels JA, McMaster P, Mayer D: Ten-year results of a randomised prospective study of FK506 versus cyclosporine in management of primary orthotopic liver transplantation. *Transplant.Proc.* 2002, 34:1507-1510.

[28] McAlister VC, Haddad E, Renouf E, Malthaner RA, Kjaer MS, Gluud LL: Cyclosporin versus tacrolimus as primary immunosuppressant after liver transplantation: a meta-analysis. *Am.J.Transplant.* 2006, 6:1578-1585.

[29] Jonas S, Neuhaus R, Junge G, Klupp J, Theruvat T, Langrehr JM, Settmacher U, Neuhaus P: Primary immunosuppression with tacrolimus after liver transplantation: 12-years follow-up. *Int.Immunopharmacol.* 2005, 5:125-128.

[30] Allison AC, Eugui EM: Mycophenolate mofetil and its mechanisms of action. *Immunopharmacology* 2000, 47:85-118.

[31] Kobashigawa J, Miller L, Renlund D, Mentzer R, Alderman E, Bourge R, Costanzo M, Eisen H, Dureau G, Ratkovec R, Hummel M, Ipe D, Johnson J, Keogh A, Mamelok R, Mancini D, Smart F, Valantine H: A randomized active-controlled trial of mycophenolate mofetil in heart transplant recipients. Mycophenolate Mofetil Investigators. *Transplantation* 1998, 66:507-515.

[32] Fisher RA, Ham JM, Marcos A, Shiffman ML, Luketic VA, Kimball PM, Sanyal AJ, Wolfe L, Chodorov A, Posner MP: A prospective randomized trial of mycophenolate mofetil with neoral or tacrolimus after orthotopic liver transplantation. *Transplantation* 1998, 66:1616-1621.

[33] Wiesner R, Rabkin J, Klintmalm G, McDiarmid S, Langnas A, Punch J, McMaster P, Kalayoglu M, Levy G, Freeman R, Bismuth H, Neuhaus P, Mamelok R, Wang W: A randomized double-blind comparative study of mycophenolate mofetil and azathioprine in combination with cyclosporine and corticosteroids in primary liver transplant recipients. *Liver Transpl.* 2001, 7:442-450.

[34] Klupp J, Glanemann M, Bechstein WO, Platz KP, Langrehr JM, Keck H, Settmacher U, Radtke C, Neuhaus R, Neuhaus P: Mycophenolate mofetil in combination with tacrolimus versus Neoral after liver transplantation. *Transplant.Proc.* 1999, 31:1113-1114.

[35] Jain AB, Hamad I, Rakela J, Dodson F, Kramer D, Demetris J, McMichael J, Starzl TE, Fung JJ: A prospective randomized trial of tacrolimus and prednisone versus tacrolimus, prednisone, and mycophenolate mofetil in primary adult liver transplant recipients: an interim report. *Transplantation* 1998, 66:1395-1398.

[36] Langrehr JM, Klupp J, Glanemann M, Junge G, Pfitzmann R, Bahra M, Radtke C, Neumann U, Neuhaus R, Neuhaus P: Long-term results of mycophenolate mofetil as part of immunosuppressive induction therapy after liver transplantation. *Clin.Transplant.* 2006, 20:272-283.

[37] Pfitzmann R, Klupp J, Langrehr JM, Uhl M, Neuhaus R, Settmacher U, Steinmuller T, Neuhaus P: Mycophenolatemofetil for immunosuppression after liver transplantation: a follow-up study of 191 patients. *Transplantation* 2003, 76:130-136.

[38] Raimondo ML, Dagher L, Papatheodoridis GV, Rolando N, Patch DW, Davidson BR, Rolles K, Burroughs AK: Long-term mycophenolate mofetil monotherapy in combination with calcineurin inhibitors for chronic renal dysfunction after liver transplantation. *Transplantation* 2003, 75:186-190.

[39] Barkmann A, Nashan B, Schmidt HH, Boker KH, Emmanouilidis N, Rosenau J, Bahr MJ, Hoffmann MW, Manns MP, Klempnauer J, Schlitt HJ: Improvement of acute and chronic renal dysfunction in liver transplant patients after substitution of calcineurin inhibitors by mycophenolate mofetil. *Transplantation* 2000, 69:1886-1890.

[40] Schlitt HJ, Barkmann A, Boker KH, Schmidt HH, Emmanouilidis N, Rosenau J, Bahr MJ, Tusch G, Manns MP, Nashan B, Klempnauer J: Replacement of calcineurin inhibitors with mycophenolate mofetil in liver-transplant patients with renal dysfunction: a randomised controlled study. *Lancet* 2001, 357:587-591.

[41] Sehgal SN: Sirolimus: its discovery, biological properties, and mechanism of action. *Transplant.Proc.* 2003, 35:7S-14S.

[42] Trotter JF: Sirolimus in liver transplantation. *Transplant.Proc.* 2003, 35:193S-200S.

[43] Dunkelberg JC, Trotter JF, Wachs M, Bak T, Kugelmas M, Steinberg T, Everson GT, Kam I: Sirolimus as primary immunosuppression in liver transplantation is not associated with hepatic artery or wound complications. *Liver Transpl.* 2003, 9:463-468.

[44] McAlister VC, Peltekian KM, Malatjalian DA, Colohan S, MacDonald S, Bitter-Suermann H, MacDonald AS: Orthotopic liver transplantation using low-dose tacrolimus and sirolimus. *Liver Transpl.* 2001, 7:701-708.

[45] Trotter JF, Wachs M, Bak T, Trouillot T, Stolpman N, Everson GT, Kam I: Liver transplantation using sirolimus and minimal corticosteroids (3-day taper). *Liver Transpl.* 2001, 7:343-351.

[46] MacDonald AS: A worldwide, phase III, randomized, controlled, safety and efficacy study of a sirolimus/cyclosporine regimen for prevention of acute rejection in recipients of primary mismatched renal allografts. *Transplantation* 2001, 71:271-280.

[47] Fung J, Marcos A: Rapamycin: friend, foe, or misunderstood? *Liver Transpl.* 2003, 9:469-472.

[48] McAlister VC, Gao Z, Peltekian K, Domingues J, Mahalati K, MacDonald AS: Sirolimus-tacrolimus combination immunosuppression. *Lancet* 2000, 355:376-377.

[49] Neff GW, Ruiz P, Madariaga JR, Nishida S, Montalbano M, Meyer D, Levi DM, Tzakis AG, O'Brien CB: Sirolimus-Associated Hepatotoxicity in Liver Transplantation. *Ann.Pharmacother.* 2004, 38:1593-1596.

[50] Qi S, Xu D, Peng J, Vu MD, Wu J, Bekersky I, Fitzsimmons WE, Peets J, Sehgal S, Daloze P, Chen H: Effect of tacrolimus (FK506) and sirolimus (rapamycin) mono- and combination therapy in prolongation of renal allograft survival in the monkey. *Transplantation* 2000, 69:1275-1283.

[51] Vu MD, Qi S, Xu D, Wu J, Fitzsimmons WE, Sehgal SN, Dumont L, Busque S, Daloze P, Chen H: Tacrolimus (FK506) and sirolimus (rapamycin) in combination are not antagonistic but produce extended graft survival in cardiac transplantation in the rat. *Transplantation* 1997, 64:1853-1856.

[52] Barten MJ, Streit F, Boeger M, Dhein S, Tarnok A, Shipkova M, Armstrong VW, Mohr FW, Oellerich M, Gummert JF: Synergistic effects of sirolimus with cyclosporine and tacrolimus: analysis of immunosuppression on lymphocyte proliferation and activation in rat whole blood. *Transplantation* 2004, 77:1154-1162.

[53] van Mourik ID, Kelly DA: Immunosuppressive drugs in paediatric liver transplantation. *Paediatr.Drugs* 2001, 3:43-60.

[54] Casas-Melley AT, Falkenstein KP, Flynn LM, Ziegler VL, Dunn SP: Improvement in renal function and rejection control in pediatric liver transplant recipients with the introduction of sirolimus. *Pediatr.Transplant.* 2004, 8:362-366.

[55] Fisher RA, Stone JJ, Wolfe LG, Rodgers CM, Anderson ML, Sterling RK, Shiffman ML, Luketic VA, Contos MJ, Mills AS, Ferreira-Gonzalez A, Posner MP: Four-year follow-up of a prospective randomized trial of mycophenolate mofetil with cyclosporine microemulsion or tacrolimus following liver transplantation. *Clin.Transplant.* 2004, 18:463-472.

[56] Glanemann M, Klupp J, Langrehr JM, Platz KP, Schroer G, Raakow R, Stange B, Settmacher U, Bechstein WO, Neuhaus P: Mycophenolate mofetil is superior in combination with tacrolimus compared to cyclosporine for immunosuppressive therapy after liver transplantation. *Transplant.Proc.* 2001, 33:1069-1070.

[57] Koch RO, Graziadei IW, Schulz F, Nachbaur K, Konigsrainer A, Margreiter R, Vogel W: Long-term efficacy and safety of mycophenolate mofetil in liver transplant recipients with calcineurin inhibitor-induced renal dysfunction. *Transpl.Int.* 2004.

[58] Chang GJ, Mahanty HD, Quan D, Freise CE, Ascher NL, Roberts JP, Stock PG, Hirose R: Experience with the use of sirolimus in liver transplantation--use in patients for whom calcineurin inhibitors are contraindicated. *Liver Transpl.* 2000, 6:734-740.

[59] Kniepeiss D, Iberer F, Grasser B, Schaffellner S, Tscheliessnigg KH: Sirolimus and mycophenolate mofetil after liver transplantation. *Transpl.Int.* 2003, 16:504-509.

[60] Neff GW, Montalbano M, Slapak-Green G, Berney T, Bejarano PA, Joshi A, Icardi M, Nery J, Seigo N, Levi D, Weppler D, Pappas P, Ruiz J, Schiff ER, Tzakis AG: A retrospective review of sirolimus (Rapamune) therapy in orthotopic liver transplant recipients diagnosed with chronic rejection. *Liver Transpl.* 2003, 9:477-483.

[61] Papatheodoridis GV, O'Beirne J, Mistry P, Davidson B, Rolles K, Burroughs AK: Mycophenolate mofetil monotherapy in stable liver transplant patients with cyclosporine-induced renal impairment: a preliminary report. *Transplantation* 1999, 68:155-157.

[62] Stewart SF, Hudson M, Talbot D, Manas D, Day CP: Mycophenolate mofetil monotherapy in liver transplantation. *Lancet* 2001, 357:609-610.
[63] Fairbanks KD, Thuluvath PJ: Mycophenolate mofetil monotherapy in liver transplant recipients: A single center experience. *Liver Transpl.* 2004, 10:1189-1194.
[64] Neff GW, Montalbano M, Slapak-Green G, Meyer D, Berney T, Safdar K, Schiff ER, Tzakis AG: Sirolimus therapy in orthotopic liver transplant recipients with calcineurin inhibitor related chronic renal insufficiency. *Transplant.Proc.* 2003, 35:3029-3031.
[65] Fairbanks KD, Eustace JA, Fine D, Thuluvath PJ: Renal function improves in liver transplant recipients when switched from a calcineurin inhibitor to sirolimus. *Liver Transpl.* 2003, 9:1079-1085.
[66] Nair S, Eason J, Loss G: Sirolimus monotherapy in nephrotoxicity due to calcineurin inhibitors in liver transplant recipients. *Liver Transpl.* 2003, 9:126-129.
[67] Everson GT, Trouillot T, Wachs M, Bak T, Steinberg T, Kam I, Shrestha R, Stegall M: Early steroid withdrawal in liver transplantation is safe and beneficial. *Liver Transpl.Surg.* 1999, 5:S48-S57.
[68] Tisone G, Angelico M, Palmieri G, Pisani F, Anselmo A, Baiocchi L, Negrini S, Orlando G, Vennarecci G, Casciani CU: A pilot study on the safety and effectiveness of immunosuppression without prednisone after liver transplantation. *Transplantation* 1999, 67:1308-1313.
[69] Rolles K, Davidson BR, Burroughs AK: A pilot study of immunosuppressive monotherapy in liver transplantation: tacrolimus versus microemulsified cyclosporin. *Transplantation* 1999, 68:1195-1198.
[70] Trotter JF, Wallack A, Steinberg T: Low incidence of cytomegalovirus disease in liver transplant recipients receiving sirolimus primary immunosuppression with 3-day corticosteroid taper. *Transpl.Infect.Dis.* 2003, 5:174-180.
[71] Reding R, Gras J, Sokal E, Otte JB, Davies HF: Steroid-free liver transplantation in children. *Lancet* 2003, 362:2068-2070.
[72] Bourdeaux C, Darwish A, Jamart J, Tri TT, Janssen M, Lerut J, Otte JB, Sokal E, de Ville de GJ, Reding R: Living-related versus deceased donor pediatric liver transplantation: a multivariate analysis of technical and immunological complications in 235 recipients. *Am.J.Transplant.* 2007, 7:440-447.
[73] Reding R: Long-term complications of immunosuppression in pediatric liver recipients. *Acta Gastroenterol.Belg.* 2005, 68:453-456.
[74] Crispe IN, Giannandrea M, Klein I, John B, Sampson B, Wuensch S: Cellular and molecular mechanisms of liver tolerance. *Immunol.Rev.* 2006, 213:101-118.
[75] Shapiro AM, Ricordi C, Hering BJ, Auchincloss H, Lindblad R, Robertson RP, Secchi A, Brendel MD, Berney T, Brennan DC, Cagliero E, Alejandro R, Ryan EA, DiMercurio B, Morel P, Polonsky KS, Reems JA, Bretzel RG, Bertuzzi F, Froud T, Kandaswamy R, Sutherland DE, Eisenbarth G, Segal M, Preiksaitis J, Korbutt GS, Barton FB, Viviano L, Seyfert-Margolis V, Bluestone J, Lakey JR: International trial of the Edmonton protocol for islet transplantation. *N.Engl.J.Med.* 2006, 355:1318-1330.
[76] Matsumoto S, Okitsu T, Iwanaga Y, Noguchi H, Nagata H, Yonekawa Y, Liu X, Kamiya H, Ueda M, Hatanaka N, Kobayashi N, Yamada Y, Miyakawa S, Seino Y, Shapiro AM, Tanaka K: Follow-up study of the first successful living donor islet transplantation. *Transplantation* 2006, 82:1629-1633.

[77] Calne RY, Watson CJ, Brons IG, Makisalo H, Metcalfe SM, Sriwatanawongsa V, Davies HS: Tolerance of porcine renal allografts induced by donor spleen cells and seven days' treatment with cyclosporine. *Transplantation* 1994, 57:1433-1435.

[78] Starzl TE, Murase N: Microchimerism, macrochimerism, and tolerance. *Clin.Transplant.* 2000, 14:351-354.

[79] Fechner JH, Jr., Vargo DJ, Geissler EK, Wang J, Neville DM, Jr., Knechtle SJ: Mechanisms of tolerance induced by an immunotoxin against CD3 epsilon in a rhesus kidney allograft model. *Transplant.Proc.* 1997, 29:1158.

[80] Calne RY: Prope tolerance: a step in the search for tolerance in the clinic. *World J Surg.* 2000, 24:793-796.

[81] Starzl TE, Murase N, Abu-Elmagd K, Gray EA, Shapiro R, Eghtesad B, Corry RJ, Jordan ML, Fontes P, Gayowski T, Bond G, Scantlebury VP, Potdar S, Randhawa P, Wu T, Zeevi A, Nalesnik MA, Woodward J, Marcos A, Trucco M, Demetris AJ, Fung JJ: Tolerogenic immunosuppression for organ transplantation. *Lancet* 2003, 361:1502-1510.

[82] Rao AS, Fontes P, Zeevi A, Trucco M, Dodson FS, Rybka WB, Shapiro R, Jordan M, Pham SM, Rilo HL, .: Augmentation of chimerism in whole organ recipients by simultaneous infusion of donor bone marrow cells. *Transplant.Proc.* 1995, 27:210-212.

[83] Tzakis AG, Tryphonopoulos P, Kato T, Nishida S, Levi DM, Madariaga JR, Gaynor JJ, De Faria W, Regev A, Esquenazi V, Weppler D, Ruiz P, Miller J: Preliminary experience with alemtuzumab (Campath-1H) and low-dose tacrolimus immunosuppression in adult liver transplantation. *Transplantation* 2004, 77:1209-1214.

[84] Tector AJ, Fridell JA, Mangus RS, Shah A, Milgrom M, Kwo P, Chalasani N, Yoo H, Rouch D, Liangpunsakul S, Herring S, Lumeng L: Promising early results with immunosuppression using rabbit anti-thymocyte globulin and steroids with delayed introduction of tacrolimus in adult liver transplant recipients. *Liver Transpl.* 2004, 10:404-407.

[85] Eason JD, Loss GE, Blazek J, Nair S, Mason AL: *Steroid-free liver transplantation using rabbit antithymocyte globulin induction: results of a prospective randomized trial.* 2001, 7:693-697.

[86] Bishop GA, McCaughan GW: Immune activation is required for the induction of liver allograft tolerance: implications for immunosuppressive therapy. *Liver Transpl.* 2001, 7:161-172.

[87] Koshiba T, Van Damme B, Ji P, Lu Y, Sefrioui H, Overbergh L, Tanaka K, Mathieu C, Waer M, Pirenne J: Addition of steroids blocks the tolerogenic potential of donor-specific blood transfusion. *Transplant.Proc.* 2001, 33:375-376.

[88] Eason JD, Nair S, Cohen AJ, Blazek JL, Loss GE, Jr.: Steroid-free liver transplantation using rabbit antithymocyte globulin and early tacrolimus monotherapy. *Transplantation* 2003, 75:1396-1399.

[89] Vincenti F, Nashan B, Light S: Daclizumab: outcome of phase III trials and mechanism of action. Double Therapy and the Triple Therapy Study Groups. *Transplant.Proc.* 1998, 30:2155-2158.

[90] Kovarik JM, Rawlings E, Sweny P, Fernando O, Moore R, Griffin PJ, Fauchald P, Albrechtsen D, Sodal G, Nordal K, Amlot PL: Pharmacokinetics and immunodynamics of chimeric IL-2 receptor monoclonal antibody SDZ CHI 621 in renal allograft recipients. *Transpl.Int.* 1996, 9 Suppl 1:S32-S33.

[91] Kaufman DB, Shapiro R, Lucey MR, Cherikh WS, Bustami T, Dyke DB: Immunosuppression: practice and trends. *Am.J.Transplant.* 2004, 4 Suppl 9:38-53.
[92] Hirose R, Roberts JP, Quan D, Osorio RW, Freise C, Ascher NL, Stock PG: Experience with daclizumab in liver transplantation: renal transplant dosing without calcineurin inhibitors is insufficient to prevent acute rejection in liver transplantation. *Transplantation* 2000, 69:307-311.
[93] Eckhoff DE, McGuire B, Sellers M, Contreras J, Frenette L, Young C, Hudson S, Bynon JS: The safety and efficacy of a two-dose daclizumab (zenapax) induction therapy in liver transplant recipients. *Transplantation* 2000, 69:1867-1872.
[94] Heffron TG, Smallwood GA, de Vera ME, Davis L, Martinez E, Stieber AC: Daclizumab induction in liver transplant recipients. *Transplant.Proc.* 2001, 33:1527.
[95] Emre S, Gondolesi G, Polat K, Ben Haim M, Artis T, Fishbein TM, Sheiner PA, Kim-Schluger L, Schwartz ME, Miller CM: Use of daclizumab as initial immunosuppression in liver transplant recipients with impaired renal function. *Liver Transpl.* 2001, 7:220-225.
[96] Washburn K, Speeg KV, Esterl R, Cigarroa F, Pollack M, Tourtellot C, Maxwell P, Halff G: Steroid elimination 24 hours after liver transplantation using daclizumab, tacrolimus, and mycophenolate mofetil. *Transplantation* 2001, 72:1675-1679.
[97] Figueras J, Bernardos A, Prieto M, Gomez M, Rimola A, Ortiz dU, Cuervas-Mons V, de la MM, Dominguez-Granados R: Steroid-free regimen with daclizumab, mycophenolate mofetil, and tacrolimus in liver transplant recipients. *Transplant.Proc.* 2002, 34:1511-1513.
[98] Neuhaus P, Clavien PA, Kittur D, Salizzoni M, Rimola A, Abeywickrama K, Ortmann E, Chodoff L, Hall M, Korn A, Nashan B: Improved treatment response with basiliximab immunoprophylaxis after liver transplantation: results from a double-blind randomized placebo-controlled trial. *Liver Transpl.* 2002, 8:132-142.
[99] Ganschow R, Lyons M, Grabhorn E, Venzke A, Broering DC, Rogiers X, Hellwege HH, Burdelski M: Experience with basiliximab in pediatric liver graft recipients. *Transplant.Proc.* 2001, 33:3606-3607.
[100] Heffron TG, Pillen T, Smallwood GA, Welch D, Oakley B, Romero R: Pediatric liver transplantation with daclizumab induction. *Transplantation* 2003, 75:2040-2043.
[101] Aw MM, Taylor RM, Verma A, Parke A, Baker AJ, Hadzic D, Muiesan P, Rela M, Heaton ND, Mieli-Vergani G, Dhawan A: Basiliximab (Simulect) for the treatment of steroid-resistant rejection in pediatric liver transpland recipients: a preliminary experience. *Transplantation* 2003, 75:796-799.
[102] Charlton M, Seaberg E: Impact of immunosuppression and acute rejection on recurrence of hepatitis C: results of the National Institute of Diabetes and Digestive and Kidney Diseases Liver Transplantation Database. *Liver Transpl.Surg.* 1999, 5:S107-S114.
[103] Gane EJ, Naoumov NV, Qian KP, Mondelli MU, Maertens G, Portmann BC, Lau JY, Williams R: A longitudinal analysis of hepatitis C virus replication following liver transplantation. *Gastroenterology* 1996, 110:167-177.
[104] Sheiner PA: Hepatitis C after liver transplantation. *Semin.Liver Dis.* 2000, 20:201-209.
[105] Sreekumar R, Gonzalez-Koch A, Maor-Kendler Y, Batts K, Moreno-Luna L, Poterucha J, Burgart L, Wiesner R, Kremers W, Rosen C, Charlton MR: Early identification of

recipients with progressive histologic recurrence of hepatitis C after liver transplantation. *Hepatology* 2000, 32:1125-1130.

[106] Berenguer M, Prieto M, Cordoba J, Rayon JM, Carrasco D, Olaso V, San Juan F, Gobernado M, Mir J, Berenguer J: Early development of chronic active hepatitis in recurrent hepatitis C virus infection after liver transplantation: association with treatment of rejection. *J Hepatol.* 1998, 28:756-763.

[107] Ben Ari Z, Mor E, Bar-Nathan N, Shaharabani E, Shapira Z, Tur-Kaspa R: Comparison of tacrolimus with cyclosporin as primary immunosuppression in patients with hepatitis C virus infection after liver transplantation. *Transplant.Proc.* 2003, 35:612-613.

[108] Nelson DR, Soldevila-Pico C, Reed A, Abdelmalek MF, Hemming AW, Van der Werf WJ, Howard R, Davis GL: Anti-interleukin-2 receptor therapy in combination with mycophenolate mofetil is associated with more severe hepatitis C recurrence after liver transplantation. *Liver Transpl.* 2001, 7:1064-1070.

[109] Calmus Y, Scheele JR, Gonzalez-Pinto I, Jaurrieta EJ, Klar E, Pageaux GP, Scudamore CH, Cuervas-Mons V, Metselaar HJ, Prestele H, Girault D: Immunoprophylaxis with basiliximab, a chimeric anti-interleukin-2 receptor monoclonal antibody, in combination with azathioprine-containing triple therapy in liver transplant recipients. *Liver Transpl.* 2002, 8:123-131.

[110] Ben-Ari Z: Role of cytokine gene polymorphism in recurrent HCV infection after liver transplantation. *Liver Transpl.* 2006, 12:1723-1724.

[111] Kimball P, Baker M, Fisher RA: Allograft TNFbeta and IL16 polymorphisms influence HCV recurrence and severity after liver transplantation. *Liver Transpl.* 2006, 12:247-252.

[112] Ben Ari Z, Pappo O, Druzd T, Sulkes J, Klein T, Samra Z, Gadba R, Tambur AR, Tur-Kaspa R, Mor E: Role of cytokine gene polymorphism and hepatic transforming growth factor beta1 expression in recurrent hepatitis C after liver transplantation. *Cytokine* 2004, 27:7-14.

[113] Gane EJ, Portmann BC, Naoumov NV, Smith HM, Underhill JA, Donaldson PT, Maertens G, Williams R: Long-term outcome of hepatitis C infection after liver transplantation. *N.Engl.J Med.* 1996, 334:815-820.

[114] Zekry A, Whiting P, Crawford DH, Angus PW, Jeffrey GP, Padbury RT, Gane EJ, McCaughan GW: Liver transplantation for HCV-associated liver cirrhosis: predictors of outcomes in a population with significant genotype 3 and 4 distribution. *Liver Transpl.* 2003, 9:339-347.

In: Immunosuppression: New Research
Editor: Charles B. Taylor, pp. 153-166
ISBN: 978-1-60692-102-9

Chapter 6

The Role of Pharmacogenomics in Tailoring Immunosuppressive Therapy for Liver Transplant Recipients

Nyingi Kemmer[1,2,*], *Pankaj B. Desai*[1] *and Guy W. Neff*[1]
[1]University of Cincinnati, USA;
[2]Cincinnati VA Medical Center, USA.

Abstract

Improvements in the field of transplant immunosuppression have led to a dramatic improvement in long-term survival of liver transplant recipients. The art of immunosuppression involves maintaining a fine balance between optimizing efficacy and minimizing adverse effects. Application of pharmacogenomics in immunotherapy has paved the way towards the concept of individualized therapy. Integrating the knowledge from pharmacogenomics technology with individual factors such as ethnicity and etiology of liver disease may achieve our goals of optimizing immunotherapy. This review will discuss the changing landscape of modern immunosuppression and the clinical application of pharmacogenomics in liver transplantation.

Keywords: Pharmacogenomics, Immunosuppression.

Introduction

Since the introduction of liver transplantation in 1960's this life saving procedure has been extended to individuals with end-stage kidney, heart, lung and heart disease with favorable outcomes. Currently, transplantation provides excellent long-term survival for carefully selected patients with end-stage disease of the respective solid organs. Although

* E-mail address: Nyingi.Kemmer@uc.edu. Phone: 513-558-7200; Fax: 513-558-1744; Correspondence concerning this article should be addressed to: Nyingi Kemmer, MD, MPH, Division of Digestive Diseases, University of Cincinnati, 231 Albert Sabin Way, MSB Room 6363, Cincinnati, Ohio 45267-0595.

advances in surgical techniques in the field of organ transplantation have improved in the last two decades, the untoward effects of the currently available immunosuppressive (IS) drugs hamper the overall survival of transplant recipients. The art of immunosuppressive therapy involves maintaining a fine balance between optimizing efficacy and minimizing adverse or untoward effects. These untoward effects of IS therapy are a consequence of the inter-individual differences in drug effectiveness and susceptibility to toxicity among transplant recipients, which inadvertently tilts the balance towards the latter in some recipients

After surgical implantation of donor organ into a recipient, the normal immunologic response is recognition of the donor organ as "foreign" by the recipients T- and B-lymphocyte and this leads to a cascade of events [1]. This adaptive immune response post-implantation involves the release of cytokines that are specifically targeted toward the graft resulting in destruction and rejection of the organ. In liver transplantation, there are three main types of graft rejection, namely: (i) hyperacute or humoral), (ii) acute or cellular and (iii) chronic or ductopenic rejection. Each of these forms of rejection involve the immune system and are capable of progressing to graft loss if identification is delayed and treatment with IS therapy not initiated promptly [2,3]. Thus, the primary goal of IS therapy in liver transplant recipients is to prevent graft rejection.

Differences in IS protocols exist and in general are dependent on the immunologic risk for rejection of the transplanted organ. The immunogenicity of transplanted organ varies and the risk of rejection in the order of increased intensity is lung-heart followed by kidney and then liver. The liver is the least immunogenic and therefore requires the least immune suppression in comparison to the other organs. Current IS regimens for liver transplantation includes an induction and maintenance phase.

Induction Phase

The induction phase is of short duration and typically designed to prevent hyperacute rejection via the humoral arm of the immune response. Immunosuppression during this phase is intensified due to the increased risk of rejection and though there is no standardized induction regimen, most centers utilize biologic agents such as humanized or non-humanized monoclonal or polyclonal antibodies for recipients with high immunologic risk. The existence of inter-individual differences for these biologic agents is yet to be determined, and there is paucity of literature pertaining to individualized therapy with these agents. Since their route of administration is parenteral and the treatment duration during this period is brief, identification of mechanisms responsible for intra or inter-individual differences in efficacy or toxicity is unlikely to translate into a significant improvement in long-term outcome of transplant recipients. Thus utilization of these agents in transplant recipients in relation to pharmacogenomics and individualized therapy is not addressed in this report.

Maintenance Phase

The maintenance phase is the prolonged or life-long treatment period and involves the use of agents that are considered the corner stone of immunosuppressive therapy. During this phase, the goal of IS therapy is to prevent acute and chronic rejection, and at the same time creating a fine balance between optimizing efficacy and minimizing adverse drug reaction.

The IS agents used during this phase include Calcineurin inhibitors (Cyclosporine and Tacrolimus), Antimetabolites (Azathioprine and Mycophenolate mofetil) and the newer Mammalian target of rapamycin (mTOR) inhibitors (Everolimus and Sirolimus). They are used in varying combinations as single, dual or triple therapy combinations with or without corticosteroids. Implementation of pharmacogenomics during this phase is of key interest.

Current Immunosuppressive Drugs

Drug discovery in transplantation therapeutics began in 1978 with the introduction of cyclosporine into the field of immunosuppression. Since its inception, FDA has approved several potent agents with different mechanisms of action for use as anti-rejection medications. The classification of currently used IS drugs (maintenance regimen) according to the mechanism of action are as follows [4-6]:

- Corticosteroids: Prednisone and Prednisolone
- Immunophilin binding agents: Calcineurin inhibitors (cyclosporine and tacrolimus) and mTOR inhibitors (Everolimus and Sirolimus)
- Antimetabolites: Azathioprine and Mycophenolate mofetil

Corticosteroids

Prednisone, is the most commonly used corticosteroid for maintenance therapy It is an inactive pro-drug that is hydrolyzed into prednisolone, its active form. Although it is a key component of IS regimens, its mechanism is not completely understood. In general, they bind to cytosolic glucocorticoid receptors, which initiate a sequence of events that effectively blocks B and T-cell activation thereby inducing a generalized state of lymphopenia. Despite its generalized effect, few cases of glucocorticoid resistance in association with polymorphism of the glucocorticoid receptor gene have been reported. Additional studies are required to confirm this association and its possible clinical implication in transplant recipients.

Antimetabolites

Azathioprine, an imidazoyl derivative of mercaptopurine was the first antimetabolite used as an IS drug in organ transplantation. With the introduction of the newer antimetabolite-mycophenolate mofetil (MMF) as an IS drug, the use of azathioprine has decreased remarkably and currently < 5% of recent transplant recipients are maintained on azathioprine. MMF is the ester pro-drug of mycophenolic acid (MPA), a potent inhibitor of inosine monophosphate dehydrogenase (IMDPH), which is required for de novo guanosine synthesis thus inhibiting lymphocyte proliferation. After oral administration, MMF is hydrolyzed to MPA, which is subsequently metabolized to MPA glucuronide via UDP-glucuronyltransferase (*UDPGT*). After absorption, MPA is converted to the inactive metabolite MPA glucuronide (MPAG) by *UGT1A9*. The MPAG is then converted to its active metabolite AcMPAG predominantly by the hepatic *UGT2B7*. In contrast to the other IS drugs used in maintenance regimens, routine therapeutic drug monitoring (TDM) is not useful for MMF due to the poor correlation between AUC and trough levels [7]. The exact role of genetic polymorphism of *UDPGT* in liver transplant recipients receiving MMF is unknown, and to date there are no published studies addressing this issue.

Immunophilin Binding Agents

The Calcineurin inhibitors (CNI) inhibit Interleukin-2 mediated T-cell activation and proliferation by binding to their respective immunophilin proteins: Cyclophilin (Cyclosporine) and FK-binding protein (Tacrolimus) [1]. After oral administration, the rate of absorption of CNI is regulated by P-glycoprotein (P-gp), a counter-transport protein located in the small intestine brush border. Once the drug is absorbed, subsequent metabolism is primarily by isoenzymes of the cytochrome P450 (*CYP3A*). Sirolimus and Everolimus bind to mTOR via the FK-binding protein, thereby blocking T-cell activation. The mTOR inhibitors have similar pharmacokinetic parameters as the CNI with involvement of P-gp and CYP3A [8]. The immunophilin binding agents have a narrow therapeutic index and exhibit highly variable pharmacokinetics, thus routine TDM is essential.

Despite aggressive TDM with adequate trough levels some recipients experience adverse effects, suggesting that there are other factors that play a role in the inter-individual differences in pharmacokinetic parameters. One of the factors implicated in the observed inter-individual variability is genetic polymorphism of the drug transport proteins and the drug metabolism enzymes. Therefore, understanding the relationship between genetic polymorphism and therapeutic outcomes of IS therapy is of great importance.

In recent years, better understanding of the efficacy and toxicity profile of the various IS drugs has led to a change in prescription pattern at transplant centers in United States. The IS drugs of liver transplant recipients in the United States is captured in the Scientific Registry of Transplantation Recipients (SRTR). Based on the SRTR, in 1998 the most common maintenance regimens at 2-year post transplantation was tacrolimus monotherapy (29.1%) followed by tacrolimus and prednisone (23.8%), cyclosporine and prednisone (10.3%), cyclosporine monotherapy (6.8%) in contrast to 2003, in which tacrolimus monotherapy accounted for 37.9%, tacrolimus and mycophenolate mofetil (16%), tacrolimus and prednisone (13.8%) and triple therapy with tacrolimus, mycophenolate mofetil and prednisone in (9.4%) [9]. This trend reflects a changing landscape in transplantation therapeutics in response to the noted imbalance between toxicity and efficacy of IS drugs as well as the additive/synergistic effect of the various drug combinations.

This change in drug utilization pattern by transplant centers does not take into consideration the existing inter-individual differences but focuses on the 'one-size fits all concept' of pharmacotherapy. Thus, although the current IS drugs have led to a dramatic decrease in the incidence of graft rejection, their long-term use in some recipients contributes immensely to morbidity associated with liver transplantation. Therefore understanding the role of genomics and drug metabolism enzymes in the mechanisms underlying the individual differences in drug efficacy and toxicity is the focus of this report.

Pharmacogenomics and Drug Metabolism

A key role of pharmacogenomics is the application of genetic information in the clinical decision involved in appropriate selection of drug therapy. Therefore the identified genetic variations in the main drug metabolism enzymes and drug transporters that are associated with IS drugs are reviewed below.

The cytochrome P450 (CYP450) enzymes are involved in 75% of phase I-dependent drug metabolism [10]. In the classification scheme of the CYP450 enzymes, a family number, a subfamily letter and a number for an individual enzyme within the subfamily designates each individually. To date there are 50 identified CYP450 enzymes, and of these *CYP3A4*, *CYP3A5*, *CYP2D6*, *CYP2C19* and *CYP2C9* enzymes are involved with the metabolism of 90% of all currently marketed drugs [11]. Genetic polymorphisms of CYP450 enzymes have been implicated in the development of a significant number of adverse drug reactions and non-responsiveness to therapy [12].

The drug transport proteins (DTP) facilitate the movement of drugs across cell membranes. There are two main families of DTP, namely those involved in passive process (solute linked carrier) and those involved in active transport (e.g. P-glycoprotein) [13]. The P-glycoprotein (P-gp), a product of the multidrug resistance gene (MDR1) is involved in the transportation of the Calcineurin and mTOR inhibitors at the cellular level by acting as an efflux pump. The functional importance and impact of genetic polymorphism of the CYP450 and MDR1 (also known as *ABCB1* gene) in the metabolism of immunosuppressive medications specifically in liver transplant recipients is not clearly understood.

In addition to MDR1 and the CYP450 enzymes, another important enzyme involved in metabolism of immunosuppressive drugs is the UDP-glucoronosyl transferases (*UDP-GT*), which are typically involved in phase II dependent drug metabolism [14]. The *UDP-GT* enzymes have not been extensively investigated in relation to IS drug metabolism. Additional studies to elucidate the importance of genetic polymorphism of *UDP-GT* enzymes and its clinical application in liver transplant recipients are warranted.

Genetic Polymorphism and Immunosuppressive Drugs

The current immunosuppressive drugs in use for liver transplantation have narrow therapeutic windows with wide inter-individual variations in PK parameters. These variations have led to deleterious clinical outcomes ranging from allograft rejection to long-term drug-specific adverse effect such as nephrotoxicity, hypertension and new-onset Diabetes Mellitus after transplantation (NODAT). To date TDM is the only tool in use as a surrogate marker for PK parameters of IS drugs. Despite our experience with TDM, its limited utility in drugs with narrow therapeutic index hampers its reliability and predictive capability. Therefore, to optimize IS therapy and decrease the related adverse effects additional tools to supplement TDM are desirable. Since drug metabolism is a key determinant of the observed interindividual variability in PK parameters, understanding the therapeutic implications of genetic polymorphism of the CYP450 enzymes and transport proteins involved in IS drug metabolism is invaluable information. In a meta-analysis by Phillips et al, the investigators found a high association between polymorphic CYP450 genes and the occurrence of adverse drug reactions [15]. Though this study was not specifically designed to evaluate IS drugs, the findings provide a rationale for the utilization of PG as a predictive tool in liver transplant recipients receiving immunosuppressive therapy.

Multidrug Resistance Gene (MDR1)

Several SNP's of the MDR1 gene have been identified and found to play a role in the metabolism of the Calcineurin inhibitors. The three most common that have been studied extensively are located in exon 12 (*C1236T*), exon 21 (*G2677T/A*), exon 26 (*C3435T*) and promoter region (*T-129-C*) [16-18]. Similar to the SNP's of *CYP3A*, there is an ethnic variation in frequency of occurrence and it is present in 15% of individuals of African descent and 40-60% in Caucasians and Asians [19]. Clinical studies evaluating the effect of SNP of MDR1 gene have not shown a consistent alteration of PK parameters in recipients taking Tacrolimus, Cyclosporine or Sirolimus.

Cytochrome P450 3A Enzymes

The contribution of *CYP3A4* and *CYP3A5* to the metabolism of the Calcineurin inhibitors has been widely studied. Although, single nucleotide polymorphism in the *CYP3A4* gene is uncommon, *CYP3A4*1*, *CYP3A4*1B* and *CYP3A4*3* have been identified in its promotor region [8]. Of these, *CYP3A4*1B* is the most frequent and has been extensively studied in relation to immunosuppressive therapy. The *CYP3A4*1B* is common in individuals of African descent (35-67%), relatively infrequent in Caucasians (2-9%) and absent in Asians [20]. The SNP's identified in the CYP3A5 gene (*CYP3A5*1, CYP3A5*3 and CYP3A5*6*), have also been investigated in clinical trials and found to occur in varying frequencies that are dependent on the ethnic population. The *CYP3A5*1* is the most common, with a prevalence of 55% in African Americans, 10-40% in Caucasians and 33% in those of Asian ethnicity [20].

CYP3A4 Genotype

Although in vitro studies have shown increase in *CYP3A4* gene transcription in those with SNP in the promotor region, in vivo studies have failed to support these findings showing no alterations in the metabolism of its substrates such as Calcineurin and mTOR inhibitor. To date, the published studies on genetic polymorphism of *CYP3A4* gene (*CYP3A4*1, CYP3A4*1B and CYP3A4*3*) in transplant recipients receiving tacrolimus; cyclosporine and sirolimus have failed to identify an association with the PK parameters obtained [21-24]. The exact reason for the discrepancy in the findings of the in vitro and in vivo studies is unclear. Based on these findings, the currently identified SNP's of *CYP3A4* gene are not useful as predictive tools for liver transplant recipients on immunosuppressive therapy.

CYP3A5 Genotype

In contrary, to the reports in reference to *CYP3A4* gene polymorphism, there is accumulating evidence suggesting an association between Tacrolimus, Sirolimus and *CYP3A5* gene [25]. There is so far, no convincing evidence linking SNP of *CYP3A5* gene to Cyclosporine [21,26,27]. The clinical observations from several studies have confirmed the association between *CYP3A5* expression and altered PK parameters consistent with higher clearance and lower trough levels for a given Tacrolimus dose [28-30]. Additionally, the tacrolimus trough level is lower in recipients with *CYP3A5*1* in comparison to those with *CYP3A5*3* genotype, translating to a 2.3 fold difference in dose requirement [31]. Regarding Sirolimus, alterations in PK parameters that are similar to that described with Tacrolimus have been reported. Accordingly, lower trough levels of sirolimus are reported in recipients with *CYP3A5* expressers in comparison to non-expressers [32]. If these findings are confirmed in large randomized controlled prospective trials, the presence of *CYP3A5* polymorphism will be a useful pre-transplant risk-stratification tool, as it will aid dose selection and pave the way towards individualized therapy.

Limitations of Clinical application of Pharmacogenomics

On the basis of these studies focusing on drug metabolism enzymes, the *CYP3A5* genotype appears to be the most promising candidate for pharmacogenetic-guided dose selection for recipients receiving tacrolimus based therapy. Implementation and integration of PG technology into routine clinical practice requires an understanding of the limitations of this strategy. Several factors present unique challenges that impede reliable interpretation and application in the liver transplant recipient. Firstly, the ethnic variation in *CYP3A5* genotype independently adds to the complexity of its clinical application in an ethnically diverse population. Secondly, the impact of donor genotype on tacrolimus metabolism though not fully understood further complicates PG application and the logistics of obtaining urgent donor genotype prior to liver transplantation [29]. Thirdly the ethical, social, cultural, and economic implications of genetic profiling are real issues that deserve further investigation prior to its acceptance among medical and non-medical professionals [33-35]. Thus, though the overall expectation of PG application in clinical practice is to shift medical care from *"trial-and-error"* and *"one-size-fits-all"* to personalized or individualized therapy, failure to address and understand the factors outlined above will to a great extent hinder its success as well as its wide spread acceptance in the transplant community.

The limitations of PG application into clinical practice today, raises the issue of the role of alternate strategies that take into consideration non-genetic factors such as liver disease etiology. Several clinical studies have identified liver disease etiology as an independent predictor of long-term survival post transplantation [36]. In particular, among liver transplant recipients; those with underling Hepatitis C have a lower survival in comparison to non-HCV recipients [37]. Since Hepatitis C (HCV) and its sequelae Hepatocellular Carcinoma (HCC) are the most frequent indications for liver transplantation, immunosuppressive strategies that will influence individual patient outcome in relation to these disease entities are important

[38,39]. Additionally, with the improving survival of Human Immunodeficiency virus (HIV) infected individuals in the HAART era, end-stage liver disease has emerged as a significant cause of morbidity and mortality in HCV-HIV co-infected individuals [40]. Thus, the demand for liver transplantation in these individuals is on the rise, and tailoring IS therapy is critical given their immunocompromised state and anticipated drug-drug interaction.

Hepatitis C

Though there is no definite or direct correlation between immunosuppression and HCV and/or HCV recurrence, several studies have suggested that the type and intensity of IS in relation to the timing post-transplantation influences recipient outcomes. The impact of corticosteroids on severity and rate of progression of HCV recurrence has been extensively investigated. Despite the lack of consensus on the optimal or preferred protocol, the following findings have been reported: (i) steroid boluses increase HCV viremia (ii) slow taper is better than abrupt or rapid tapering of steroids (iii) steroid free protocols appear to have no beneficial impact in comparison to steroid based protocols [41-44]. The role of MMF as an antiviral agent has been controversial with conflicting results from different studies [45-48]. In the case of Calcineurin inhibitors, while cyclosporine has been found to have potent antiviral effect in HCV replicon models, published studies have found no clinically significant difference between Tacrolimus and Cyclosporine [49-54]. In a North American survey study of liver transplant centers, Khalili et al found a change in clinical practice in relation to IS utilization for HCV recipients [55]. In particular, they report a trend towards tapering prednisone dose to 5mg/d or less at 3 months post-transplant from 36% in 1998 to 67% in 2003. Thus in North American transplant centers, individualized IS therapy for HCV recipients is increasing though its impact on long-term patient and graft survival is yet to be determined.

Hepatocellular Carcinoma

Among recipients with a pre-transplant diagnosis of HCC, the concern of tumor recurrence has been the subject of great debate. Aggressive IS therapy is known to be associated with tumor recurrence in non-transplant settings. Translation of this clinical information to the transplant recipient has led to attempts geared towards tailoring IS therapy for these recipients with the goal of modifying their post-transplant course. In recent years, there has been a growing interest in the role of Sirolimus-based IS therapy in recipients with pre-transplant HCC. Sirolimus has been shown both *in vivo* and *in vitro* studies to inhibit HCC tumor cell lines presumably due to its known anti-proliferative effect [56]. Despite the findings of the pre-clinical studies, the role of Sirolimus in decreasing tumor recurrence or improving disease-free survival is yet to be determined [57].

Human Immunodeficiency Virus

Immunosuppressive therapy in the HIV infected transplant recipient on antiretroviral therapy is complicated by the altered pharmacokinetic parameters that are a direct consequence of similar metabolic pathway via the cytochrome P450 system [58]. The most commonly used antiretroviral therapies used in HIV therapeutics include protease inhibitors, nonnucleoside reverse transcriptase inhibitors (NNRTI) and nucleoside reverse transcriptase inhibitors (NRTI). The protease inhibitors (PI) are substrates of the CYP3A enzymes while the NNRTI are inducers and thus have a propensity to decrease or increase drug metabolism respectively. Thus recipients receiving concomitant PI have a 3-fold to 7-fold increase in AUC of cyclosporine and tacrolimus respectively, necessitating a 50-85% reduction in dose with accompanying increase in dosing interval [59,60]. For those using concomitant NNRTI in particular efavirenz, the reverse effect occurs due to its inducer role, and a corresponding higher dose of cyclosporine and tacrolimus is required to maintain non-toxic trough levels. In contrary to PI and NNRTI, the NRTI are excreted via the renal system and have no interaction with the CYP450 enzymes. Thus in general, liver transplant recipients on PI require lower doses while those on NRTI need higher doses of Calcineurin inhibitors. Due to the complexity of the drug-drug interactions in the HIV infected recipient, aggressive therapeutic drug monitoring is crucial in order to optimize therapy and maintain a fine balance between efficacy and toxicity.

Conclusion

Immune suppression has transcended over the last four decades with introduction of Calcineurin inhibitors and steroid therapy. Several agents have entered the field of post liver transplantation through research yet have not impacted the field in the same level as the Calcineurin inhibitors. Efforts geared towards chimerism and immune tolerance are ongoing but are yet to impact the clinical practice of transplantation medicine. Thus to achieve the goal of improving long-term outcome of liver transplant recipients, genetic and non-genetic factors have to be addressed and evaluated in large prospective clinical studies. Inclusion of genomic studies from the outset and adequate representation of all ethnic groups in sufficient sample size will serve, as the first step towards the realization of personalized therapy.

References

[1] Rosen HR (2008) Transplantation immunology: what the clinician needs to know for immunotherapy. *Gastroenterology* **134**: 1789-1801. DOI S0016-5085(08)00300-4 [pii] 10.1053/j.gastro.2008.02.062

[2] Wiesner RH, Batts KP, Krom RA (1999) Evolving concepts in the diagnosis, pathogenesis, and treatment of chronic hepatic allograft rejection. *Liver Transpl Surg* **5:** 388-400. DOI S1527646599000830 [pii] 10.1002/lt.500050519

[3] Eksteen B, Neuberger JM (2008) Mechanisms of Disease: the evolving understanding of liver allograft rejection. *Nat Clin Pract Gastroenterol Hepatol* **5:** 209-219. DOI ncpgasthep1070 [pii] 10.1038/ncpgasthep1070

[4] Danesi R, Mosca M, Boggi U, Mosca F, Del Tacca M (2000) Genetics of drug response to immunosuppressive treatment and prospects for personalized therapy. *Mol Med Today* **6:** 475-482. DOI S1357431000018220 [pii]

[5] Post DJ, Douglas DD, Mulligan DC (2005) Immunosuppression in liver transplantation. *Liver Transpl* **11**: 1307-1314. DOI 10.1002/lt.20614

[6] Gaston RS (2006) Current and evolving immunosuppressive regimens in kidney transplantation. *Am J Kidney Dis* **47**: S3-21. DOI S0272-6386(06)00017-5 [pii] 10.1053/j.ajkd.2005.12.047

[7] Arns W, Cibrik DM, Walker RG, Mourad G, Budde K, Mueller EA, Vincenti F (2006) Therapeutic drug monitoring of mycophenolic acid in solid organ transplant patients treated with mycophenolate mofetil: review of the literature. *Transplantation* **82**: 1004-1012. DOI 10.1097/01.tp.0000232697.38021.9a 00007890-200610270-00002 [pii]

[8] Anglicheau D, Legendre C, Beaune P, Thervet E (2007) Cytochrome P450 3A polymorphisms and immunosuppressive drugs: an update. *Pharmacogenomics* **8**: 835-849. DOI 10.2217/14622416.8.7.835

[9] www.unos.org

[10] Lynch T, Price A (2007) The effect of cytochrome P450 metabolism on drug response, interactions, and adverse effects. *Am Fam Physician* **76**: 391-396

[11] Wojnowski L (2004) Genetics of the variable expression of CYP3A in humans. *Ther Drug Monit* **26**: 192-199

[12] Hustert E, Haberl M, Burk O, Wolbold R, He YQ, Klein K, Nuessler AC, Neuhaus P, Klattig J, Eiselt R, Koch I, Zibat A, Brockmoller J, Halpert JR, Zanger UM, Wojnowski L (2001) The genetic determinants of the CYP3A5 polymorphism. *Pharmacogenetics* **11**: 773-779

[13] Sakaeda T, Nakamura T, Okumura K (2004) Pharmacogenetics of drug transporters and its impact on the pharmacotherapy. *Curr Top Med Chem* **4**: 1385-1398

[14] Picard N, Ratanasavanh D, Premaud A, Le Meur Y, Marquet P (2005) Identification of the UDP-glucuronosyltransferase isoforms involved in mycophenolic acid phase II metabolism. *Drug Metab Dispos* **33**: 139-146. DOI dmd.104.001651 [pii] 10.1124/dmd.104.001651

[15] Phillips KA, Veenstra DL, Oren E, Lee JK, Sadee W (2001) Potential role of pharmacogenomics in reducing adverse drug reactions: a systematic review. *JAMA* **286**: 2270-2279. DOI jrv10032 [pii]

[16] Marzolini C, Paus E, Buclin T, Kim RB (2004) Polymorphisms in human MDR1 (P-glycoprotein): recent advances and clinical relevance. *Clin Pharmacol Ther* **75**: 13-33. DOI 10.1016/j.clpt.2003.09.012 S0009923603003011 [pii]

[17] Sakaeda T, Nakamura T, Okumura K (2003) Pharmacogenetics of MDR1 and its impact on the pharmacokinetics and pharmacodynamics of drugs. *Pharmacogenomics* **4**: 397-410. DOI PGS040408 [pii] 10.1517/phgs.4.4.397.22747

[18] Song P, Li S, Meibohm B, Gaber AO, Honaker MR, Kotb M, Yates CR (2002) Detection of MDR1 single nucleotide polymorphisms C3435T and G2677T using real-time polymerase chain reaction: MDR1 single nucleotide polymorphism genotyping assay. *AAPS PharmSci* **4**: E29. DOI 10.1208/ps040429

[19] Ameyaw MM, Regateiro F, Li T, Liu X, Tariq M, Mobarek A, Thornton N, Folayan GO, Githang'a J, Indalo A, Ofori-Adjei D, Price-Evans DA, McLeod HL (2001) MDR1 pharmacogenetics: frequency of the C3435T mutation in exon 26 is significantly influenced by ethnicity. *Pharmacogenetics* **11**: 217-221

[20] Lamba JK, Lin YS, Schuetz EG, Thummel KE (2002) Genetic contribution to variable human CYP3A-mediated metabolism. *Adv Drug Deliv Rev* **54**: 1271-1294. DOI S0169409X02000662 [pii]

[21] Hesselink DA, van Schaik RH, van der Heiden IP, van der Werf M, Gregoor PJ, Lindemans J, Weimar W, van Gelder T (2003) Genetic polymorphisms of the CYP3A4, CYP3A5, and MDR-1 genes and pharmacokinetics of the calcineurin inhibitors cyclosporine and tacrolimus. *Clin Pharmacol Ther* **74**: 245-254. DOI 10.1016/S0009-9236(03)00168-1 S0009923603001681 [pii]

[22] Roy JN, Barama A, Poirier C, Vinet B, Roger M (2006) Cyp3A4, Cyp3A5, and MDR-1 genetic influences on tacrolimus pharmacokinetics in renal transplant recipients. *Pharmacogenet Genomics* **16**: 659-665. DOI 10.1097/01.fpc.0000220571.20961.dd 01213011-200609000-00005 [pii]

[23] von Ahsen N, Richter M, Grupp C, Ringe B, Oellerich M, Armstrong VW (2001) No influence of the MDR-1 C3435T polymorphism or a CYP3A4 promoter polymorphism (CYP3A4-V allele) on dose-adjusted cyclosporin A trough concentrations or rejection incidence in stable renal transplant recipients. *Clin Chem* **47**: 1048-1052

[24] Rivory LP, Qin H, Clarke SJ, Eris J, Duggin G, Ray E, Trent RJ, Bishop JF (2000) Frequency of cytochrome P450 3A4 variant genotype in transplant population and lack of association with cyclosporin clearance. *Eur J Clin Pharmacol* **56**: 395-398

[25] MacPhee IA, Holt DW (2008) A pharmacogenetic strategy for immunosuppression based on the CYP3A5 genotype. *Transplantation* **85**: 163-165. DOI 10.1097/TP.0b013e3181609054 00007890-200801270-00001 [pii]

[26] Haufroid V, Mourad M, Van Kerckhove V, Wawrzyniak J, De Meyer M, Eddour DC, Malaise J, Lison D, Squifflet JP, Wallemacq P (2004) The effect of CYP3A5 and MDR1 (ABCB1) polymorphisms on cyclosporine and tacrolimus dose requirements and trough blood levels in stable renal transplant patients. *Pharmacogenetics* **14**: 147-154. DOI 00008571-200403000-00002 [pii]

[27] Zhao Y, Song M, Guan D, Bi S, Meng J, Li Q, Wang W (2005) Genetic polymorphisms of CYP3A5 genes and concentration of the cyclosporine and tacrolimus. *Transplant Proc* **37**: 178-181. DOI S0041-1345(05)00106-5 [pii] 10.1016/j.transproceed.2005.01.077

[28] Goto M, Masuda S, Kiuchi T, Ogura Y, Oike F, Okuda M, Tanaka K, Inui K (2004) CYP3A5*1-carrying graft liver reduces the concentration/oral dose ratio of tacrolimus in recipients of living-donor liver transplantation. *Pharmacogenetics* **14**: 471-478. DOI 00008571-200407000-00010 [pii]

[29] Wei-lin W, Jing J, Shu-sen Z, Li-hua W, Ting-bo L, Song-feng Y, Sheng Y (2006) Tacrolimus dose requirement in relation to donor and recipient ABCB1 and CYP3A5 gene polymorphisms in Chinese liver transplant patients. *Liver Transpl* **12**: 775-780. DOI 10.1002/lt.20709

[30] Uesugi M, Masuda S, Katsura T, Oike F, Takada Y, Inui K (2006) Effect of intestinal CYP3A5 on postoperative tacrolimus trough levels in living-donor liver transplant recipients. *Pharmacogenet Genomics* **16**: 119-127. DOI 01213011-200602000-00006 [pii]

[31] MacPhee IA, Fredericks S, Tai T, Syrris P, Carter ND, Johnston A, Goldberg L, Holt DW (2004) The influence of pharmacogenetics on the time to achieve target tacrolimus

concentrations after kidney transplantation. *Am J Transplant* **4:** 914-919. DOI 10.1111/j.1600-6143.2004.00435.x AJT435 [pii]

[32] Anglicheau D, Le Corre D, Lechaton S, Laurent-Puig P, Kreis H, Beaune P, Legendre C, Thervet E (2005) Consequences of genetic polymorphisms for sirolimus requirements after renal transplant in patients on primary sirolimus therapy. *Am J Transplant* **5**: 595-603. DOI AJT745 [pii] 10.1111/j.1600-6143.2005.00745.x

[33] van Delden J, Bolt I, Kalis A, Derijks J, Leufkens H (2004) Tailor-made pharmacotherapy: future developments and ethical challenges in the field of pharmacogenomics. *Bioethics* **18**: 303-321

[34] Norbert PW, Roses AD (2003) Pharmacogenetics and pharmacogenomics: recent developments, their clinical relevance and some ethical, social, and legal implications. *J Mol Med* **81**: 135-140

[35] Paul NW, Fangerau H (2006) Why should we bother? Ethical and social issues in individualized medicine. *Curr Drug Targets* **7**: 1721-1727

[36] Roberts MS, Angus DC, Bryce CL, Valenta Z, Weissfeld L (2004) Survival after liver transplantation in the United States: a disease-specific analysis of the UNOS database. *Liver Transpl* **10**: 886-897. DOI 10.1002/lt.20137

[37] Forman LM, Lewis JD, Berlin JA, Feldman HI, Lucey MR (2002) The association between hepatitis C infection and survival after orthotopic liver transplantation. *Gastroenterology* **122**: 889-896. DOI S0016508502603853 [pii]

[38] O'Leary JG, Lepe R, Davis GL (2008) Indications for liver transplantation. *Gastroenterology* **134**: 1764-1776. DOI S0016-5085(08)00258-8 [pii] 10.1053/j.gastro.2008.02.028

[39] Murray KF, Carithers RL, Jr. (2005) AASLD practice guidelines: Evaluation of the patient for liver transplantation. *Hepatology* **41**: 1407-1432. DOI 10.1002/hep.20704

[40] Samuel D, Weber R, Stock P, Duclos-Vallee JC, Terrault N (2008) Are HIV-infected patients candidates for liver transplantation? *J Hepatol* **48**: 697-707. DOI S0168-8278(08)00128-1 [pii] 10.1016/j.jhep.2008.02.009

[41] Segev DL, Sozio SM, Shin EJ, Nazarian SM, Nathan H, Thuluvath PJ, Montgomery RA, Cameron AM, Maley WR (2008) Steroid avoidance in liver transplantation: meta-analysis and meta-regression of randomized trials. *Liver Transpl* **14**: 512-525. DOI 10.1002/lt.21396

[42] Vivarelli M, Burra P, Barba GL, Canova D, Senzolo M, Cucchetti A, D'Errico A, Guido M, Merenda R, Neri D, Zanello M, Giannini FM, Grazi GL, Cillo U, Pinna AD (2007) Influence of steroids on HCV recurrence after liver transplantation: A prospective study. *J Hepatol* **47**: 793-798. DOI S0168-8278(07)00474-6 [pii] 10.1016/j.jhep.2007.07.023

[43] Klintmalm GB, Washburn WK, Rudich SM, Heffron TG, Teperman LW, Fasola C, Eckhoff DE, Netto GJ, Katz E (2007) Corticosteroid-free immunosuppression with daclizumab in HCV(+) liver transplant recipients: 1-year interim results of the HCV-3 study. *Liver Transpl* **13**: 1521-1531. DOI 10.1002/lt.21182

[44] Berenguer M, Aguilera V, Prieto M, San Juan F, Rayon JM, Benlloch S, Berenguer J (2006) Significant improvement in the outcome of HCV-infected transplant recipients by avoiding rapid steroid tapering and potent induction immunosuppression. *J Hepatol* **44**: 717-722. DOI S0168-8278(06)00021-3 [pii] 10.1016/j.jhep.2006.01.005

[45] Firpi RJ, Nelson DR, Davis GL (2003) Lack of antiviral effect of a short course of mycophenolate mofetil in patients with chronic hepatitis C virus infection. *Liver Transpl* **9**: 57-61. DOI 10.1053/jlts.2003.50003

[46] Wiesner RH, Shorr JS, Steffen BJ, Chu AH, Gordon RD, Lake JR (2005) Mycophenolate mofetil combination therapy improves long-term outcomes after liver transplantation in patients with and without hepatitis C. *Liver Transpl* **11**: 750-759. DOI 10.1002/lt.20453

[47] Henry SD, Metselaar HJ, Lonsdale RC, Kok A, Haagmans BL, Tilanus HW, van der Laan LJ (2006) Mycophenolic acid inhibits hepatitis C virus replication and acts in synergy with cyclosporin A and interferon-alpha. *Gastroenterology* **131**: 1452-1462. DOI S0016-5085(06)01786-0 [pii] 10.1053/j.gastro.2006.08.027

[48] Jain A, Kashyap R, Demetris AJ, Eghstesad B, Pokharna R, Fung JJ (2002) A prospective randomized trial of mycophenolate mofetil in liver transplant recipients with hepatitis C. *Liver Transpl* **8**: 40-46. DOI S1527646502733327 [pii] 10.1053/jlts.2002.29763

[49] Berenguer M, Royuela A, Zamora J (2007) Immunosuppression with calcineurin inhibitors with respect to the outcome of HCV recurrence after liver transplantation: results of a meta-analysis. *Liver Transpl* **13**: 21-29. DOI 10.1002/lt.21035

[50] Firpi RJ, Zhu H, Morelli G, Abdelmalek MF, Soldevila-Pico C, Machicao VI, Cabrera R, Reed AI, Liu C, Nelson DR (2006) Cyclosporine suppresses hepatitis C virus in vitro and increases the chance of a sustained virological response after liver transplantation. *Liver Transpl* **12**: 51-57. DOI 10.1002/lt.20532

[51] Berenguer M, Aguilera V, Prieto M, San Juan F, Rayon JM, Benlloch S, Berenguer J (2006) Effect of calcineurin inhibitors on survival and histologic disease severity in HCV-infected liver transplant recipients. *Liver Transpl* **12**: 762-767. DOI 10.1002/lt.20655

[52] Margarit C, Bilbao I, Castells L, Lopez I, Pou L, Allende E, Escartin A (2005) A prospective randomized trial comparing tacrolimus and steroids with tacrolimus monotherapy in liver transplantation: the impact on recurrence of hepatitis C. *Transpl Int* **18**: 1336-1345. DOI TRI217 [pii] 10.1111/j.1432-2277.2005.00217.x

[53] Martin P, Busuttil RW, Goldstein RM, Crippin JS, Klintmalm GB, Fitzsimmons WE, Uleman C (2004) Impact of tacrolimus versus cyclosporine in hepatitis C virus-infected liver transplant recipients on recurrent hepatitis: a prospective, randomized trial. *Liver Transpl* **10**: 1258-1262. DOI 10.1002/lt.20222

[54] Watashi K, Hijikata M, Hosaka M, Yamaji M, Shimotohno K (2003) Cyclosporin A suppresses replication of hepatitis C virus genome in cultured hepatocytes. *Hepatology* **38**: 1282-1288. DOI 10.1053/jhep.2003.50449 S0270913903008322 [pii]

[55] Khalili M, Vardanian AJ, Hamerski CM, Wang R, Bacchetti P, Roberts JP, Terrault NA (2006) Management of hepatitis C-infected liver transplant recipients at large North American centres: changes in recent years. *Clin Transplant* **20**: 1-9. DOI CTR449 [pii] 10.1111/j.1399-0012.2005.00449.x

[56] Zhang JF, Liu JJ, Lu MQ, Cai CJ, Yang Y, Li H, Xu C, Chen GH (2007) Rapamycin inhibits cell growth by induction of apoptosis on hepatocellular carcinoma cells in vitro. *Transpl Immunol* **17**: 162-168. DOI S0966-3274(06)00203-6 [pii] 10.1016/j.trim.2006.12.003

[57] Zimmerman MA, Trotter JF, Wachs M, Bak T, Campsen J, Skibba A, Kam I (2008) Sirolimus-based immunosuppression following liver transplantation for hepatocellular carcinoma. *Liver Transpl* **14**: 633-638. DOI 10.1002/lt.21420

[58] Izzedine H, Launay-Vacher V, Baumelou A, Deray G (2004) Antiretroviral and immunosuppressive drug-drug interactions: an update. *Kidney Int* **66**: 532-541. DOI 10.1111/j.1523-1755.2004.00772.x KID772 [pii]

[59] Teicher E, Vincent I, Bonhomme-Faivre L, Abbara C, Barrail A, Boissonnas A, Duclos-Vallee JC, Taburet AM, Samuel D, Vittecoq D (2007) Effect of highly active antiretroviral therapy on tacrolimus pharmacokinetics in hepatitis C virus and HIV co-infected liver transplant recipients in the ANRS HC-08 study. *Clin Pharmacokinet* **46**: 941-952. DOI 46112 [pii]

[60] Frassetto LA, Browne M, Cheng A, Wolfe AR, Roland ME, Stock PG, Carlson L, Benet LZ (2007) Immunosuppressant pharmacokinetics and dosing modifications in HIV-1 infected liver and kidney transplant recipients. *Am J Transplant* **7**: 2816-2820. DOI AJT2007 [pii] 10.1111/j.1600-6143.2007.02007.x

In: Immunosuppression: New Research
Editor: Charles B. Taylor, pp. 167-183

ISBN: 978-1-60692-102-9

Chapter 7

Immunosuppression Caused by Photochemo- and Photodynamic Therapy: Focus on Photosensitizer Photoproducts

A.A. Kyagova*[*], *M.V. Malakhov and A.Ya. Potapenko
Russian State Medical University, Moscow, 117997, Ostrovityanova Street 1, Russia

Abstract

Application of photosensitizers (PSs) in medicine [Psoralen+UVA-therapy (PUVA) or Photodynamic Therapy (PDT)] is frequently accompanied by induction of systemic immunosuppression. Taking advantage of this immunosuppressive capacity, PUVA and PDT have been used as immunosuppressive therapies in a variety of diseases. Photosensitized damage of biological targets responsible for immunosuppression can proceed via Type II (singlet oxygen) or Type I (free radicals) mechanisms. Due to the limited lifetime of singlet oxygen or free radical species, the simultaneous exposure to light of both the biological target and the PS is required when Type I or II mechanisms are realized. Exposure to light induces not only the damage of biological targets but also photodegradation of PS molecules with generation of stable PS photooxidation products. Addition of these photoproducts to biosystems in the dark can induce multiple biological effects, including modulation (suppression/activation) of T cell immunity. In this review, the authors summarize their experimental data on modulation of Delayed Type and Contact Hypersensitivity responses in animals by photooxidation products of psoralens, porphyrins and merocyanine 540 as well as preliminary human clinical studies. Immune mechanisms of immunosuppression caused by PUVA and PDT are compared with those induced by products of PS photooxidation. Development of a new method of photochemotherapy, which is based on application of PS photoproducts to patients without irradiation of their tissues, is discussed.

[*] E-mail address: kyagova_alla@front.ru

Introduction

Photochemotherapy with psoralens is widely used for the treatment of psoriasis, T cell lymphoma, alopecia areata, atopic dermatitis and other inflammatory skin and autoimmune diseases [1-4]. This therapy is based on the oral or topical application of psoralens (Ps), which serve as photosensitizers, with subsequent UVA-irradiation of a patient's skin (PUVA-therapy) or blood (photopheresis). The therapeutic effects of PS photochemotherapy are frequently accompanied by a variety of side effects, such as erythema, hyperpigmentation and carcinogenesis [5]. However, these adverse reactions, although of concern, do not seem to override the efficacy and usefulness of this photochemotherapy.

The vast majority of skin diseases that show a favourable response to psoralen photochemotherapy are immunologic in nature and mediated by T cells. It has been suggested that Ps photochemotherapy exerts its beneficial effects via suppression of the T cell immune response [4]. This modulation can be realized through: activation of antigen-presenting cells [2], alteration in the cytokine production by T cells [6, 7], induction of programmed cell death (apoptosis) in activated T lymphocytes [2, 8, 9], activation of specific regulatory T cells [9], and selective cytotoxic effect on tissue-infiltrating inflammatory cells [10].

Photodynamic therapy (PDT) is presumably used as a treatment of various malignant tumors [11, 12]. PDT is based on administration of an exogenous photosensitizer (PS), which selectively accumulates in tumors, followed by exposure of the tumor area to the light. Photoactivation of the PS leads to production of reactive oxygen species, which mediate oxidative damage of biological targets [11, 12]. PDT is frequently accompanied by induction of systemic immunosuppression that has been detected primarily as a reduction in the T cell-mediated immune response [13-15]. Depending on the type of photosensitizer applied and on the site of the PDT application, this immunosuppression can be due to various causes, among them i) inhibition of antigen-presenting activity of macrophages and dendritic cells, presumably by altering their surface molecules [13, 14]; ii) induction of non-specific suppressor cells that belong to the macrophage lineage [15]; iii) activation of specific $CD4^+$ T cells responsible for the immunosuppression [16]; or iv) alteration in the cytokine production by activated T lymphocytes [17, 18].

The photochemical mechanism underlying the development of PDT- and PUVA-induced immunosuppression is questionable. It is conventional to classify the photochemical reactions of photosensitizers by four types (Figure 1). The consensus of opinion is that all PDT-photosensitizers act via the so-called type II photochemical mechanism, i.e., by transferring energy from triplet excited states of PS to molecular oxygen leading to generation of singlet oxygen ($^1O_2$), which mediates damage (oxidation) of biological targets, as well as photooxidation of the photosensitizer itself [19, 20]. Another mechanism exists involving generation of radical species and is generally grouped in the type I reaction [21]. Due to the limited lifetime of $^1O_2$ or other free radical species, photogenerated from the PS molecules [22, 23], the simultaneous exposure of both the biological target and the photosensitizer to light is required. The contribution of the Type II reaction to PUVA-therapy or photopheresis was considered to be irrelevant. The involvement of the Type I photoreaction in the induction of skin erythema has been confirmed [24, 25]. The Type III reaction consists of photoaddition of psoralens to DNA and unsaturated fatty acids without participation of molecular oxygen. The Type III mechanism, i.e., the formation of photooadducts of psoralens with DNA, for a long time was considered the basis for PUVA-therapy and photopheresis. This mechanism provided an excellent explanation of the antiproliferative effects of Ps photochemotherapy; however, it could not explain the immunosuppressive action of PUVA. In the type IV photochemical reactions, the Ps molecules are photooxidized to give relatively persistent Ps photooxidation products, which then react in the dark with biological substrates, resulting in multiple biological effects, including immunosuppression [26].

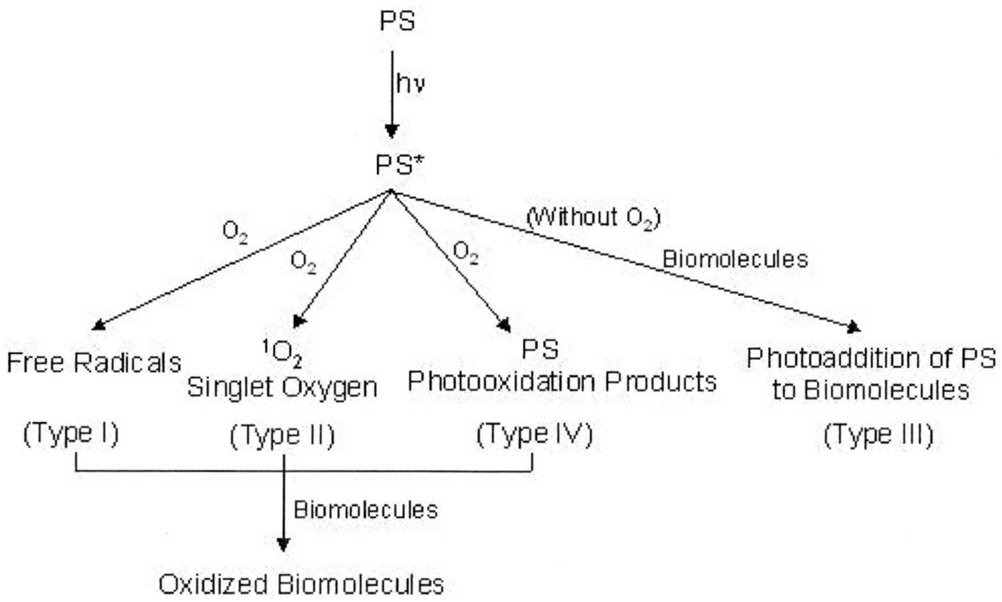

Figure 1. Photochemical reactions of photosensitizers. PS and PS* are ground and electronically excited states of photosensitizer.

Suppression of Delayed Type Hypersensitivity (DTH) Reaction by Products of Photosensitizer Photooxidation

The first observation that photoproducts of PS photooxidation can modulate (activate/suppress) the T-cell immune response in vivo was revealed in the experiments on the application (i/v injection or per os administration) of solution of psoralen, 8-methoxypsoralen (8-MOP) (Figure 2) or peucedanin previously exposed to light instead of irradiation of mice stained with photosensitizer [25, 27]. The model of delayed type hypersensitivity (DTH) response in vivo to sheep red blood cells (SRBC) was employed for these studies. Figure 3 shows the DTH response in mice as a function of the fluence applied for the psoralen pre-irradiation. It is evident that application of non-irradiated Ps did not result in the alteration of the DTH response. In contrast, when mice were treated with pre-irradiated Ps, the DTH response was significantly decreased in a fluence-dependent manner: the greater the fluence the higher was the decrease. Figure 3 also shows that the suppressive effect of the pre-irradiated psoralen was dependent on the fluence rate during irradiation: this suppressive effect shifted toward lower fluences if psoralen solution was photodecomposed at low fluence rate (20.8 W/m^2). The kinetic analysis of photochemical reactions, which led to formation of Ps photoproducts with immunosuppressive activity, revealed that the labile intermediate was produced as a result of Ps molecule excitation [27]. This intermediate might either convert to a stable psoralen photoproduct with immunosuppressive activity or recombine to form membranotoxic Ps photoproduct. It was suggested that PUVA-therapy conditions were more favorable for the formation of immunosuppressive rather than membranotoxic psoralen photooxidation products [27]. It was demonstrated that immunosuppressive Ps photooxidation products preserved their activity for 3 days at room temperature but were thermolabile and destroyable with ferrous ions, suggesting their peroxidic nature [25]. However, the exact chemical structure of psoralen photoproducts with immunosuppressive activity is still elusive.

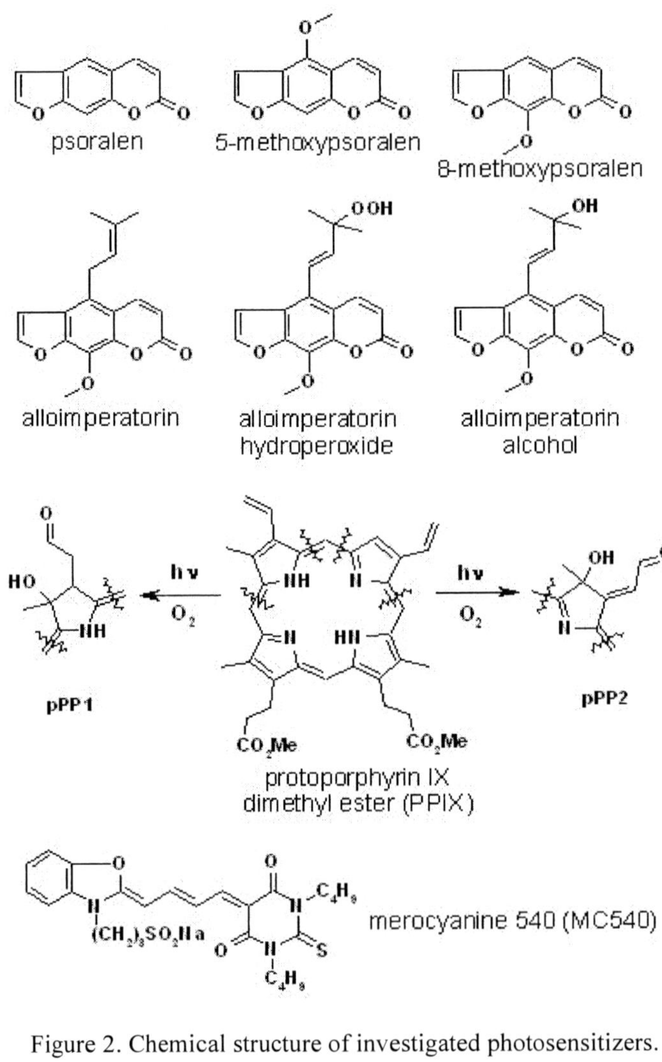

Figure 2. Chemical structure of investigated photosensitizers.

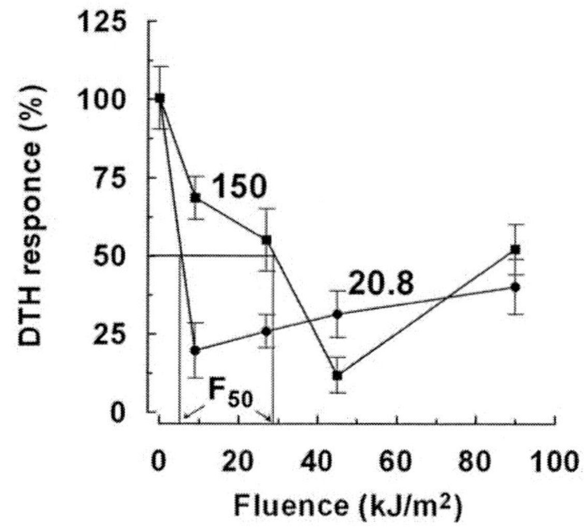

Figure 3. Suppression of the DTH response to sheep red blood cells (SRBC) induced by pre-irradiated psoralen (POP): the effect of fluence rate. Psoralen solution (10^{-4} M in PBS with 1% ethanol) was UVA-irradiated (365 nm) at two fluence rates (150 and 20.8 W/m^2). Irradiation was carried out at 6°C under continuous agitation with a magnetic stirrer. The mice were injected intravenously with 0.5 mL of POP solution 72 h after sensitization with SRBC. In the positive (P) and negative (N) control groups 0.5 mL PBS was injected instead of POP. The DTH response (%) was calculated as: DTH% = [(E - N)/(P - N)]×100%, were E, N, and P are the footpad swelling in mice from experimental, negative and positive control groups, respectively. The numbers beside the curves indicate the fluence rate of UVA (W/m^2). Each point is the mean of the footpad swelling for 10 mice ± SEM.

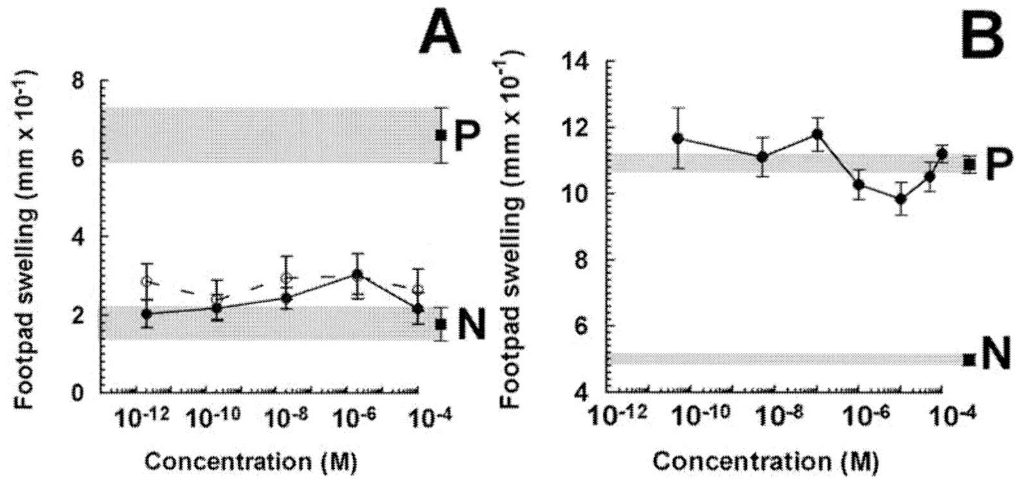

Figure 4. Effect of alloimperatorin hydroperoxide (A) and its corresponding alcohol (B) on the DTH to SRBC in mice. The SRBC-sensitized mice were injected i/v (solid curve) or per os (dashed curve) with 0.5 mL of tested photoproduct solution at different concentrations. Application of photoproducts was carried out 24 h prior to the challenge with SRBC. Mice from the positive (P) and negative (N) control groups were injected i/v with the vehicle (PBS + 1% ethanol) without hydroperoxide or alcohol. Each point is the mean of the footpad swelling for 9-10 mice ±SEM.

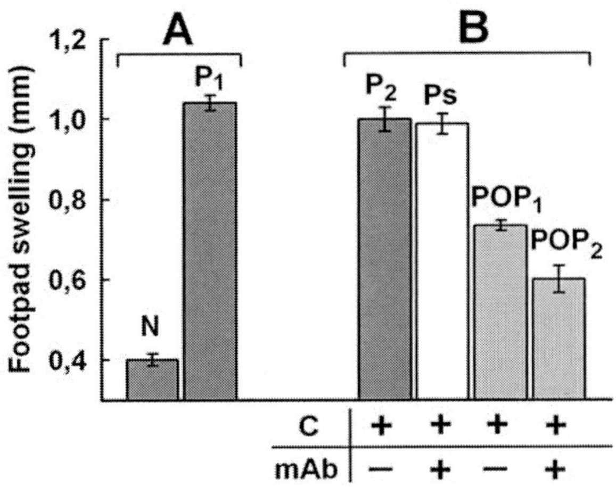

Figure 5. Adoptive transfer of spleen cells from mice treated with pre-irradiated psoralen (POP) results in suppression of the DTH response in SRBC-sensitized mice. This suppression is augmented after treatment of transferred cells with anti-Thy 1.2mAb and Complement. Panel A: positive (P_1) and negative (N) DTH-controls without cell transfer. Panel B: one day after the sensitization with SRBC, mice-donors were injected i/v with 0,5 mL either non-irradiated (Ps, 10^{-4} M in PBS with 1% ethanol) or pre-irradiated (POP, 365 nm, 10 kJ/m^2) psoralen solution. One part of spleen cells from mice-donors was treated with anti-Thy 1.2 mAb (mAb) and incubated with complement (C), and second part was incubated with complement only. After the treatment, 10^8 splenocytes were transferred i/v to mice-recipients that have been sensitized with SRBC 4 days prior to the transfer. Recipient mice were footpad-challenged with SRBC 2 h after the cell transfer. SRBC-sensitized recipient mice, to which spleen cells were transferred from the vehicle-treated (PBS with 1% ethanol) donors, served as positive control P_2. Bars are the mean of the ear swelling for 8 recipient mice ± SEM.

Another point in support of the contribution of the Type IV photoreactions in immunosuppressive effects of psoralens emerged from studies in which suppression of the DTH induced by solution of pre-irradiated alloimperatorin was demonstrated [28]. The photochemical oxygenation of the alloimperatorin has been studied, the photooxidation products were isolated and their structures were determined [29]. The chemical structures of alloimperatorin and its photoproducts (namely, alloimperatorin hydroperoxide and alcohol) are presented in Figure 2. Application of the alloimperatorin hydroperoxide resulted in the DTH suppression, while the corresponding alcohol was not active (Figure 4).

To explore the immune mechanism by which psoralen and alloimperatorin photoproducts can suppress the DTH, adoptive cell transfer experiments were performed [25, 28, 30]. In these studies, mice-donors that have been previously sensitized with SRBC were treated i.v. with pre-irradiated psoralen (POP). Then, spleen cells from donor mice were isolated and i.v. transferred to recipient syngeneic mice that had been sensitized with SRBC prior to the cell transfer. As shown in Figure 5, transfer of cells from POP-treated mice-donors reduced the DTH-response in the recipient animals. Elimination of T-cells by anti-Thy1.2-mAb and complement from transferred cell suspensions from POP-treated donor-mice lead to increase in POP-induced suppression. These data indicate that suppression of the DTH by photoproducts of psoralen and alloimperatorin is adoptively transferred by cells that are of a different nature than T lymphocytes [25, 30].

Suppression of Contact Hypersensitivity (CHS) by PUVA-Treatment and by Photosensitizer Photoproducts

Immunosuppressive activity of PUVA-therapy or PDT in vivo have been accessed by applying presumably the model contact hypersensitivity (CHS) response to different haptens in vivo [8, 10, 13-16]. The CHS response in contrast to the DTH response is mediated by CD8+ T cytotoxic 1 (Tc 1) cells, but not by CD4+ T cells [31-33]. In addition, the CHS response to haptens in mice represents an experimental murine model of human allergic contact dermatitis [32, 33].

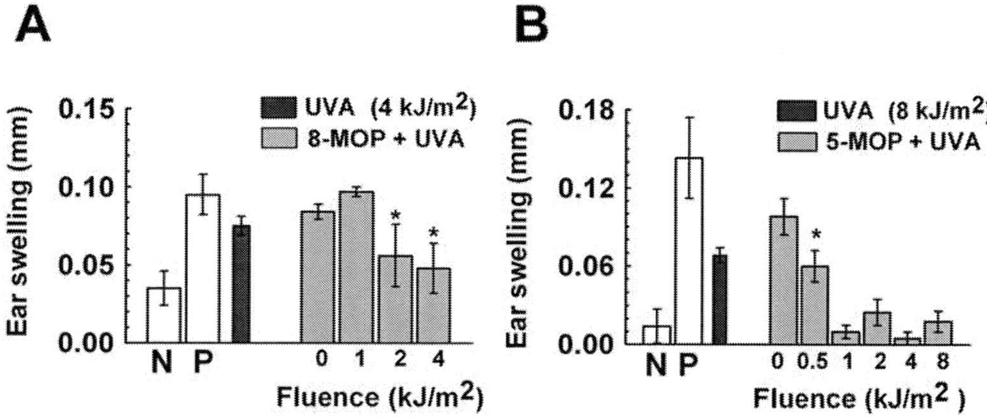

Figure 6. Suppression of the CHS induced by PUVA-treatment with 8-MOP or 5-MOP. DNFB-sensitized mice were treated orally with 0.5mL solution of either 8-MOP (Panel A) or 5-MOP (Panel B) (10^{-4} M in PBS with 1% ethanol). Two hours later, the mice were exposed to UVA (365 nm) at different fluencies on their dorsal shaved skin. The mice were ear-challenged with DNFB 24 h after the UVA-exposure and the ear swelling was registered 24 h later. Mice from the positive (P) and negative (N) control groups were treated per os with the vehicle without psoralens. Mice from the UVA-control group were exposed to UVA after per os application of the vehicle. Bars are the mean of the ear swelling for 9 recipient mice ± SEM. *$p<0.05$ versus positive control.

It was affirmed that PUVA-therapy induces suppression of the afferent but not the effector phase of the CHS [34]. We found that PUVA-treatment (oral application of psoralens with subsequent UVA-irradiation of skin) of mice with 8-MOP or 5-MOP efficiently suppresses the effector phase of the CHS to 2,4-dinitrofluorobenzene (DNFB) (Figure 6). Suppression of the CHS induced by PUVA-treatment with 5-MOP or 8-MOP was fluence dependent. Immunosuppressive efficacy of PUVA with 5-MOP was higher than that for 8-MOP (Figure 6).

Suppressive effect of the PUVA-treatment on the effector phase of the CHS was compared with those of treatment with photoproducts of psoralen, 8-MOP and 5-MOP [35]. It was revealed that orally administered photolysis products of Ps, 8-MOP and 5-MOP induced suppression of the CHS to DNFB in mice (Figure 7). The CHS suppression induced by photolysis products of all studied psoralens was fluence dependent: the more was the fluence applied for the photosensitiser photodecomposition the higher was the CHS suppression. Immunosuppressive efficacy of PS photoproducts was different: 5-MOP=8-MOP>Ps (Figure 7).

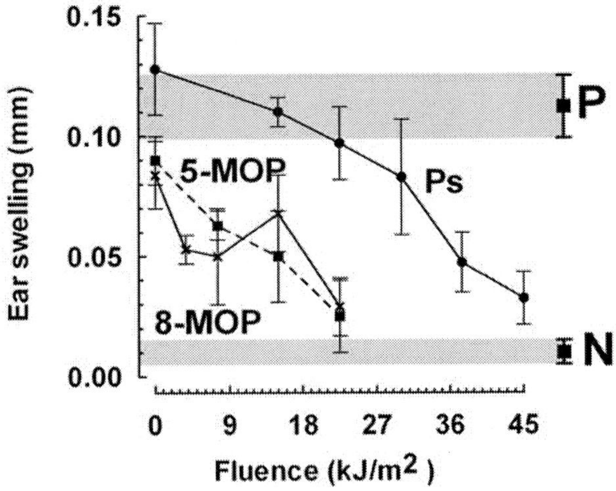

Figure 7. Dependence of the CHS-response to DNFB on the fluence applied for pre-irradiation of psoralen (Ps), 8-methoxypsoralen (8-MOP) and 5-methoxypsoralen (5-MOP). Half milliliter of pre-irradiated (365 nm, fluence rate 23 W/m^2) or non-irradiated solution of each psoralen (10 mM in PBS with 1 % ethanol) was administered per os to DNFB-sensitized mice 24 h prior to the ear challenge with DNFB. Mice from the positive (P) and negative (N) control groups were treated per os with the vehicle without psoralens. Each point represents the mean of the ear swelling for 7 mice ±SEM.

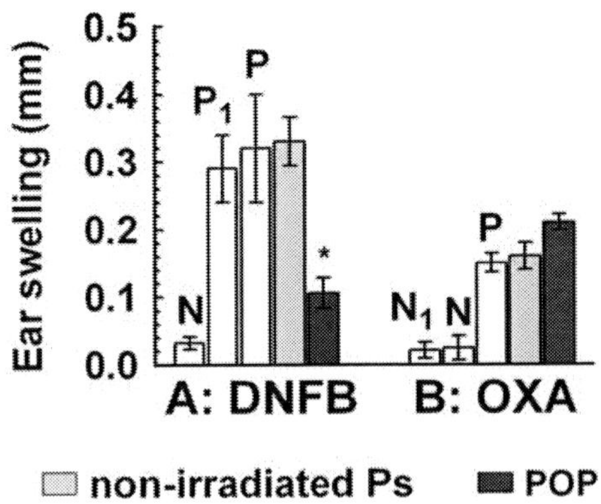

Figure 8. Suppression of the CHS induced by pre-irradiated psoralen (POP) is adoptively transferable and antigen-specific. Four days after the sensitization with DNFB, mice-donors were per os treated with 0,5 mL either non-irradiated (Ps) or pre-irradiated (POP, 365 nm, 27 W/m^2, 20 kJ/m^2) solution of psoralen (1 mM in PBS with 1 % ethanol). One day later, spleen cells (10^8 cells) from these animals were transferred i/v to recipient mice that have been sensitized ether with DNFB (A) or OXA (B) 6 days prior to the transfer. Two hours after the transfer, recipient mice were ear-challenged against either DNFB (A) or OXA (B). DNFB-sensitized or OXA-sensitized recipient mice, to which spleen cells were transferred from the DNFB-sensitized donors, served as positive controls P to the corresponding antigen. Positive control P_1 mice were DNFB-sensitized and DNFB-challenged without the cell transfer. Mice from negative control N were ear challenged with the corresponding antigen (DNFB or OXA) only. Negative control N_1 - naïve recipient mice received spleen cells from DNFB-sensitized donors and then ear-challenged with OXA. Mice from all positive and negative control groups were treated per os with the vehicle (PBS + 1% ethanol). Bars represent the mean of the ear swelling for 8 recipient mice ± SEM. *$p<0.001$ versus corresponding positive control P.

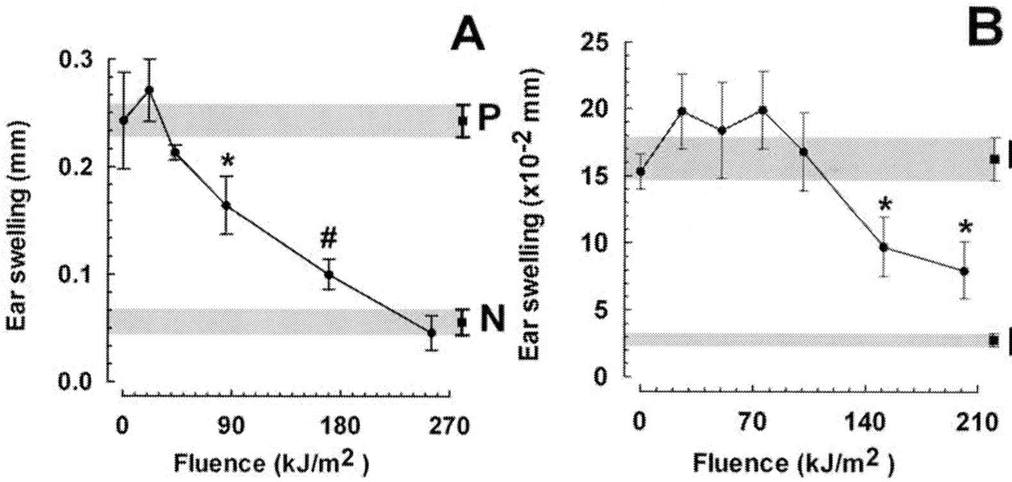

Figure 9. Suppression of the CHS by pre-irradiated MC540 and PPIX. **Panel A:** DNFB-sensitized mice were injected i/v with 0.5 mL of either non-irradiated or pre-irradiated (546 nm, fluence rate 23.6 W/m^2, 170 kJ/m^2) solution of MC540 (17.6 μM in PBS with 0.5% ethanol) 24 h prior to the ear challenge with DNFB. **Panel B:** Half milliliter of pre-irradiated (365 nm, fluence rate 28 W/m^2) or non-irradiated solution of PPIX (10 μM in PBS with 0.4% ethanol and 0.6% PEG-400) was injected i/v to naïve mice 24 h prior to sensitization with DNFB. In the positive (P) and negative (N) controls 0.5 mL of the corresponding vehicle was injected instead of tested PS solution. Each point designates the mean of the ear swelling for 9-10 mice ± SEM. *$p<0.01$ and #$p<0.001$ versus positive control, respectively.

It was reported that PUVA-treatment downregulates the CHS response by activation of specific T-regulatory/suppressive cells [8]. These regulatory cells can be revealed in experiments on the adoptive cell transfer of the CHS suppression. To determine whether the PS photoproducts can induces cells with suppressive activity, adoptive transfer experiments of the CHS suppression were performed (Figure 8). In these studies, mice-donors that have been previously sensitized with DNFB were treated orally either with non-irradiated Ps or photodecomposed Ps solution (POP). Then spleen cells were obtained and i.v. transferred to recipient syngeneic mice that had been sensitized with either DNFB or oxazolone (OXA) prior to the cell transfer. As shown in Figure 8, transfer of spleen cells from Ps-treated donors did not influence the CHS-response either in DNFB- or OXA-sensitized recipients. In contrast, transfer of cells from POP-treated mice-donors reduced the CHS-response in the DNFB-recipient animals and did not influence it in OXA-sensitized recipients. These data indicate that POP-induced suppression of the CHS is: i) adoptively transferrable, ii) realized through activation of cells with specific suppressive functions. The nature of these suppressor cells is still unclear.

Our later studies showed that immunosuppressive effect on the CHS can be initiated by photoproducts of photosensitizers, which are applied in the PDT [36, 37]. Figure 9 shows that intravenous injection of pre-irradiated solution of either merocyanine 540 (MC540) or protoporphyrin IX (PPIX) resulted in suppression of the CHS-response in fluence-dependent manner. The samples of photodecomposed PPIX with suppressive effect on the CHS contained chlorin-type products, namely, two isomers of photoprotoporphyrin (pPP1 and pPP2, Figure 2) as main photoproducts. Concentration dependent suppression of the CHS was also induced when purified pPP1 or pPP2 were injected to mice intravenously [37]. These purified photoproducts exerted equal immunosuppressive activity. Adoptive transfer experiments revealed that suppression of the CHS induced by either pPP1 or pre-irradiated MC540 was adoptively transferable and was associated with generation of cells with non-specific suppressive potential (Figure 10).

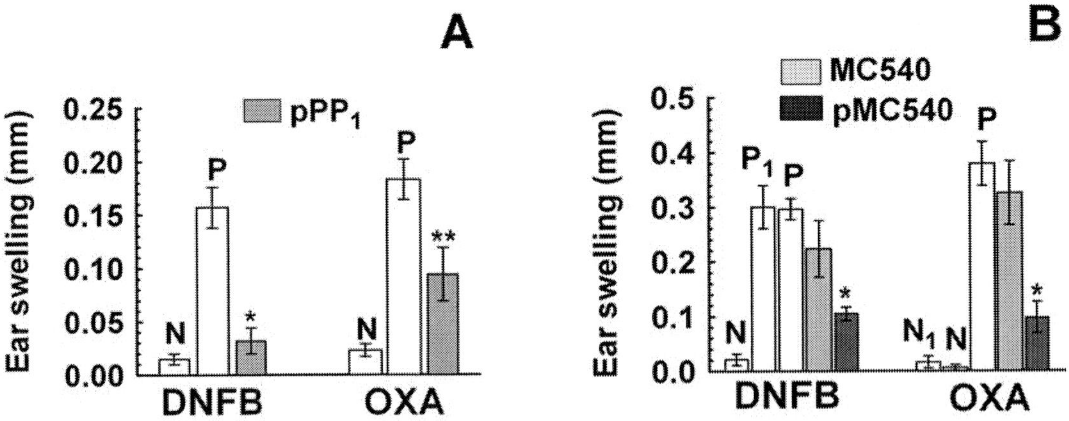

Figure 10. Both photoproduct of PPIX (pPP1) or pre-irradiated MC540 generate in vivo cells with non-specific suppressive effect on the CHS. **Panel A:** Twenty-one hour prior to the sensitization with DNFB, mice-donors were injected i/v with 0.5 mL either pPP1 (0.1 μM in PBS with 0.4% ethanol and 0.6% PEG-400) or with the vehicle alone. Six days later, spleen cells (10^8 cells) from these animals were transferred i/v to mice-recipients that have been sensitized either with DNFB or OXA 6 days prior to the transfer. **Panel B**: Four days after the sensitization with DNFB, mice-donors were injected i/v with either non-irradiated (MC540) or pre-irradiated (pMC540, 170 kJ/m^2) solution of MC540 (17.6 μM in PBS with 0.5% ethanol). One day later, spleen cells (10^8 cells) from these animals were transferred i/v to recipient mice that have been sensitized ether with DNFB or OXA 6 days prior to the transfer. Recipient mice were ear-challenged with the corresponding antigen 2 h after the cell transfer. Positive control P_1 mice were DNFB-sensitized and DNFB-challenged without the cell transfer. Negative control N_1 - naïve recipient mice received spleen cells from DNFB-sensitized donors and then ear-challenged with OXA. DNFB-sensitized or OXA-sensitized recipient mice, to which spleen cells were transferred from the DNFB-sensitized donors, served as positive controls P to the corresponding antigen. Mice from negative control N were ear-challenged with the corresponding antigen (DNFB or OXA) only. Mice from all positive and negative control groups were treated per os with the corresponding vehicle. Bars represent the mean of the ear swelling for 8 recipient mice ± SEM; *$p<0.001$ and **<0.003 versus corresponding positive control P, respectively.

POP Therapy Is a New Patient-Friendly Photochemotherapy That Requires No UV-A Irradiation of Skin or Blood

It is acknowledged that psoralen photochemotherapy is immunotherapy directed to modulation of T cell immunity [38]. T cell immunity is responsible for delayed type reactions: DTH and CH [31]. Our data evidence that immunosuppression can be induced by photooxidized psoralens (POP) which are produced in Type IV photoreactions. For example, POP suppressed DTH and CH in mice presumably due to suppression of antigen-specific T cells [27, 28, 39]. These data strongly indicated that POP could be a potential therapeutic agent. Our preliminary clinical trials have shown that orally applied POP-induced clinical effects in patients with diseases which were known to be sensitive to PUVA or photopheresis, like cutaneous T cell lymphoma, psoriasis, alopecia areata, eczema, acna and rheumatoid arthritis [40]. Topical application of photooxidized 8-methoxypsoralen induced a limited therapeutic effect in psoriatic patients [41].

Evidence-based medicine demands that clinical trials must be done by the double-blind method. We studied the efficiency of POP therapy using this method in patients with eczema due to two reasons: mechanistic and ethical.

Mechanistic reason implies that eczema is associated with impaired T cell-mediated immunity [42], namely T cell activation [43]. Psoralen photochemotherapy suppresses T cell immune system [44]. Probably this effect is the basis of successful PUVA-therapy of eczema [45]. POP is known to be an efficient suppressor of T cell immunity [26], thus positive effect of POP therapy is likely in the case of eczema. There were the following ethical considerations. Control patients must receive placebo in the double blind method. So they remain without treatment during trial. Our preliminary results indicated that the clinical effect of POP was the quickest in the case of eczema in comparison with other nosologies tested. Thus, we could limit the placebo experiment to a one-week period.

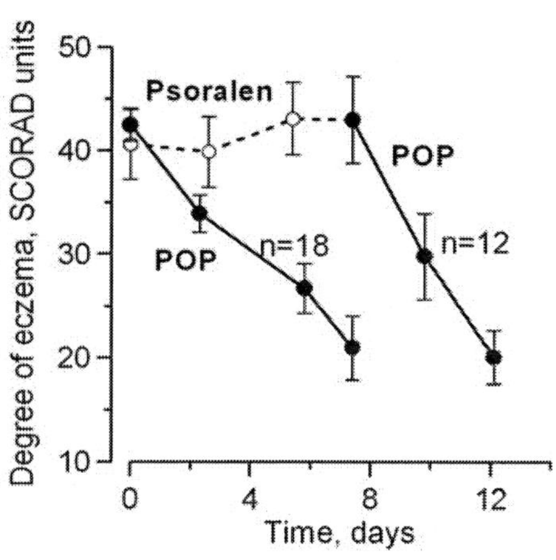

Figure 11. A double-blind control clinical trial of photooxidized psoralen (POP) for eczema. Patients received either non-irradiated psoralen (empty circles, placebo) or POP (black circles) 3 times per a week. Each intake consisted of 1 mg of psoralen diluted in 50 mL of PBS. To produce POP, this solution was preirradiated at 365 nm on air in a dose of 24 kJ/m^2. SCORAD units were used to estimate a degree of eczema. Points are mean ± SEM.

Thirty patients with moderate and mainly hand eczema were divided into two groups. The experimental group of 18 patients received orally aqueous POP solution, while 12 patients (placebo) received non-irradiated psoralen during the first week of trial and then they were passed on to POP (Figure 11) [46]. POP was given every other day for a period of 7 to 10 days. SCORAD was used to estimate the severity of the disease [47]. The value of SCORAD before the treatment was 42±3 (mean±SEM). During a week of POP-therapy it decreased to 21±3. Itching disappeared after second application of POP. The state of the patients continued to improve during 1.5 months after the end of POP applications, SCORAD being decreased to 9±2. The mean remission duration made about 8 months. DTH to tuberculin (Mantoux test) was ca. two times suppressed ($p<0.02$) after one week of POP treatment in comparison with non-treated eczema patients.

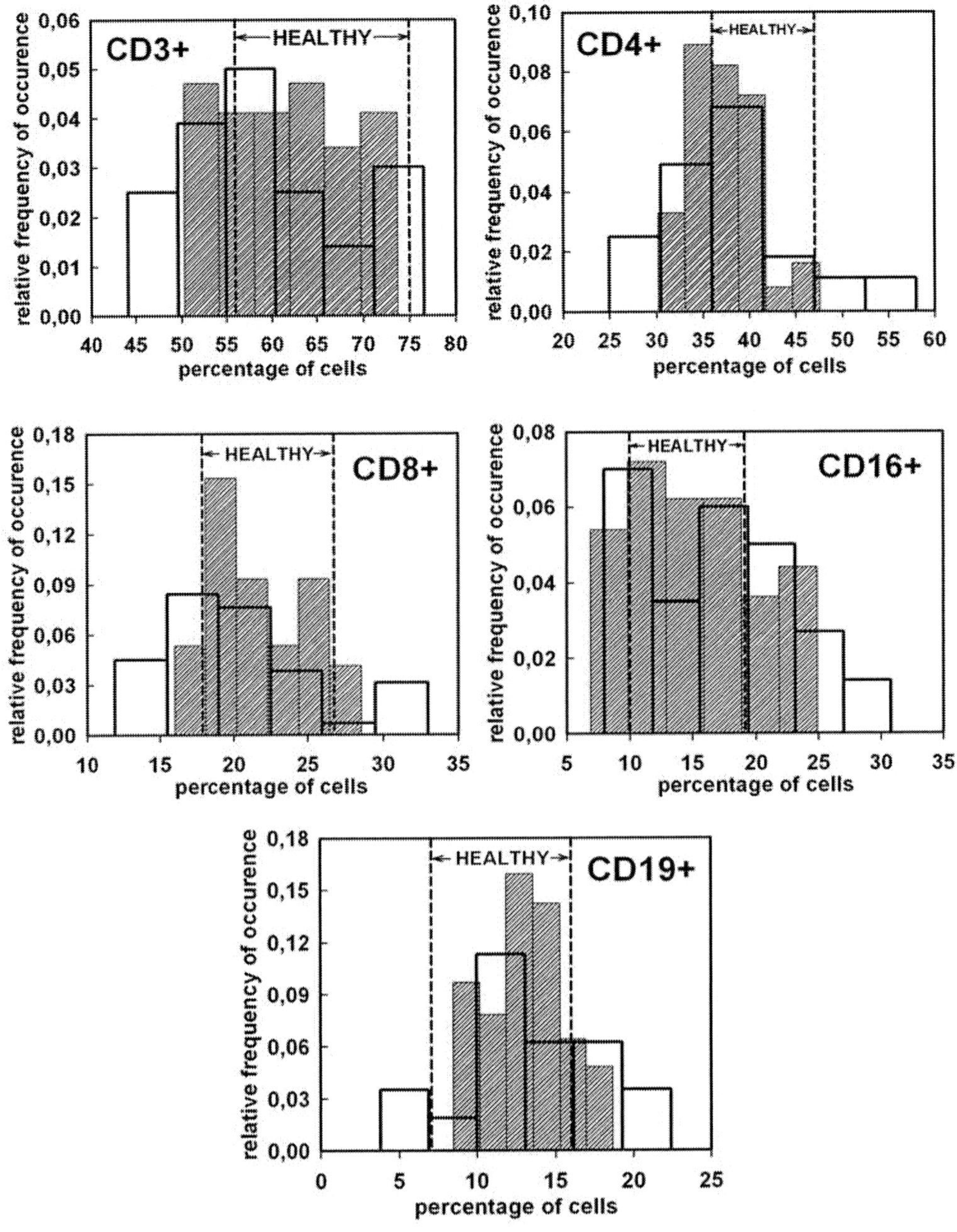

Figure 12. Distribution bar chart of lymphocyte subpopulations before (white bars) and one month after (dashed bars) POP therapy of patients with hand eczema. Relative frequencies of occurrence of total T cells (CD3+), T helper cells (CD4+), cytotoxic T cells (CD8+), total B cells (CD19+) and NK cells (CD16+) in blood were assessed as compared to healthy donors (vertical dotted lines cut down interval: mean ± 2 sd for healthy volunteers).

Phenotyping of peripheral blood mononuclear cells (PBMC) from healthy volunteers and from eczema patients before and one month after POP therapy was done. The percent content of CD3+, CD4+, CD8+, CD16+ and CD19+ lymphocyte subpopulations was estimated with fluorescent-labeled monoclonal antibodies and fluorescent flow cytometry. There was no significant difference in mean values of cell counts for all subpopulations studied in healthy volunteers and eczema patients before and after POP therapy. But the dispersion of the investigated lymphocyte population counts was two to three times higher in eczema patients as compared to healthy volunteers, and approached the normal counts one month after POP-therapy (Fig. 12) [48]. The obtained results show that POP therapy had immunotropic effect that was manifested in the normalization of the variability of the contents of the main lymphocyte populations in eczema patients.

These preliminary results suggest that products of psoralen photooxidation may play a crucial role in psoralen photochemotherapy. Oral application of photooxidized psoralens (POP) may be efficient in the treatment of skin diseases, sensitive to PUVA-treatment.

Psoralen photochemotherapy, although first reported in 1974 [49], is in fact thousands of years old, having been used in Egypt and India since 1200-2000 B.C. [50]. Ancient physicians and herbalists prepared boiled extracts (like tea) of certain umbelliferous or leguminous plants. These preparations were either applied to the skin or ingested as an "infusion"; the patients then exposed the skin to the intense Egyptian or Indian sunlight [50]. In the case of topical application of extracts, the ancient therapy was very close to modern topical PUVA. But it is difficult to explain why oral application of extracts was efficient. Psoralens exhibit low water solubility. A saturated solution of 8-MOP contains approximately 2 mg of a sensitizer per 100 ml. It is known that photochemotherapy efficiency depends on sensitizer concentration in plasma. For 8-MOP, the threshold dose is about 0.23 mg per 1 kg of the body weight [51]. Below this dose, 8-MOP is completely metabolized and does not produce any detectable plasma levels. As a result, the patient's photosensitivity does not change. When a saturated 8-MOP solution is administered orally, and when the body weight is approximately 70 kg, the minimal (threshold) extract volume should be 800 ml. To achieve the optimal therapeutic concentration of 0.6 $mg \cdot kg^{-1}$, this volume should amount to approximately 2,100 ml. Could patients drink such volumes of extract to make therapy efficient? Probably not. Nevertheless, oral therapy was efficient. The explanation can be simple. It is doubtful that plant extracts were prepared in the dark—surely this was done in sunlight, and thus psoralens were photooxidized and contained POP. Thus, ancient physicians could practically use POP therapy.

Conclusion

Products of photosensitizer photooxidation are able to affect T cell immunity in vivo and can contribute to PUVA- and PDT-induced immunosuppression. A new method of photochemotherapy for the treatment of diseases associated with hyperreactivity of T-cell immune system may be developed. This method is based on administration of photosensitizer photoproducts to patients without irradiation of their skin or blood. Among photosensitizers studied (PPIX, MC540 and psoralens), products of psoralens photooxidation (POP) attract special attention because their suppressive action is immunospecific. POP therapy has significant advantages over PUVA therapy and photopheresis because it is much more friendly to patients. Photoaddition of psoralens to DNA as well as attack of biotissues by singlet oxygen and free radicals of psoralens are excluded. Thus, the deleterious effects of UVA/PUVA can be avoided.

References

[1] Hönigsmann, H., (2001) Phototherapy for Psoriasis., *Clin. Exp. Dermatol., 26*, 343-350.

[2] Oliven, A., & Shechter, Y., (2001) Extracorporeal Photopheresis: A Review., *Blood Rev.,* **15**, 103-108.

[3] Meidan, V. M., & Touitou, E., (2001) Treatments for Androgenetic Alopecia and Alopecia Areata: Current Options and Future Prospects., *Drugs,* **61**, 53-69.

[4] Krutmann, J., (2000) Phototherapy for Atopic Dermatitis., *Clin. Exp. Dermatol.,* **25**, 552-558.

[5] Averbeck, D., (1989) Recent Advances in Psoralen Phototoxicity Mechanism., *Photochem. Photobiol.,* **50**, 859-889.

[6] Tokura, Y., Seo, N., Yagi, H., Wakita, H., Moriwaki, S., F., F., & Takigawa, M., (1999) Treatment of T Lymphocytes with 8-Methoxypsoralen Plus Ultraviolet a Induces Transient but Biologically Active Th1-Skewing Cytokine Production., *J. Invest. Dermatol.,* **113**, 202-208.

[7] Klosner, G., Trautinger, F., Knobler, R., & Neuner, P., (2001) Treatment of Peripheral Blood Mononuclear Cells with 8-Methoxypsoralen Plus Ultraviolet a Radiation Induces a Shift in Cytokine Expression from a Th1 to a Th2 Response., *J. Invest. Dermatol.,* **116**, 459-462.

[8] Tambur, A. R., Ortegel, J. W., Morales, A., Klingemann, H., Gebel, H. M., & Tharp, M. D., (2000) Extracorporeal Photopheresis Induces Lymphocyte but Not Monocyte Apoptosis., *Transplant. Proc.,* **32**, 747-748.

[9] Maeda, A., Schwarz, A., Kernebeck, K., Gross, N., Aragane, Y., Peritt, D., & Schwarz, T., (2005) Intravenous Infusion of Syngeneic Apoptotic Cells by Photopheresis Induces Antigen-Specific Regulatory T Cells., *J. Immunol.,* **174**, 5968-5976.

[10] Edelson, R. L., (1991) Photopheresis: Present and Future Aspects., *J. Photochem. Photobiol. B: Biol.,* **10**, 165-174.

[11] Dougherty, T. J., (2002) An Update on Photodynamic Therapy Applications., *J. Clin. Laser Med. Surg.,* **20**, 3-7.

[12] Moan, J., & Peng, Q., (2003) An Outline of the Hundred-Year History of PDT., *Anticancer Res.,* **23**, 3591-3600.

[13] King, D. E., Jiang, H., Simkin, G. O., Obochi, M. O., Levy, J. G., & Hunt, D. W., (1999) Photodynamic Alteration of the Surface Receptor Expression Pattern of Murine Splenic Dendritic Cells., *Scand. J. Immunol.,* **49**, 184-192.

[14] Obochi, M. O., Ratkay, L. G., & Levy, J. G., (1997) Prolonged Skin Allograft Survival after Photodynamic Therapy Associated with Modification of Donor Skin Antigenicity., *Transplantation,* **63**, 810-817.

[15] Lynch, D. H., Haddad, S., King, V. J., Ott, M. J., Straight, R. C., & Jolles, C. J., (1989) Systemic Immunosuppression Induced by Photodynamic Therapy (PDT) Is Adoptively Transferred by Macrophages., *Photochem. Photobiol.,* **49**, 453-458.

[16] Musser, D. A., & Oseroff, A. R., (2001) Characteristics of the Immunosuppression Induced by Cutaneous Photodynamic Therapy: Persistence, Antigen Specificity and Cell Type Involved., *Photochem. Photobiol.,* **73**, 518-524.

[17] Gollnick, S. O., Liu, X., Owczarczak, B., Musser, D. A., & Henderson, B. W., (1997) Altered Expression of Interleukin 6 and Interleukin 10 as a Result of Photodynamic Therapy *in vivo., Cancer Res.,* **57**, 3904-3909.

[18] Gollnick, S. O., Musser, D. A., Oseroff, A. R., Vaughan, L., Owczarczak, B., & Henderson, B. W., (2001) IL-10 Does Not Play a Role in Cutaneous Photofrin Photodynamic Therapy-Induced Suppression of the Contact Hypersensitivity Response., *Photochem. Photobiol.,* **74**, 811-816.

[19] Ochsner, M., (1997) Photophysical and Photobiological Processes in the Photodynamic Therapy of Tumours., *J. Photochem. Photobiol. B. Biol.,* **39**, 1-18.

[20] Konan, Y. N., Gurny, R., & Allemann, E., (2002) State of the Art in the Delivery of Photosensitizers for Photodynamic Therapy., *J. Photochem. Photobiol. B. Biol.,* **66**, 89-106.

[21] Foote, C. S., (1991) Definition of Type I and Type II Photosensitized Oxidation., *Photochem. Photobiol.,* **54**, 659.

[22] Ando, T., Yoshikawa, T., Tanigawa, T., Kohno, M., Yoshida, N., & Kondo, M., (1997) Quantification of Singlet Oxygen from Hematoporphyrin Derivative by Electron Spin Resonance., *Life Sci.,* **61**, 1953-1959.

[23] Moan, J., & Berg, K., (1991) The Photodegradation of Porphyrins in Cells Can Be Used to Estimate the Lifetime of Singlet Oxygen., *Photochem. Photobiol.,* **53**, 549-553.

[24] Potapenko, A. Y., Abijev, G. A., Pistsov, M. Y., Roshchupkin, D. I., Vladimirov, Y. A., Pliquett, F., Ermolajev, A. V., Sarycheva, I. K., & Evstigneeva, R. P., (1984) PUVA-Induced Erythema and Changes in Mechanoelectrical Properties of Skin. Inhibition by Tocopherols., *Arch. Dermatol. Res.,* **276**, 12-16.

[25] Potapenko, A. Y., & Kyagova, A. A., (1998) The Application of Antioxidants in Investigation and Optimization of Photochemotherapy., *Membr. Cell Biol.,* **12**, 269-278.

[26] Potapenko, A. Y., Kyagova, A. A., Bezdetnaya, L. N., Lysenko, E. P., Chernyakhovskaya, I. Y., Bekhalo, V. A., Nagurskaya, E. V., Nesterenko, V. A., Korotky, N. G., Akhtyamov, S. N., & Lanshchikova, T. M., (1994) Products of Psoralen Photooxidation Possess Immunomodulative and Antileukemic Effects, *Photochem. Photobiol.,* **60**, 171-174.

[27] Kyagova, A. A., Zhuravel, N. N., Malakhov, M. V., Lysenko, E. P., Adam, W., Saha-Möller, C. R., & Potapenko, A. Y., (1997) Suppression of Delayed-Type Hypersensitivity and Hemolysis Induced by Previously Photooxidized Psoralen: Effect of Fluence Rate and Psoralen Concentration., *Photochem. Photobiol.,* **65**, 694-700.

[28] Andina, E. S., Kyagova, A. A., Yurikova, N. A., Neklyukova, M. B., Potapenko, A. Y., Adam, W., & Saha-Möller, C. R., Immunosuppression Induced by the Photooxidation Products of Furocoumarins (Psoralens). In: ed. by Holick, M. F. & Jung, E. G., *Biologic Effects of Light.* (Boston, London, Dordrecht:: Kluger Academic Publishers, 1999), pp. 213-216.

[29] Abou-Elzahab, M., Adam, W., Saha-Möller, C. R., & (), (1991) Photooxidation of Some Potentially Skin-Photosensitizing Furocoumarins: Imperatorin, Alloimperatorin and Its Methyl Ether and Acetate Derivatives., *Liebigs Ann. Chem.,* 967-970.

[30] Kyagova, A. A., Kozir, L. A., Mansurova, G. V., Zorin, V. P., Bezdetnaya, L. N., Guillemin, F., & Potapenko, A. Y., (2002) Modulation of Delayed Type Hypersensitivity in Mice Treated with Photoproducts of Various Photosensitizers Used in Photodynamic Therapy., *Russ. J. Immunol.,* **7**, 327-334.

[31] Grabbe, S., & Schwarz, T., (1998) Immunoregulatory Mechanisms Involved in Elicitation of Allergic Contact Hypersensitivity., *Immunol.Today,* **19**, 37-44.

[32] Girolomoni, G., Gisondi, P., Ottaviani, C., & Cavani, A., (2004) Immunoregulation of Allergic Contact Dermatitis., *J. Dermatol.,* **31**, 264-270.

[33] Saint-Mezard, P., Berard, F., Dubois, B., Kaiserlian, D., & Nicolas, J. F., (2004) The Role of CD4+ and CD8+ T Cells in Contact Hypersensitivity and Allergic Contact Dermatitis., *Eur. J. Dermatol.,* **14**, 131-138.

[34] Kripke, M. L., Morison, W. L., & Parrish, J. A., (1983) Systemic Suppression of Contact Hypersensitivity in Mice by Psoralen Plus UVA Radiation (PUVA). *J. Invest. Dermatol.,* **81**, 87-92.

[35] Kyagova, A., Moshnina, Z., Kozir, L., Glazunova, O., Moshnin, M., & Potapenko, A., (2006) Specific Suppression of Contact Hypersensitivity in Mice by Photolysis Products of Psoralens., *J. Invest. Dermatol.,* **126**, s79.

[36] Kyagova, A. A., Kozir, L. A., Mansurova, G. V., Moshnina, Z. I., Kozhiniva, E. A., Ponomarev, G. V., & Potapenko, A. Y., (2007) Immunosuppresive Effects of Psoralen Photochemotherapy and Photodynamic Therapy May Be Realized through Production of Photosensitizer Photooxidation Products., *J. Invest. Dermatol.,* **127**, S42.

[37] Kyagova, A. A., Mansurova, G. V., Kozir, L. A., Ponomarev, G. V., Pavlov, V. Y., Konstantinov, I. O., & Potapenko, A. Y., (2005) Systemic Suppression of Contact Hypersensitivity by Products of Protoporphyrin IX Photooxidation., *Photochem Photobiol.,* **81**, 1380-1385.

[38] Heald, P. W., & Edelson, R. L., (1988) Photopheresis for T Cell Mediated Diseases. , *Adv. Dermatol.,* **3,** 25-40.

[39] Kyagova, A. A., Nagurskaya, E. V., Bekhalo, V. A., Chernyakhovskaya, I. Y., Belichenko, I. V., & Potapenko, A. Y., (1996) The Attenuation of Effectors and Induction of Suppressors of Delayed Type Hypersensitivity Reaction under the Treatment with Psoralen Photooxidation Products., *Russian J. Immunol.,* **1**, 61-68.

[40] Potapenko, A. Y., Kyagova, A. A., Bezdetnaya, L. N., Lysenko, E. P., Chernyakhovskaya, I. Y., Bekhalo, V. A., Nagurskaya, E. V., Nesterenko, V. G., Korotky, N. G., Akhtyamov, S. N., & Lanshchikova, T. M., (1993) Immunologic and Therapeutic Efficacy of Photooxidized Psoralen *in vivo*., *Photochem. Photobiol.,* **57,** *Suppl.*, 29S.

[41] Mizuno, N., (1980) Topical PUVA - Review on Basic and Clinical Problems., *The Korean J. Dermatol.,* **18**, 5-26.

[42] Reinhold, U., Atopic Dermatitis. In: ed. by Burg, G. & Dummer, R. G., *Strategies for Immunointerventions in Dermatology.* (Berlin, Heidelberg: Springer-Verlag, 1997), pp. 243-251.

[43] Thestrup-Pedersen, K., Ellingsen, A. R., Olesen, A. B., Lund, M., & Kaltoft, K., (1997) Atopic Dermatitis May Be a Genetically Determined Dysmaturation of Ectodermal Tissue, Resulting in Disturbed T-Lymphocyte Maturation. A Hypothesis., *Acta Derm. Venereol.,* **77**, 20-21.

[44] Aubin, F., & Humbert, P., (1998) Immunomodulation Induced by Psoralen Plus Ultraviolet a Radiation., *Eur. J. Dermatol.* , **8**, 212-213.

[45] Sheehan, M. P., Atherton, D. J., Norris, P., & Hawk, J., (1993) Oral Psoralen Photochemotherapy in Severe Childhood Atopic Eczema: An Update., *Br. J. Dermatol.*, **129**, 431-436.

[46] Levinzon, E. S., Butov, Y. S., Yurikova, N. A., Andina, E. S., Neklyukova, M. B., S.N., A., Mamedov, I. S., Kyagova, A. A., & Potapenko, A. Y., (1998) Treatment of Eczema with Photooxidized Psoralen in Randomized Double Blind Clinical Trial. (in Russian), *Rus. J. Skin Venereol. Diseases*, 14-18.

[47] Consensus Report of the European Task Force on Atopic Dermatitis. Severity Scoring of Atopic Dermatitis: The SCORAD Index., (1993) *Dermatol.,* **186**, 23-31.

[48] Levinzon, E. S., Therapeutic and Immune Effects of Photooxidized Psoralen in Eczema, (Thesis, Candidate of Medical Sciences, Russian State Medical University, 1999), p. 137.

[49] Parrish, J. A., Fitzpatrick, T. B., Tanenbaum, L., & Pathak, M. A., (1974) Photochemotherapy of Psoriasis with Oral Methoxalen and Longwave Ultraviolet Light., *N. Engl. J. Med.,* **291**, 1207-1211.

[50] Fitzpatrick, T. B., & Pathak, M. A., Research and Development of Oral Psoralen and Longwave Radiation Photochemotherapy: 2000 B.C. - 1982 A.D. In: Pathak, M. A. & Dunnick, J. K. editors. *Natl. Cancer Inst. Monogr.* Bethesda: Natl. Cancer Inst.; 1984; pp. 3-11.

[51] Brickl, R., Schmid, J., & Koss, F. W., Pharmacokinetics and Pharmacodynamics of Psoralens after Oral Administration: Considerations and Conclusions. In: Pathak, M. A. & Dunnick, J. K. editors. *Natl. Cancer Inst. Monogr.* Bethesda: Natl. Cancer Inst.; 1984; pp. 63-67.

In: Immunosuppression: New Research
Editor: Charles B. Taylor, pp. 185-207

ISBN: 978-1-60692-102-9

Chapter 8

Sunlight Induced Immunosuppression: A Role for Inflammatory Mediators in the Induction of Suppressor Cells

Scott N. Byrne and Gary M. Halliday
Dermatology Research Laboratories,
University of Sydney, Australia

Abstract

It has been known for some time that the ultraviolet (UV) component of the solar spectrum is immunosuppressive. This, combined with the DNA damaging properties of UV is the reason why sunlight is such a potent carcinogen. While it is well established that one way UV causes immunosuppression is via the induction of regulatory T cells, recent studies have demonstrated that UV also induces a suppressor B cell population. Furthermore, it has been suggested that inflammatory cytokines and oxidised lipids play a key role in the activation of these regulatory populations. We will review the most recent evidence that elucidate the mechanisms by which UV causes immunosuppression focusing on the activation of regulatory cells and the potential for therapeutic intervention.

Introduction

Sunlight is one of the most potent and significant environmental carcinogens humans are exposed to. Exposure to the ultraviolet (UV) wavelengths in sunlight gives rise to skin cancer which is more common than all the other cancers combined (1). The UVA (320-400nm) and UVB (290-320nm) wavebands in sunlight damage DNA (2) although via different mechanisms. UVB has sufficient energy to be directly absorbed by DNA while UVA primarily damages DNA via production of reactive oxygen species (ROS) (3). Both wavebands also suppress the host anti-tumour immune response (12). These two forms of damage are required for the development of skin tumours. More than three decades ago using immunogenic skin tumours that would normally be rejected by naïve recipients, Fisher and Kripke demonstrated that exposure to UV radiation prior to tumour inoculation would cause tumours to grow progressively (5). The conclusion was that UV had *immunosuppressive* properties that could inhibit the host anti-tumour response, the importance of which can now be seen in the abnormally high incidence of skin cancer in immunosuppressed transplant patients (6). It has since been shown that the mechanism of this UV-induced immunosuppression is via the activation of regulatory cell populations (7, 9, 90). However, the early and intermediary steps that lead to the activation of these suppressor cells is still not known, and the cells themselves have been inadequately characterised. Understanding the mechanisms involved in regulatory cell activation, and how they mediate immunosuppression will hopefully lead to novel immunotherapeutics designed to treat a wide variety of conditions including cancer, allergies, autoimmunity and transplantation tolerance.

Immunosuppression Only Requires Exposure to Low Doses of UV Radiation

Exposure of humans to 144 $mJcm^{-2}$ UVB, which is about one-third the dose required to cause barely detectable sunburn in pale skinned humans is immunosuppressive (10,11). UVA is also highly immunosuppressive in humans and mice. As UVA has little effect on sunburn, it is not realistic to relate these doses to the amount required to cause sunburn, however the UVA dose can be related to the amount present in sunlight that would cause sunburn, as UVB within sunlight would cause sunburn. Irradiation with 1900 $mJcm^{-2}$ UVA is immunosuppressive in humans and mice (10,12). As UVA is about 20 times more abundant than UVB in sunlight, this dose could be achieved with half the amount of sunlight required to cause sunburn.

Sunlight Is Immunosuppressive

It is now well accepted that the UV wavelengths in sunlight are the prime aetiological cause of skin cancer. However, in order to understand carcinogenesis, one needs to have an appreciation for the two facets that make this biological process a possibility; genetic damage *and* immune suppression. Sunlight causes both and so is considered a complete carcinogen. Sunlight causes immunosuppression in part via the activation of suppressor cells and while the exact pathways leading to the activation of these populations remains unknown, a wide variety of immune cells (Table 1) and secreted factors (Table 2) are known to be involved in UV-immune suppression and tolerance.

UV-Induced Regulatory Cells

The suppressor cell populations induced by UV are often thought of as obstacles to an effective anti-tumour immune response with their activation preferably avoided. However there are many conceivable situations including allograft tolerance (61), treatment of the autoimmune disorder psoriasis (62), and photophoresis therapy for controlling graft versus host disease (63) where UV-induced regulatory cells could be considered beneficial. While a number of different suppressor cells have been described, including T cells, B cells, NKT cells and macrophages, little is known about the mechanism of their regulatory activity. More importantly, the factors that lead to their induction remain unresolved, delaying the development of novel therapeutics designed to either curtail or enhance their activation. We do know that relatively high, inflammatory doses of sunlight are required for the induction of regulatory T cells (64, 65) and skin infiltrating suppressor macrophages (66), while exposure to lower subinflammatory doses of UV leads to regulatory B cell activation (9) and suppression of immunity by inhibiting effector and memory T cell activation (67). This latter point is perhaps more relevant because these doses of UV are less than what is required to cause a barely detectable sunburn and are easily obtained by humans during regular non-recreational daily activities.

Table 1. Cells of the Immune System Involved in UV-immunosuppression

Cell	Function/Comment	References
Dendritic Cells	1. Migrate from irradiated skin to lymph nodes, 2. Skin derived lymph node DC harbour DNA damage, 3. Antigen presenting function adversely affected	(13) (14) (15,16)
Macrophages	1. Infiltrate skin following exposure to UV, 2. Source of anti-inflammatory cytokines	(17-19)
Mast Cells	1. Absence renders host resistant to UV-immunosuppression 2. Transmits suppressive signal to the immune system by migrating from irradiated skin to lymph nodes 3. Responsible for secreting anti-inflammatory cytokines (e.g. IL-10) locally in response to UV 4. Dermal density correlates with skin cancer susceptibility	(20,21) (22) (23) (24,25)
Regulatory B cells	1. Activated early (hours to days) after UV exposure and suppress DC activation of systemic immunity 2. Upregulate surface expression of B220 (CD45R) and MHC II 2. Activation mediated by UVB wavelengths 3. One pathway of activation is dependent on UV-inflammatory mediators such as PAF and 5HT 5. Mediate suppression via IL-10	(9) (9) (26) (27) (27)
Suppressor T cells	1. Control the development of skin tumours 2. CTLA-4+ suppressor cells activated 3. One population is $CD4^{+}CD25^{+}FoxP3^{+}CTLA\text{-}4^{+}GITR^{+}neuropilin\text{-}1^{+}$	(4,7) (29) (8, 83, 84)
Natural killer T cells	1. IL-4 secreting CD1d-restricted NKT cell activated in spleen is responsible for suppressing anti-tumour immunity	(90)

Table 2. Some of the Known Secreted Factors Involved in UV-immunosuppression

Factor	Function/Comment	References
IL-4	1. Blocking IL-4 inhibits UV-immunosuppression 2. IL-4 knockout mice are resistant to the suppressive effect of UV	(30,28) (31,32)
IL-10	1. Produced by keratinocytes after UV exposure 2. Regulatory B cells activated by UV secrete IL-10 3. Blocking IL-10 inhibits UV-immunosuppression 4. Mast cell derived IL-10 required for suppressing UVB inflammation 5. IL-10 knockout mice are resistant to the carcinogenic effects of long term UV irradiation	(33) (27) (30,28) (23) (34)
IL-12	1. Rescues the host from UV-immunosuppression and tolerance 2. Blocks the induction of suppressor T cells 3. Enhances DNA repair after UV exposure 4. IL-12 knockout mice are more susceptible to UV-photocarcinogenesis 5. UV causes antigen presenting cells to secrete antagonistic IL-12p40 homodimers	(35,36) (37) (38,39) (40) (41)
IL-18	1. Enhances DNA repair after UV exposure and rescues the host from UV-immunosuppression	(42)
TNF	1. UV induces TNF release from keratinocytes 2. UV-induced TNF responsible for alteration to skin DC 3. Blocking TNF inhibits UV-immunosuppression	(43) (44) (30)
Prostaglandin E_2 (PGE_2)	1. Increased prostaglandin synthesis following UV exposure 2. COX-2 is enhanced by UV while inhibiting COX-2 protects from UV-induced skin tumours 3. PGE_2 receptor knockout mice are resistant to the carcinogenic effects of long term UV irradiation	(45,46) (47,48) (49)
Platelet Activating Factor (PAF)	1. Phospholipid released from keratinocytes following UV exposure 2. Blocking PAF binding to its receptor inhibits UV and Psoralen UVA–induced immunosuppression 3. Together with serotonin is responsible for the activation of UV-regulatory B cells 4. Mediates Langerhans Cell migration from the skin to lymph nodes 5. PAF receptor expression required on the surface of haematopoeitc cells	(50-52) (53,54) (27) (55) (56)
cis-Urocanic (UCA) (5HT; serotonin)	1. UV converts the endogenous *trans* isomer of urocanic acid in skin to the immunosuppressive *cis* form 2. Binds to and mediates its immunosuppressive function via serotonin receptors 3. Signalling through cis-UCA receptors responsible for the activation of immunoregulatory B cells	(57,58) (59) (27)
RANKL	1. Receptor activator of NF-kappa B (RANK) Ligand is upregulated in UV-irradiated epidermis 2. RANKL activates DC to control T-reg numbers	(60) (60)

1. Suppressor Macrophages

Innate immunity is mediated by neutrophils, granulocytes, mast cells, basophils, eosinophils and macrophages. This type of immune response is one of the earliest to respond to danger signals and is characterised by a lack of specificity to the antigen together with the absence of immunological memory. It is now well established that one of the first cells to infiltrate UV-irradiated skin are a subset of suppressor macrophages (68, 69). The appearance of these CD1a(T6)$^-$HLA-DR$^+$ cells is dose and wavelength dependent as increasing amounts of UVB but not UVA results in greater infiltration into the irradiated epidermis, reaching a maximum at 2-3 days post UVB exposure (70). Moreover, these CD11b$^+$ cells are able to activate suppressor T cell populations (71, 72) via an IL-10 (18) and TGFβ (73) dependent mechanism. Confirming a role for these suppressor macrophages was the observation that anti-CD11b therapy prevents UV-immunosuppression *in vivo* (74).

The epidermal infiltration and acquisition of suppressor activity by these macrophages depends on two factors. The first is the release and deposition of complement component 3b (C3b) from irradiated keratinocytes (75), and the second is the binding of the stable form of C3b (iC3b) to its receptor CD11b on the surface of the infiltrating macrophages (76). Using mice deficient in C3 or mice treated with sCR1 (which inhibits C3 cleavage to C3b) Hammerberg et al. demonstrated that this pathway was important for both blocking the recruitment of suppressor macrophages and preventing UV-induced immunosuppression. More recently this group has demonstrated that suppressor macrophages from UV-irradiated skin migrate to the draining lymph nodes following contact with antigen where they produce IL-10 for immune modulation (77).

A number of reports have described a role for macrophages in suppressing anti-tumour immunity (for a review please see (78)) and we have recently shown that macrophages infiltrating UV-induced skin tumours are associated with tumour progression (79, 80). Whether UV-induced suppressor macrophages and tumour associated macrophages are related however, remains to be determined.

2. Suppressor T cells

Recent research efforts have greatly increased our understanding of the role of UV-induced regulatory T cells (UV-Tregs) in modulating immune responses (for an overview of UV-Tregs please see (81)). Similar to conventional regulatory T cells, UV-Tregs express a wide variety of surface and intracellular markers that characterise them as suppressor populations, including CD4 (82), CD25 (65), CD152 (CTLA-4) (29) and the transcription factor FoxP3 (8, 83). Recently, Maeda et al. extended the range of regulatory markers that UV-Tregs express to include the glucocorticoid-induced TNF family-related receptor (GITR) and the surface molecule neuropilin-1 (84). CD4$^+$CD25$^+$ T regs are defined, in part, by their expression of surface markers such as GITR (85) and neuropilin-1 (86). This expression is of functional significance because depleting GITR$^+$ cells *in vivo* results in deadly autoimmunne gastritis (87) while treatment of virally infected mice with anti-GITR antibodies improves the disease outcome by suppressing the activity of T regs (88). Additionally, T reg activation can be prevented with antibodies against neuropilin-1 which interfere with neuropilin-1 mediated DC interaction with T regs (89). While it is not yet clear whether expression of these markers on UV-Tregs is of similar functional significance, understanding the phenotype of UV-Tregs is important if we are to design specific therapeutic targets.

UV-Induced NK-T Cells

In 2000, Moodycliffe and colleagues demonstrated the UV-induced activation of a unique subset of DX5-expressing, CD1d-restricted T cells (90). Adoptive transfer of these Natural Killer-T (NKT) cells from the spleen of chronically UV-irradiated mice into naïve recipients suppressed both the delayed type hypersensitivity (DTH) response in an antigen specific manner, and the anti-tumour immune response to transplanted tumour cells. While these UV-NK-Tregs produce significant amounts of IL-4, the exact mechanism of this immune suppression remains to be determined. In addition, it is not yet clear whether the $CD4^+CD25^+CD152^+GITR^+$neuroplin-1^+FoxP3^+ T cells described above are a separate UV-Treg population or are generated in parallel and in addition to these UV-NKT cells.

It is important to determine the mechanism by which UV-Tregs exert their suppressive function. Cytokines such as interleukin-4 have been firmly established as key mediators of UV-immunosuppression (28, 30-32) and as discussed above, UV-induced $CD3^+CD4^+DX5^+$ NK-T cells secrete significant amounts of IL-4 (90). Meanwhile, the CTLA-4^+CD4^+ UV-Tregs described by Schwarz and colleagues exert their suppressive function principally via IL-10 secretion, a feature essential to their ability to suppress anti-tumour immune responses (34). This same group demonstrated that UV-Tregs also secrete high levels of transforming growth factor ®$_1$ (TGF®$_1$) and IFN© but low levels of IL-2 and no IL-4 (29). This would be consistent with UV-Tregs being closely related to T regulatory 1 (Tr1) cells (91). However, unlike Tr1 cells that require IL-10 for their activation and regulate immunity in an antigen specific manner, UV-Tregs are not dependent on IL-10 and control immune responses via bystander suppression (84). In contrast to these findings, Ghoreishi and Dutz found that while UV-Treg production of IL-10 was not a feature of UV-immunosuppression in a trans-cutaneous antigen model, expression of IL-10 by the host was required (92). These confusing and contradictory findings from different experiments suggest that UV-Tregs could represent a unique and distinct subset of T regs and that their activation and subsequent phenotype is dependent on a number of factors including UV dose, kinetics and mode of antigen delivery.

A Unique Role ror Transforming Growth Factor B_1 (Tgfβ_1)

Mice deficient in the immune modulating cytokine TGF®$_1$ develop severe inflammatory disease resulting in premature death (93,94). This observation lead researchers to postulate that the anti-inflammatory and immunosuppressive properties of TGF®$_1$ is one mechanism by which T-regs modulate immune outcomes. A definitive role for T-reg production of TGF®$_1$ however is still to be confirmed and is somewhat controversial. Early reports suggested that Tregs mediated immune suppression via TGF®$_1$ production (95-98), while others dispute some of these findings (99). More recently, $CD4^+CD25^+$ Tregs have been shown to restore self-tolerance in autoimmune diabetes (100) and suppress CD8 anti-tumour T cell responses (101) via TGF®$_1$-dependent mechanisms. Therefore, a role for TGF®$_1$ in T-reg mediated immune suppression probably depends on the type of response that is being regulated and whether the T-regs are naturally occurring thymic originating CD25$^+$ or inducible CD25$^-$ T cells in the periphery (102, 103).

While T-reg production of TGF®$_1$ might not be absolutely required for suppression under all circumstances, it does appear to be critically important for the activation of inducible Tregs (104). TGF®$_1$ converts CD4$^+$CD25$^-$ cells into CD25$^+$FoxP3-expressing Tregs (105,106) and influences the peripheral pool of T-regs (107). TGF® is also responsible for maintaining both Foxp3 expression and the suppressor function of peripheral T-regs (103). This is of functional significance because TGF®$_1$-induced Tregs are capable of suppressing the development of various inflammatory conditions (108, 109) and autoimmune diseases (110). Indeed, it has recently been shown that TGF®$_1$-latency-associated peptide (LAP)-expressing T-regs suppress EAE in mice via TGF®$_1$ production (111, 112).

The availability of TGF®$_1$ for signalling to CD4$^+$CD25$^+$ T cells is important for the continued maintenance of T-regs in secondary lymphoid tissues, as withdrawal of TGF®$_1$ stimulation results in a loss of Foxp3 expression and the associated regulatory function after approximately 4 days (113). We have previously shown that one of the ways UV-induced skin tumours evade immunological destruction is via TGFβ$_1$-secretion (114). Indeed, TGFβ$_1$-overexpressing skin tumours alter the anti-tumour immune outcome by altering DC migration patterns (115) and recruiting suppressor macrophages to the tumour micro environment (80). Unfortunately, results from experiments designed to assess the ability of UV radiation to directly alter TGF®$_1$ levels in skin are conflicting. Direct exposure of human skin to UV *in vivo* (116) and human keratinocytes *in vitro* (117, 118) has been shown to significantly upregulate TGF®$_1$, while others show either no effect (119), or a decrease in expression (120). Using human skin fibroblasts as a model, *in vitro* exposure to UVB has been shown to both increase (119, 121, 122,) and decrease TGF®$_1$ expression (123). It is likely that a combination of different UV spectra, dose, experimental kinetics and cell type used would explain these apparent contradictions.

While UV-Tregs isolated from lymph nodes can produce TGF®$_1$ (29), and TGF®$_1$ is required for the induction of Tregs, it is not yet known whether TGF®$_1$ is involved in the induction or maintenance of *UV-induced* Tregs. While antibodies against TGF®$_1$ were found to be ineffective in blocking UV-induced immunosuppression in one study (29), it remains to be determined whether the recently described peptide inhibitors of TGFβ$_1$ would be more effective in blocking the activity of UV-Tregs (124). Hopefully, future investigations into the expression of TGF®$_1$-LAP on UV-Tregs, together with a more detailed analysis of the source of any upregulated TGF®$_1$ in skin or elsewhere following UV exposure might help answer some of these questions.

3. Immunoregulatory B Sells

B cells have the capacity to exert both effector and suppressive actions on the immune system (125, 126) inducing tolerance when presenting antigen to naïve T cells (127). While research into regulatory T cells has intensified over the last decade, suppressor B cells have remained a relatively unexplored subset of regulatory cells (for recent reviews on regulatory B cells please see (128-130). An important role for B cells in the recovery from experimental autoimmune encephalomyelitis (EAE; a mouse model of multiple sclerosis) has been demonstrated (131). In this study, B cell deficient mice failed to spontaneously enter disease remission. This suggested that the absence of B cells precluded the eventual activation of T helper 2 (Th2) cells, resulting in hyperactivity of the $CD4^+$ Th1 cells that were ultimately responsible for mediating disease progression. While the mechanism of B cell-mediated immune regulation was unknown at that time, it has since been shown that in addition to their more traditional role of antibody secretion, B cells have the capacity to regulate immune outcomes via cytokine secretion. Similar to helper T cell subsets (132), "effector" Be1 and Be2 cells directed an IFN©/IL-12 or IL-4/6/10 dominant response respectively (133). Around the same time Moulin et al. demonstrated that B cells could suppress DC induction of Th1-immunity (possibly via IL-10 secretion) and were therefore essential for IL-4 mediated Th2 immune responses (134). It has since been confirmed that B cell secretion of IL-10 is a key feature of the ability of these cells to suppress immune responses and is important for controlling chronic intestinal inflammation (135), tempering the severity of autoimmune diseases (136-139) and limiting contact dermatitis (140). Regulatory B cells also participate in transplantation tolerance (141) and allow the outgrowth of tumours by suppressing anti-tumour immunity (142). Recently it has been demonstrated that in addition to IL-10, B cells may regulate T cell responses via secretion of other cytokines such as IL-13 (143) and $TGF\beta_1$ (144). B cells may also regulate immunity via immunoglobulin (Ig) production. For example, B cell derived IgM antibodies are required for augmenting the contact sensitivity response (146). Whether cytokine and Ig-secreting suppressor B cells are a discreet antigen-specific subset of the wider B cell population (140, 145) or conventional B cells activated by specific stimuli still remains to be determined.

We have recently discovered that within hours (24-72h) of exposure to UV radiation, the total B cell pool in skin-draining lymph nodes expands by over 40%. These B cells have an activated phenotype, characterised by an increase in the surface expression of MHC II and B220 antigens. When these B cells are isolated from the lymph nodes and transferred into naïve, unirradiated syngeneic hosts, they suppress dendritic cell induction of immune responses (9). Similar to the B cells described above, these UV-regulatory B cells secrete significant amounts of IL-10, which was necessary for their immune-inhibiting function as B cells isolated from UV-irradiated IL-10 deficient mice were unable to transfer suppression (27).

Factors Involved in the Activation of UV-Regulatory Cells

DNA damage, together with urocanic acid isomerisation and membrane lipid oxidation occurs within minutes of exposure to UV radiation. One consequence of this is the release of inflammatory mediators such as platelet activating factor (PAF) (52) and *cis*-UCA (57), both of which are immunosuppressive (53, 147). The UV-induced release of these factors occurs primarily in the irradiated skin site, but how this immunosuppressive signal is then transmitted to the secondary lymphoid tissues where lymphocyte activation occurs has been a mystery. One possibility is that soluble factors such as PAF, cis-UCA and cytokines flow freely to the draining lymph nodes where they bind to receptors on the surface of regulatory lymphocyte populations. While this is indeed feasible there has so far been no evidence to support this assertion. Both PAF and serotonin are required for the activation of regulatory B cells (27), and while B cells express PAF (148) and serotonin (149) receptors it is not clear whether lymph node B cells are the ultimate target of these inflammatory mediators. Interestingly, *in vitro* studies have confirmed that exposure to PAF induces IL-4 and IL-13 secretion by B cells (150), however considering that PAF is degraded within minutes (151), it is more likely that the cellular target of oxidised lipids such as PAF reside in the skin. This is likely to be important because it has recently been shown that blocking both the PAF and serotonin receptor pathways prevents UV-induced skin cancer formation (152).

Dendritic Cells as Mediators of Regulatory T Cell Activation

The skin contains a number of cellular candidates that could be targets of UV indued factors. Dendritic cells (DC) express PAF receptors (153) and migrate from the skin to local lymph nodes in response to PAF (55). Because DC have the unique capacity to activate both primary immunity (154) and induce antigen specific tolerance (155, 156), many studies have focused on understanding the effects of UV on DC function. Exposing skin to UV induces Langerhans cell migration from the epidermis to the draining lymph nodes (157). It is believed that these DNA-damaged, migrating subset of DC, are responsible for inducing immunological tolerance (14, 158-160). While this certainly occurs during *local* UV-immunosuppression; where the antigen is applied directly to the site of irradiation, it does not appear to be the case for *systemic* immunosuppression (13, 161). This is observed as suppression to an antigen applied to a site distant to that receiving the UV. Using this model, antigen-bearing DC isolated from skin-draining lymph nodes have the same capacity to activate immunity as those from control un-irradiated groups (9, 162). This suggests that another skin derived cell transports the *systemically* immunosuppressive effects of UV radiation from the skin to lymph nodes.

Mast Cells and the Activation of Regulatory Populations in Secondary Lymphoid Tissues

Using mice with a mutation in the cKit gene that renders them mast cell deficient, Hart et al. demonstrated an absolute requirement for mast cells in systemic UV-immunosuppression (20). It has been suggested that TNF (21), histamine (20) and more recently IL-10 (23) are responsible for the suppressive effects induced by mast cells, although it remained unclear how suppressive signals acting on mast cells in the skin could alter the activation of lymphocytes in distant lymphoid tissues. Because mast cells have the capacity to migrate from the skin to the draining lymph nodes following antigen contact (163), we investigated the possibility that UV is a mast cell migratory trigger. To that end we recently demonstrated that one way UV causes systemic immunosuppression is by inducing mast cells to migrate from the site of irradiation to the local draining lymph nodes (22). This migration was facilitated by the establishment of a UV induced CXCL12 chemokine gradient directing $CXCR4^+$ cells towards draining lymph nodes. Skin resident mast cells expressed CXCR4 (the specific receptor for CXCL12) and migrated to the lymph node B cell areas which was found to be the source of the increased CXCL12. This event was critical to the downstream immunosuppressive pathway because when mast cell migration was blocked using the specific CXCR4 inhibitor AMD3100, UV immunosuppression was inhibited (22). Our work supports the findings of others that mast cell migration to lymph nodes is an important prelude to altering and influencing immune outcomes. In a mouse model of multiple sclerosis (EAE), mast cells migrate from the spleen to lymph nodes only after the induction of disease (164). More recently using a model of glomerulonephritis it was shown that mast cell accumulation in lymph nodes (but not the kidneys) was an essential feature of the ability of mast cells to inhibit Th1-mediated disease progression (165). While it has previously been demonstrated that mast cells have the capacity to regulate lymphocyte activation *in vitro* (166, 167) and participate in maintaining regulatory T cells in the periphery (168), our studies demonstrate the mechanism by which mast cells could potentially alter lymphocyte activation and differentiation *in vivo*. Considering the demonstrated *in vitro* potential for mast cell mediated growth and differentiation of B cells (169-171) together with their localisation to B cell areas within lymphoid tissues (22) our current work is aimed at investigating what role these migrating mast cells play in the subsequent generation of effector and regulatory populations.

Regulatory B Cells as Facilitators of UV-Immunosuppression

Regulatory T cells can easily be identified by flow cytometry in the lymph nodes and spleens of UV-irradiated, antigen sensitised mice. We now know that the ultimate UV suppressor population activated *in vivo* that is responsible for regulating the immune response is a $CD4^+$ T cell because when isolated, these populations transfer immune suppression when injected into naive syngeneic hosts. Surprisingly, it still remains to be determined exactly how these UV-Tregs become activated, and while all of the cytokines mentioned above including IL-4, IL-10, TGFβ and RANKL can activate UV-Tregs, the source of these mediators remains relatively unknown. Keratinocytes in the skin and DC, at least in the context of *local* UV-immune suppression, may be a potential source of some of these inflammatory mediators, but this does not explain the ability of UV to suppress *systemic* immunity. As already discussed, UV does not alter the migration of DC from unirradiated skin sites (13) and we and others have demonstrated that draining lymph node DC are not defective in their antigen presenting capacity (9, 162). This suggests that another cell population must be responsible for the activation of UV-Tregs. We believe that mast cells are an important bridge between the UV-induced inflammatory events in irradiated skin and the immune suppressive environment established in secondary lymphoid tissues. Although a direct link between mast cells and the activation of B cells has yet to be established *in vivo*, mast cells have been demonstrated to activate B cells *in vitro* (169, 170). A number of membrane bound and soluble factors are needed for effective B cell activation including CD40-CD40L interactions (172-174) and the presence of cytokines such as IL-4, 6, 10 and 13. Mast cells have all these requisite molecules or produce them following activation. We have shown that UV activates an IL-10 secreting B cell, which when transferred into naive recipients is immunosuppressive

(9, 27). There is now considerable evidence that B cells have the capacity to profoundly alter the immune outcome through direct interactions with T cells and via the secretion of various cytokines (discussed above and summary Figure 1). We have shown that UV-induced PAF and serotonin are both required for the activation of IL-10-secreting regulatory B cells (27) and studies from the laboratory of Bruce Mazer have demonstrated that PAF induces the secretion of IL-13 in human B lymphocytes (150) which was important for IgE class switching (143). Whether an IL-13-secreting B cell is activated after UV irradiation is not known, though this could be an important mechanism of B cell mediated regulation considering the requirement of IL-13 for Th2 development to skin acquired antigens (175). It's possible that IL-13 production by B cells may serve two roles: as an autocrine B cell activating cytokine (176) and as a critical mediator of Th2 cell development (177).

Conclusion

UV radiation is likely to be the major environmental immunosuppressive agent to which most humans are exposed. Doses of sunlight that are too low to be inflammatory or cause sunburn in addition to inflammatory doses are suppressive. Therefore sunlight exposure most days of the year, during normal daily activities, in addition to the higher exposures seen during recreational activities modulates immunity but probably with different molecular mediators being involved. Therefore sunlight would modulate immunity nearly each day in the lives of most humans except perhaps during mid winter in cold climates. Sunlight alters production of soluble factors that influences cells in locally irradiated skin and establishes a cascade of events culminating in immunological alterations to skin draining lymph nodes that favour immunosuppression. Both UVB and UVA wavebands are immunosuppressive. In this way sunlight has a profound affect on many aspects of immunity in the skin, including to skin tumours, vaccinations and infectious agents.

Many aspects of how UV radiation leads to a suppressive microenvironment in skin draining lymph nodes is unknown, but many major players have been identified. A considerable amount of further research attention is required in order to fully understand these events. The multiple signals initiated by sunlight offers a range of therapeutic targets to improve immunity in humans, enhancing our ability to live healthy lives in the presence of continuous sunlight exposure.

UV radiation can cause genetic damage to cells, isomerization of trans to cis urocanic acid, production of ROS, and oxidation of membrane phospholipids, all of which can initiate immunosuppression. Oxidized lipids such as PAF, PGE_2 produced from activation of COX_2, suppressive cytokines such as IL-10, TGF$®_1$ and TNF produced by keratinocytes, fibroblasts and other cells are all involved in initiating immunosuppression. Cellular changes include suppressor macrophages and mast cells migrating to lymph nodes where suppressor B and T reg cells become activated. However, with low dose UV irradiation, suppression of T effector and memory cell development can occur in the absence of Treg (67) demonstrating that there are sunlight induced suppressive mechanisms that do not involve Treg. Regulatory B cells may be involved at these low doses.

It is likely that the importance of different mediators and cellular events is dependent on UV dose and spectrum, although the condition whereby each of these mediators is involved is under explored. However knowledge of these events is improving and eventually should contribute to our ability to prevent these deleterious effects of sunlight while hopefully enabling the health benefits of sunlight such as vitamin D production to be maintained.

References

[1] Tracey, E., D. Baker, W. Chen, E. Stavrou, and J. Bishop. 2007. Cancer in New South Wales: Incidence, Mortality and Prevalence, 2005. *Cancer Institute NSW* .

[2] Agar, N. S., G. M. Halliday, R. S. Barnetson, H. N. Ananthaswamy, M. Wheeler, and A. M. Jones. 2004. The basal layer in human squamous tumors harbors more UVA than UVB fingerprint mutations: a role for UVA in human skin carcinogenesis. *Proc Nat Acad Sci USA* **101**: 4954-4959.

[3] Halliday, G. M. 2005. Inflammation, gene mutation and photoimmunosuppression in response to UVR-induced oxidative damage contributes to photocarcinogenesis. *Mutat Res* **571**: 107-120.

[4] Shreedhar, V. K., M.W. Pride, Y. Sun, M.L. Kripke, and FM.Strickland 1998. Origin and characteristics of ultraviolet-B radiation-induced suppressor T lymphocytes *J Immunol* **161**: 520-530.

[5] Fisher, M. S., and M. L. Kripke. 1977. Systemic alteration induced in mice by ultraviolet light irradiation and its relationship to ultraviolet carcinogenesis. *Proc Nat Acad Sci USA* **74**: 1688-1692.

[6] Moloney, F. J., H. Comber, P. O'Lorcain, P. O'Kelly, P. J. Conlon, and G. M. Murphy. 2006. A population-based study of skin cancer incidence and prevalence in renal transplant recipients. *Br J Dermatol* **154**: 498-504.

[7] Fisher, M. S., and M. L. Kripke. 1982. Suppressor T lymphocytes control the development of primary skin cancers in ultraviolet-irradiated mice. *Science* **216**: 1133-1134.

[8] Gorman, S, J. W. Tan, S. T. Yerkovich, J. J. Finlay-Jones, P. H. Hart. 2007. CD4+ T cells in lymph nodes of UVB-irradiated mice suppress immune responses to new antigens both in vitro and in vivo. *J Immunol* **127**: 915-924.

[9] Byrne, S. N., and G. M. Halliday. 2005. B Cells activated in lymph nodes in response to ultraviolet irradiation or by interleukin-10 inhibit dendritic cell induction of immunity. *J Invest Dermatol* **124**: 570-578.

[10] Damian, D. L., R. S. Barnetson, and G. M. Halliday. 1999. Low-dose UVA and UVB have different time courses for suppression of contact hypersensitivity to a recall antigen in humans. *J Invest Dermatol* **112**: 939-944.

[11] Yoshikawa, T., and J. W. Streilein. 1990. Genetic basis of the effects of ultraviolet light B on cutaneous immunity. Evidence that polymorphism at the TNF-alpha and LPS loci governs susceptibility. *Immunogenetics* **32**: 398-405.

[12] Byrne, S. N., N. Spinks, and G. M. Halliday. 2002. Ultraviolet-A irradiation of C57BL/6 mice suppresses systemic contact hypersensitivity or enhances secondary immunity depending on dose. *J Invest Dermatol* **119**: 858-864.

[13] Noonan, F. P., C. Bucana, D. N. Sauder, and E. C. De Fabo. 1984. Mechanism of systemic immune suppression by UV irradiation in vivo. II. The UV effects on number and morphology of epidermal Langerhans cells and the UV-induced suppression of contact hypersensitivity have different wavelength dependencies. *J Immunol* **132**: 2408-2416.

[14] Sontag, Y., C. L. Guikers, A. A. Vink, F. R. de Gruijl, H. van Loveren, J. Garssen, L. Roza, M. L. Kripke, J. C. van der Leun, and W. A. van Vloten. 1995. Cells with UV-

specific DNA damage are present in murine lymph nodes after in vivo UV irradiation. *J Invest Dermatol* **104**: 734-738.

[15] Greene, M. I., M. S. Sy, M. Kripke, and B. Benacerraf. 1979. Impairment of antigen-presenting cell function by ultraviolet radiation. *Proc Nat Acad Sci USA* **76**: 6591-6595.

[16] Stingl, G., L. A. Gazze-Stingl, W. Aberer, and K. Wolff. 1981. Antigen presentation by murine epidermal langerhans cells and its alteration by ultraviolet B light. *J Immunol* **127**: 1707-1713.

[17] Cooper, K. D., L. Oberhelman, T. A. Hamilton, O. Baadsgaard, M. Terhune, G. LeVee, T. Anderson, and H. Koren. 1992. UV exposure reduces immunization rates and promotes tolerance to epicutaneous antigens in humans: relationship to dose, CD1a-DR+ epidermal macrophage induction, and Langerhans cell depletion. *Proc Nat Acad Sci USA* **89**: 8497-8501.

[18] Kang, K., C. Hammerberg, L. Meunier, and K. D. Cooper. 1994. CD11b+ macrophages that infiltrate human epidermis after in vivo ultraviolet exposure potently produce IL-10 and represent the major secretory source of epidermal IL-10 protein. *J Immunol* 153: 5256-5264.

[19] Stevens, S. R., A. Shibaki, L. Meunier, and K. D. Cooper. 1995. Suppressor T cell-activating macrophages in ultraviolet-irradiated human skin induce a novel, TGF-beta-dependent form of T cell activation characterized by deficient IL-2r alpha expression. *J Immunol* 155: 5601-5607.

[20] Hart, P. H., M. A. Grimbaldeston, G. J. Swift, A. Jaksic, F. P. Noonan, and J. J. Finlayjones. 1998. Dermal mast cells determine susceptibility to ultraviolet B-induced systemic suppression of contact hypersensitivity responses in mice. *J Exp Med* **187**: 2045-2053.

[21] Alard, P., H. Niizeki, L. Hanninen, and J. W. Streilein. 1999. Local ultraviolet B irradiation impairs contact hypersensitivity induction by triggering release of tumor necrosis factor-alpha from mast cells. Involvement of mast cells and Langerhans cells in susceptibility to ultraviolet B. *J Invest Dermatol* **113**: 983-990.

[22] Byrne, S. N., A. Y. Limon-Flores, and S. E. Ullrich. 2008. Mast cell migration from the skin to the draining lymph nodes upon UV-irradiation represents a key step in the induction of immune suppression. *J Immunol* **180**: 4648-4655.

[23] Grimbaldeston, M. A., S. Nakae, J. Kalesnikoff, M. Tsai, and S. J. Galli. 2007. Mast cell-derived interleukin 10 limits skin pathology in contact dermatitis and chronic irradiation with ultraviolet B. *Nat Immunol* **8**: 1095-1104.

[24] Grimbaldeston, M. A., A. Green, S. Darlington, B. O. Robertson, G. Marshman, J. J. Finlay-Jones, and P. H. Hart. 2003. Susceptibility to basal cell carcinoma is associated with high dermal mast cell prevalence in non-sun-exposed skin for an Australian population. *Photochem & Photobiol* **78**: 633-639;.

[25] Grimbaldeston, M. A., A. L. Pearce, B. O. Robertson, B. J. Coventry, G. Marshman, J. J. Finlay-Jones, and P. H. Hart. 2004. Association between melanoma and dermal mast cell prevalence in sun-unexposed skin. *Br J Dermatol* **150**: 895-903;.

[26] Byrne, S. N., J. Ahmed, and G. M. Halliday. 2005. Ultraviolet B but not A radiation activates suppressor B cells in draining lymph nodes. *Photochem & Photobiol* **81**: 1366-1370.

[27] Matsumura, Y., S. N. Byrne, D. Nghiem, Y. Miyahara, and S. E. Ullrich. 2006. A role for inflammatory mediators in the induction of immunoregulatory B cells. *J Immunol* **177**: 4810-4817.

[28] Shreedhar, V., T. Giese, V. W. Sung, and S. E. Ullrich. 1998. A cytokine cascade including prostaglandin E2, IL-4, and IL-10 is responsible for UV-induced systemic immune suppression. *J Immunol* **160**: 3783-3789.

[29] Schwarz, A., S. Beissert, K. Grosse-Heitmeyer, M. Gunzer, J. A. Bluestone, S. Grabbe, and T. Schwarz. 2000. Evidence for functional relevance of CTLA-4 in ultraviolet-radiation-induced tolerance. *J Immunol* **165**: 1824-1831.

[30] Rivas, J. M., and S. E. Ullrich. 1994. The role of IL-4, IL-10, and TNF-alpha in the immune suppression induced by ultraviolet radiation. *J Leuk Biol* **56**: 769-775.

[31] El-Ghorr, A. A., and M. Norval. 1997. The role of interleukin-4 in ultraviolet B light-induced immunosuppression. *Immunology* **92**: 26-32.

[32] Hart, P. H., M. A. Grimbaldeston, A. Jaksic, J. E. Tan, G. J. Swift, E. K. Hosszu, G. M. Halliday, and J. J. Finlay-Jones. 2000. Ultraviolet B-induced suppression of immune responses in interleukin-4-/-mice: Relationship to dermal mast cells. *J Invest Dermatol* **114**: 508-513.

[33] Enk, C. D., D. Sredni, A. Blauvelt, and S. I. Katz. 1995. Induction of IL-10 gene expression in human keratinocytes by UVB exposure in vivo and in vitro. *J Immunol* **154**: 4851-4856.

[34] Loser, K., J. Apelt, M. Voskort, M. Mohaupt, S. Balkow, T. Schwarz, S. Grabbe, and S. Beissert. 2007. IL-10 controls ultraviolet-induced carcinogenesis in mice. *J Immunol* **179**: 365-371.

[35] Schwarz, A., S. Grabbe, Y. Aragane, K. Sandkuhl, H. Riemann, T. A. Luger, M. Kubin, G. Trinchieri, and T. Schwarz. 1996. Interleukin-12 prevents ultraviolet B-induced local immunosuppression and overcomes UVB-induced tolerance. *J Invest Dermatol* **106**: 1187-1191.

[36] Schwarz, A., S. Grabbe, K. Mahnke, H. Riemann, T. A. Luger, M. Wysocka, G. Trinchieri, and T. Schwarz. 1998. Interleukin 12 breaks ultraviolet light induced immunosuppression by affecting CD8(+) rather than CD4(+) T cells. *J Invest Dermatol* **110**: 272-276.

[37] Schmitt, D. A., L. Owen-Schaub, and S. E. Ullrich. 1995. Effect of IL-12 on immune suppression and suppressor cell induction by ultraviolet radiation. *J Immunol* **154**: 5114-5120.

[38] Schwarz, A., S. Stander, M. Berneburg, M. Bohm, D. Kulms, H. van Steeg, K. Grosse-Heitmeyer, J. Krutmann, and T. Schwarz. 2002. Interleukin-12 suppresses ultraviolet radiation-induced apoptosis by inducing DNA repair. *Nature Cell Biol* **4**: 26-31.

[39] Schwarz, A., A. Maeda, K. Kernebeck, H. van Steeg, S. Beissert, and T. Schwarz. 2005. Prevention of UV radiation-induced immunosuppression by IL-12 is dependent on DNA repair. *J Exp Med* **201**: 173-179.

[40] Maeda, A., S. W. Schneider, M. Kojima, S. Beissert, T. Schwarz, and A. Schwarz. 2006. Enhanced photocarcinogenesis in interleukin-12-deficient mice. *Cancer Res* **66**: 2962-2969.

[41] Schmitt, D. A., and S. E. Ullrich. 2000. Exposure to ultraviolet radiation causes dendritic cells/macrophages to secrete immune-suppressive IL-12p40 homodimers. *J Immunol* **165**: 3162-3167.

[42] Schwarz, A., A. Maeda, S. Stander, H. van Steeg, and T. Schwarz. 2006. IL-18 reduces ultraviolet radiation-induced DNA damage and thereby affects photoimmunosuppression. *J Immunol* **176**: 2896-2901.

[43] Kock, A., T. Schwarz, R. Kirnbauer, A. Urbanski, P. Perry, J. C. Ansel, and T. A. Luger. 1990. Human keratinocytes are a source for tumor necrosis factor alpha: evidence for synthesis and release upon stimulation with endotoxin or ultraviolet light. *J Exp Med* **172**: 1609-1614.

[44] Vermeer, M., and J. W. Streilein. 1990. Ultraviolet B light-induced alterations in epidermal Langerhans cells are mediated in part by tumor necrosis factor-alpha. *Photoderm, Photoimmunol & Photomed* **7**: 258-265.
[45] Chung, H. T., D. K. Burnham, B. Robertson, L. K. Roberts, and R. A. Daynes. 1986. Involvement of prostaglandins in the immune alterations caused by the exposure of mice to ultraviolet radiation. *J Immunol* **137**: 2478-2484.
[46] Pentland, A. P., M. Mahoney, S. C. Jacobs, and M. J. Holtzman. 1990. Enhanced prostaglandin synthesis after ultraviolet injury is mediated by endogenous histamine stimulation. A mechanism for irradiation erythema. *J Clin Invest* **86**: 566-574.
[47] Buckman, S. Y., A. Gresham, P. Hale, G. Hruza, J. Anast, J. Masferrer, and A. P. Pentland. 1998. COX-2 expression is induced by UVB exposure in human skin: implications for the development of skin cancer. *Carcinogenesis* **19**: 723-729.
[48] Pentland, A. P., J. W. Schoggins, G. A. Scott, K. N. M. Khan, and R. J. Han. 1999. Reduction of UV-induced skin tumors in hairless mice by selective COX-2 inhibition. *Carcinogenesis.* **20**: 1939-1944.
[49] Brouxhon, S., R. L. Konger, J. VanBuskirk, T. J. Sheu, J. Ryan, B. Erdle, A. Almudevar, R. M. Breyer, G. Scott, and A. P. Pentland. 2007. Deletion of prostaglandin E2 EP2 receptor protects against ultraviolet-induced carcinogenesis, but increases tumor aggressiveness. *J Invest Dermatol* **127**: 439-446.
[50] Travers, J. B., K. A. Harrison, C. A. Johnson, K. L. Clay, and J. G. Morelli. 1996. Platelet-activating factor biosynthesis induced by various stimuli in human HaCaT keratinocytes. *J Invest Dermatol* **107**: 88-94.
[51] Alappatt, C., C. A. Johnson, K. L. Clay, and J. B. Travers. 2000. Acute keratinocyte damage stimulates platelet-activating factor production. *Arch Dermatol Res* **292**: 256-259.
[52] Marathe, G. K., C. Johnson, S. D. Billings, M. D. Southall, Y. Pei, D. Spandau, R. C. Murphy, G. A. Zimmerman, T. M. McIntyre, and J. B. Travers. 2005. Ultraviolet B radiation generates PAF-like phospholipids underlying cutaneous inflammation. *J Biol Chem* **280**: 35448-35457.
[53] Walterscheid, J. P., S. E. Ullrich, and D. X. Nghiem. 2002. Platelet-activating factor, a molecular sensor for cellular damage, activates systemic immune suppression. *J Exp Med* **195**: 171-179.
[54] Wolf, P., D. X. Nghiem, J. P. Walterscheid, S. Byrne, Y. Matsumura, Y. Matsumura, C. Bucana, H. N. Ananthaswamy, and S. E. Ullrich. 2006. platelet-activating factor is crucial in psoralen and ultraviolet A-induced immune suppression, inflammation, and apoptosis. *Am J Pathol* **169**: 795-805.
[55] Fukunaga, A., N. M. Khaskhely, C. S. Sreevidya, S. N. Byrne, and S. E. Ullrich. 2008. Dermal dendritic cells, and not langerhans cells, play an essential role in inducing an immune response. *J Immunol* **180**: 3057-3064.
[56] Zhang, Q., Y. Yao, R. L. Konger, A. L. Sinn, S. Cai, K. E. Pollok, and J. B. Travers. 2008. UVB radiation-mediated inhibition of contact hypersensitivity reactions is dependent on the platelet-activating factor system. *J Invest Dermatol* **128**: 1780-1787.
[57] De Fabo, E. C., and F. P. Noonan. 1983. Mechanism of immune suppression by ultraviolet irradiation in vivo. I. Evidence for the existence of a unique photoreceptor in skin and its role in photoimmunology. *J Exp Med* **158**: 84-98.
[58] Ross, J. A., S. E. Howie, M. Norval, J. Maingay, and T. J. Simpson. 1986. Ultraviolet-irradiated urocanic acid suppresses delayed-type hypersensitivity to herpes simplex virus in mice. *J Invest Dermatol* **87**: 630-633.
[59] Walterscheid, J. P., D. X. Nghiem, N. Kazimi, L. K. Nutt, D. J. McConkey, M. Norval, and S. E. Ullrich. 2006. Cis-urocanic acid, a sunlight-induced immunosuppressive

factor, activates immune suppression via the 5-HT2A receptor. *Proc Nat Acad Sci USA* **103**: 17420-17425.

[60] Loser, K., A. Mehling, S. Loeser, J. Apelt, A. Kuhn, S. Grabbe, T. Schwarz, J. M. Penninger, and S. Beissert. 2006. Epidermal RANKL controls regulatory T-cell numbers via activation of dendritic cells. *Nat Med* **12**: 1372-1379.

[61] Ullrich, S. E. 1986. Suppression of the immune response to allogeneic histocompatibility antigens by a single exposure to ultraviolet radiation. *Transplantation.* **42**: 287-291.

[62] Ullrich, S. E. 1991. Systemic immunosuppression of cell-mediated immune reactions by a monofunctional psoralen plus ultraviolet A radiation. *Photoderm, Photoimmunol & Photomed.* **8**: 116-122.

[63] Maeda, A., A. Schwarz, K. Kernebeck, N. Gross, Y. Aragane, D. Peritt, and T. Schwarz. 2005. Intravenous infusion of syngeneic apoptotic cells by photopheresis induces antigen-specific regulatory T cells. *J Immunol* **174**: 5968-5976.

[64] Ullrich, S. E., G. K. Yee, and M. L. Kripke. 1986. Suppressor lymphocytes induced by epicutaneous sensitization of UV-irradiated mice control multiple immunological pathways. *Immunology* **58**: 185-190.

[65] Schwarz, A., A. Maeda, M. K. Wild, K. Kernebeck, N. Gross, Y. Aragane, S. Beissert, D. Vestweber, and T. Schwarz. 2004. Ultraviolet radiation-induced regulatory T cells not only inhibit the induction but can suppress the effector phase of contact hypersensitivity. *J Immunol* **172**: 1036-1043.

[66] Baadsgaard, O., K. D. Cooper, S. Lisby, H. C. Wulf, and G. L. Wantzin. 1987. Dose response and time course for induction of T6- DR+ human epidermal antigen-presenting cells by in vivo ultraviolet A, B, and C irradiation. *J Am Acad Dermatol* **17**: 792-800.

[67] Rana, S., S. N. Byrne, L. J. Macdonald, C. Y. Chan, and G. M. Halliday. 2008. Ultraviolet B suppresses immunity by inhibiting effector and memory T cells. *Am J Pathol* **172**: 993-1004.

[68] Cooper, K. D., P. Fox, G. Neises, and S. I. Katz. 1985. Effects of ultraviolet radiation on human epidermal cell alloantigen presentation: initial depression of Langerhans cell-dependent function is followed by the appearance of T6- Dr+ cells that enhance epidermal alloantigen presentation. *J Immunol* **134**: 129-137.

[69] Cooper, K. D., G. R. Neises, and S. I. Katz. 1986. Antigen-presenting OKM5+ melanophages appear in human epidermis after ultraviolet radiation. *J Invest Dermatol* **86**: 363-370.

[70] Baadsgaard, O., H. C. Wulf, G. L. Wantzin, and K. D. Cooper. 1987. UVB and UVC, but not UVA, potently induce the appearance of T6- DR+ antigen-presenting cells in human epidermis. *J Invest Dermatol* **89**: 113-118.

[71] Baadsgaard, O., D. A. Fox, and K. D. Cooper. 1988. Human epidermal cells from ultraviolet light-exposed skin preferentially activate autoreactive CD4+2H4+ suppressor-inducer lymphocytes and CD8+ suppressor/cytotoxic lymphocytes. *J Immunol* 140: 1738-1744.

[72] Baadsgaard, O., B. Salvo, A. Mannie, B. Dass, D. A. Fox, and K. D. Cooper. 1990. In vivo ultraviolet-exposed human epidermal cells activate T suppressor cell pathways that involve CD4+CD45RA+ suppressor-inducer T cells. *J Immunol* **145**: 2854-2861.

[73] Stevens, S. R., A. Shibaki, L. Meunier, and K. D. Cooper. 1995. Suppressor T cell-activating macrophages in ultraviolet-irradiated human skin induce a novel, TGF-beta-dependent form of T cell activation characterized by deficient IL-2r alpha expression. *J Immunol* **155**: 5601-5607.

[74] Hammerberg, C., N. Duraiswamy, and K. D. Cooper. 1996. Reversal of immunosuppression inducible through ultraviolet-exposed skin by in vivo anti-CD11b treatment. *J Immunol* **157**: 5254-5261.

[75] Rauterberg, A., E. G. Jung, and E. W. Rauterberg. 1993. Complement deposits in epidermal cells after ultraviolet B exposure. *Photodermatol Photoimmunol Photomed* **9**: 135-143.

[76] Hammerberg, C., S. K. Katiyar, M. C. Carroll, and K. D. Cooper. 1998. Activated complement component 3 (C3) is required for ultraviolet induction of immunosuppression and antigenic tolerance. *J Exp Med* **187**: 1133-1138.

[77] Toichi, E., K. Q. Lu, A. R. Swick, T. S. McCormick, and K. D. Cooper. 2008. Skin-infiltrating monocytes/macrophages migrate to draining lymph nodes and produce IL-10 after contact sensitizer exposure to UV-irradiated skin. *J Invest Dermatol* (doi:10.1038/jid.2008.137)

[78] Mantovani, A., T. Schioppa, C. Porta, P. Allavena, and A. Sica. 2006. Role of tumor-associated macrophages in tumor progression and invasion. *Cancer Metastasis Rev* **25**: 315-322.

[79] Byrne, S. N., and G. M. Halliday. 2003. Phagocytosis by dendritic cells rather than MHC II(high) macrophages is associated with skin tumour regression. *Int J Cancer* **106**: 736-744.

[80] Byrne, S. N., M. C. Knox, and G. M. Halliday. 2008. TGFbeta is responsible for skin tumour infiltration by macrophages enabling the tumours to escape immune destruction. *Immunol Cell Biol* **86**: 92-97.

[81] Schwarz, and Halliday. 2007. Ch 5: Photoimmunology. *In "Photodermatology" Edited by Henry Lim, Herbert Honigsmann and John Hawk. Informa healthcare, New York* : 55-74.

[82] Ullrich, S. E., and M. L. Kripke. 1984. Mechanisms in the suppression of tumor rejection produced in mice by repeated UV irradiation. *J Immunol* . **133**: 2786-2790.

[83] Gorman, S., L. A. Kuritzky, M. A. Judge, K. M. Dixon, J. P. McGlade, R. S. Mason, J. J. Finlay-Jones, and P. H. Hart. 2007. Topically applied 1,25-dihydroxyvitamin D3 enhances the suppressive activity of CD4+CD25+ cells in the draining lymph nodes. *J Immunol* **179**: 6273-6283.

[84] Maeda, A., S. Beissert, T. Schwarz, and A. Schwarz. 2008. Phenotypic and functional characterization of ultraviolet radiation-induced regulatory T cells. *J Immunol* **180**: 3065-3071.

[85] McHugh, R. S., M. J. Whitters, C. A. Piccirillo, D. A. Young, E. M. Shevach, M. Collins, and M. C. Byrne. 2002. CD4(+)CD25(+) immunoregulatory T cells: Gene expression analysis reveals a functional role for the glucocorticoid-induced TNF receptor. *Immunity* **16**: 311-323.

[86] Bruder, D., M. Probst-Kepper, A. M. Westendorf, R. Geffers, S. Beissert, K. Loser, H. von Boehmer, J. Buer, and W. Hansen. 2004. Neuropilin-1: a surface marker of regulatory T cells. *Eur J Immunol* **34**: 623-630.

[87] Shimizu, J., S. Yamazaki, T. Takahashi, Y. Ishida, and S. Sakaguchi. 2002. Stimulation of CD25(+)CD4(+) regulatory T cells through GITR breaks immunological self-tolerance. *Nat Immunol* **3**: 135-142.

[88] Dittmer, U., H. He, R. J. Messer, S. Schimmer, A. R. M. Olbrich, C. Ohlen, P. D. Greenberg, I. M. Stromnes, M. Iwashiro, S. Sakaguchi, L. H. Evans, K. E. Peterson, G. J. Yang, and K. J. Hasenkrug. 2004. Functional impairment of CD8(+) T cells by regulatory T cells during persistent retroviral infection. *Immunity* **20**: 293-303;.

[89] Sarris, M., K. G. Andersen, F. Randow, L. Mayr, and A. G. Betz. 2008. Neuropilin-1 expression on regulatory T cells enhances their interactions with dendritic cells during antigen recognition. *Immunity* **28**: 402-413.

[90] Moodycliffe, A. M., D. Nghiem, G. Clydesdale, and S. E. Ullrich. 2000. Immune suppression and skin cancer development: regulation by NKT cells. *Nature Immunology* **1**: 521-525.

[91] Groux, H., A. Ogarra, M. Bigler, M. Rouleau, S. Antonenko, J. E. Devries, and M. G. Roncarolo. 1997. A CD4(+) T-cell subset inhibits antigen-specific T-cell responses and prevents colitis. *Nature* **389**: 737-742.

[92] Ghoreishi, M., and J. P. Dutz. 2006. Tolerance induction by transcutaneous immunization through ultraviolet-irradiated skin is transferable through CD4+CD25+ T regulatory cells and is dependent on host-derived IL-10. *J Immunol* **176**: 2635-2644.

[93] Shull, M. M., I. Ormsby, A. B. Kier, S. Pawlowski, R. J. Diebold, M. Yin, R. Allen, C. Sidman, G. Proetzel, D. Calvin, and others. 1992. Targeted disruption of the mouse transforming growth factor-beta 1 gene results in multifocal inflammatory disease. *Nature* **359**: 693-699.

[94] Kulkarni, A. B., C. G. Huh, D. Becker, A. Geiser, M. Lyght, K. C. Flanders, A. B. Roberts, M. B. Sporn, J. M. Ward, and S. Karlsson. 1993. Transforming growth factor beta 1 null mutation in mice causes excessive inflammatory response and early death. *Proc Natl Acad Sci U S A* **90**: 770-774.

[95] Miller, A., O. Lider, A. B. Roberts, M. B. Sporn, and H. L. Weiner. 1992. Suppressor T cells generated by oral tolerization to myelin basic protein suppress both in vitro and in vivo immune responses by the release of transforming growth factor beta after antigen-specific triggering. *Proc Natl Acad Sci U S A* **89**: 421-425.

[96] Chen, Y., V. K. Kuchroo, J. Inobe, D. A. Hafler, and H. L. Weiner. 1994. Regulatory T cell clones induced by oral tolerance: suppression of autoimmune encephalomyelitis. *Science* **265**: 1237-1240.

[97] Powrie, F., J. Carlino, M. W. Leach, S. Mauze, and R. L. Coffman. 1996. A critical role for transforming growth factor-beta but not interleukin 4 in the suppression of T helper type 1-mediated colitis by CD45RB(low) CD4+ T cells. *J Exp Med* **183**: 2669-2674.

[98] Nakamura, K., A. Kitani, and W. Strober. 2001. Cell contact-dependent immunosuppression by CD4(+)CD25(+) regulatory T cells is mediated by cell surface-bound transforming growth factor beta. *J Exp Med* **194**: 629-644.

[99] Piccirillo, C. A., J. J. Letterio, A. M. Thornton, R. S. McHugh, M. Mamura, H. Mizuhara, and E. M. Shevach. 2002. CD4(+)CD25(+) regulatory T cells can mediate suppressor function in the absence of transforming growth factor beta1 production and responsiveness. *J Exp Med* **196**: 237-246.

[100] Belghith, M., J. A. Bluestone, S. Barriot, J. Mégret, J. F. Bach, and L. Chatenoud. 2003. TGF-beta-dependent mechanisms mediate restoration of self-tolerance induced by antibodies to CD3 in overt autoimmune diabetes. *Nat Med* **9**: 1202-1208.

[101] Chen, M. L., M. J. Pittet, L. Gorelik, R. A. Flavell, R. Weissleder, H. von Boehmer, and K. Khazaie. 2005. Regulatory T cells suppress tumor-specific CD8 T cell cytotoxicity through TGF-beta signals in vivo. *Proc Natl Acad Sci U S A* **102**: 419-424.

[102] Fahlen, L., S. Read, L. Gorelik, S. D. Hurst, R. L. Coffman, R. A. Flavell, and F. Powrie. 2005. T cells that cannot respond to TGF-beta escape control by CD4(+)CD25(+) regulatory T cells. *J Exp Med* **201**: 737-746.

[103] Marie, J. C., J. J. Letterio, M. Gavin, and A. Y. Rudensky. 2005. TGF-beta1 maintains suppressor function and Foxp3 expression in CD4+CD25+ regulatory T cells. *J Exp Med* **201**: 1061-1067.

[104] Huber, S., C. Schramm, H. A. Lehr, A. Mann, S. Schmitt, C. Becker, M. Protschka, P. R. Galle, M. F. Neurath, and M. Blessing. 2004. Cutting edge: TGF-beta signaling is required for the in vivo expansion and immunosuppressive capacity of regulatory CD4+CD25+ T cells. *J Immunol* **173**: 6526-6531.
[105] Chen, W. J., W. W. Jin, N. Hardegen, K. J. Lei, L. Li, N. Marinos, G. McGrady, and S. M. Wahl. 2003. Conversion of peripheral CD4(+)CD25(-) naive T cells to CD4(+)CD25(+) regulatory T cells by TGF-beta induction of transcription factor Foxp3. *J Exp Med* **198**: 1875-1886;
[106] Fantini, M. C., C. Becker, G. Monteleone, F. Pallone, P. R. Galle, and M. F. Neurath. 2004. Cutting edge: TGF-beta induces a regulatory phenotype in CD4(+)CD25(-) T cells through Foxp3 induction and down-regulation of Smad7. *J Immunol* **172**: 5149-5153;.
[107] Schramm, C., S. Huber, M. Protschka, P. Czochra, J. Burg, E. Schmitt, A. W. Lohse, P. R. Galle, and M. Blessing. 2004. TGF beta regulates the CD4+CD25+T-cell pool and the expression of Foxp3 in vivo. *Int Immunol* **16**: 1241-1249.
[108] Oida, T., X. Zhang, M. Goto, S. Hachimura, M. Totsuka, S. Kaminogawa, and H. L. Weiner. 2003. CD4+CD25- T cells that express latency-associated peptide on the surface suppress CD4+CD45RBhigh-induced colitis by a TGF-beta-dependent mechanism. *J Immunol* **170**: 2516-2522.
[109] Nakamura, K., A. Kitani, I. Fuss, A. Pedersen, N. Harada, H. Nawata, and W. Strober. 2004. TGF-beta 1 plays an important role in the mechanism of CD4(+)CD25(+) regulatory T cell activity in both humans and mice. *J Immunol* **172**: 834-842;.
[110] Peng, Y. F., Y. Laouar, M. O. Li, E. A. Green, and R. A. Flavell. 2004. TGF-beta regulates in vivo expansion of Foxp3-expressing CD4(+)CD25(+) regulatory T cells responsible for protection against diabetes. *Proc Natl Acad Sci USA* **101**: 4572-4577;
[111] Zhang, X., J. Reddy, H. Ochi, D. Frenkel, V. K. Kuchroo, and H. L. Weiner. 2006. Recovery from experimental allergic encephalomyelitis is TGF-beta dependent and associated with increases in CD4+LAP+ and CD4+CD25+ T cells. *Int Immunol* **18**: 495-503.
[112] Chen, M. L., B. S. Yan, Y. Bando, V. K. Kuchroo, and H. L. Weiner. 2008. Latency-associated peptide identifies a novel CD4+CD25+ regulatory T cell subset with TGF-beta-mediated function and enhanced suppression of experimental autoimmune encephalomyelitis. *J Immunol* **180**: 7327-7337.
[113] Selvaraj, R. K., and T. L. Geiger. 2007. A kinetic and dynamic analysis of Foxp3 induced in T cells by TGF-beta. *J Immunol* **178**: 7667-7677.
[114] Halliday, G. M., and S. Le. 2001. Transforming growth factor-beta produced by progressor tumors inhibits, while IL-10 produced by regressor tumors enhances, Langerhans cell migration from skin. *Int Immunol* **13**: 1147-1154.
[115] Weber, F., S. N. Byrne, S. Le, D. A. Brown, S. N. Breit, R. A. Scolyer, and G. M. Halliday. 2005. Transforming growth factor-beta(1) immobilises dendritic cells within skin tumours and facilitates tumour escape from the immune system. *Cancer Immunol Immunother* **54**: 898-906.
[116] Quan, T., T. He, S. Kang, J. J. Voorhees, and G. J. Fisher. 2002. Ultraviolet irradiation alters transforming growth factor beta/Smad pathway in human skin in vivo. *J Invest Dermatol* **119**: 499-506.
[117] Lee, H. S., F. Kooshesh, D. N. Sauder, and S. Kondo. 1997. Modulation of TGF-beta 1 production from human keratinocytes by UVB. *Exp Dermatol* **6**: 105-110.
[118] Wang, H., and I. E. Kochevar. 2005. Involvement of UVB-induced reactive oxygen species in TGF-beta biosynthesis and activation in keratinocytes. *Free Radic Biol Med* **38**: 890-897.

[119] Brenner, M., K. Degitz, R. Besch, and C. Berking. 2005. Differential expression of melanoma-associated growth factors in keratinocytes and fibroblasts by ultraviolet A and ultraviolet B radiation. *Br J Dermatol* **153**: 733-739.
[120] Murakami, T., M. Fujimoto, M. Ohtsuki, and H. Nakagawa. 2001. Expression profiling of cancer-related genes in human keratinocytes following non-lethal ultraviolet B irradiation. *J Dermatol Sci* **27**: 121-129.
[121] Chainiaux, F., J. Remacle, and O. Toussaint. 2002. Exposure of human skin diploid fibroblasts to repeated subcytotoxic doses of ultraviolet-B induces the overexpression of transforming growth factor-beta1 mRNA. *Ann N Y Acad Sci* **973**: 44-48.
[122] Debacq-Chainiaux, F., C. Borlon, T. Pascal, V. Royer, F. Eliaers, N. Ninane, G. Carrard, B. Friguet, F. de Longueville, S. Boffe, J. Remacle, and O. Toussaint. 2005. Repeated exposure of human skin fibroblasts to UVB at subcytotoxic level triggers premature senescence through the TGF-beta1 signaling pathway. *J Cell Sci* **118**: 743-758.
[123] Choi, C. P., Y. I. Kim, J. W. Lee, and M. H. Lee. 2007. The effect of narrowband ultraviolet B on the expression of matrix metalloproteinase-1, transforming growth factor-beta1 and type I collagen in human skin fibroblasts. *Clin Exp Dermatol* **32**: 180-185.
[124] Gil-Guerrero, L., J. Dotor, I. L. Huibregtse, N. Casares, A. B. López-Vázquez, F. Rudilla, J. I. Riezu-Boj, J. López-Sagaseta, J. Hermida, S. Van Deventer, J. Bezunartea, D. Llopiz, P. Sarobe, J. Prieto, F. Borrás-Cuesta, and J. J. Lasarte. 2008. In vitro and in vivo down-regulation of regulatory T cell activity with a peptide inhibitor of TGF-beta1. *J Immunol* **181**: 126-135.
[125] Katz, S. I., D. Parker, and J. L. Turk. 1974. B-cell suppression of delayed hypersensitivity reactions. *Nature.* **251**: 550-551.
[126] Zembala, M., G. L. Asherson, J. Noworolski, and B. Mayhew. 1976. Contact sensitivity to picryl chloride: the occurrence of B suppressor cells in the lymph nodes and spleen of immunized mice. *Cell Immunol* **25**: 266-278.
[127] Fuchs, E. J., and P. Matzinger. 1992. B cells turn off virgin but not memory T cells. *Science* **258**: 1156-1159.
[128] Mizoguchi, A., and A. K. Bhan. 2006. A case for regulatory B cells. *J Immunol* **176**: 705-710.
[129] Fillatreau, S., D. Gray, and S. M. Anderton. 2008. Not always the bad guys: B cells as regulators of autoimmune pathology. *Nat Rev Immunol* **8**: 391-397.
[130] Lund, F. E. 2008. Cytokine-producing B lymphocytes-key regulators of immunity. *Curr Opin Immunol* **20**: 332-338.
[131] Wolf, S. D., B. N. Dittel, F. Hardardottir, and C. A. Janeway. 1996. Experimental autoimmune encephalomyelitis induction in genetically B cell-deficient mice. *J Exp Med* **184**: 2271-2278.
[132] Fiorentino, D. F., M. W. Bond, and T. R. Mosmann. 1989. Two types of mouse T helper cell. IV. Th2 clones secrete a factor that inhibits cytokine production by Th1 clones. *J Exp Med* **170**: 2081-2095.
[133] Harris, D. P., L. Haynes, P. C. Sayles, D. K. Duso, S. M. Eaton, N. M. Lepak, L. L. Johnson, S. L. Swain, and F. E. Lund. 2000. Reciprocal regulation of polarized cytokine production by effector B and T cells. *Nat Immunol* **1**: 475-482.
[134] Moulin, V., F. Andris, K. Thielemans, C. Maliszewski, J. Urbain, and M. Moser. 2000. B lymphocytes regulate dendritic cell (DC) function in vivo: Increased interleukin 12 production by DCs from B cell-deficient mice results in T helper cell type 1 deviation. *J Exp Med* **192**: 475-482.

[135] Fillatreau, S., C. H. Sweenie, M. J. McGeachy, D. Gray, and S. M. Anderton. 2002. B cells regulate autoimmunity by provision of IL-10. *Nat Immunol* **3**: 944-950.

[136] Mizoguchi, A., E. Mizoguchi, H. Takedatsu, R. S. Blumberg, and A. K. Bhan. 2002. Chronic intestinal inflammatory condition generates IL-10-producing regulatory B cell subset characterized by CD1d upregulation. *Immunity* **16**: 219-230.

[137] Mauri, C., D. Gray, N. Mushtaq, and M. Londei. 2003. Prevention of arthritis by interleukin 10-producing B cells. *J Exp Med* **197**: 489-501.

[138] Lenert, P., R. Brummel, E. H. Field, and R. F. Ashman. 2005. TLR-9 activation of marginal zone B cells in lupus mice regulates immunity through increased IL-10 production. *J Clin Immunol* **25**: 29-40.

[139] Gray, M., K. Miles, D. Salter, D. Gray, and J. Savill. 2007. Apoptotic cells protect mice from autoimmune inflammation by the induction of regulatory B cells. *Proc Natl Acad Sci U S A* **104**: 14080-14085.

[140] Yanaba, K., J. D. Bouaziz, K. M. Haas, J. C. Poe, M. Fujimoto, and T. F. Tedder. 2008. A regulatory B cell subset with a unique CD1dhiCD5+ phenotype controls T cell-dependent inflammatory responses. *Immunity* **28**: 639-650.

[141] Deng, S., D. J. Moore, X. Huang, M. Lian, M. Mohiuddin, E. Velededeoglu, M. K. I. V. Lee, S. Sonawane, J. Kim, J. Wang, H. Chen, S. A. Corfe, C. Paige, M. Shlomchik, A. Caton, and J. F. Markmann. 2007. Cutting Edge: Transplant tolerance induced by anti-CD45RB requires B lymphocytes. *J Immunol* **178**: 6028-6032.

[142] de Visser, K. E., L. V. Korets, and L. M. Coussens. 2005. De novo carcinogenesis promoted by chronic inflammation is B lymphocyte dependent. *Cancer Cell* **7**: 411-423.

[143] Hajoui, O., R. Janani, M. Tulic, P. Joubert, T. Ronis, Q. Hamid, H. Zheng, and B. D. Mazer. 2004. Synthesis of IL-13 by human B lymphocytes: regulation and role in IgE production. *J Allergy Clin Immunol* **114**: 657-663.

[144] Singh, A., W. F. Carson, E. R. Secor, L. A. Guernsey, R. A. Flavell, R. B. Clark, R. S. Thrall, and C. M. Schramm. 2008. Regulatory role of B cells in a murine model of allergic airway disease. *J Immunol* **180**: 7318-7326.

[145] Burke, F., A. J. Stagg, P. A. Bedford, N. English, and S. C. Knight. 2004. IL-10-producing B220+CD11c- APC in mouse spleen. *J Immunol* **173**: 2362-2372.

[146] Tsuji, R. F., M. Szczepanik, I. Kawikova, V. Paliwal, R. A. Campos, A. Itakura, M. Akahira-Azuma, N. Baumgarth, L. A. Herzenberg, and P. W. Askenase. 2002. B cell-dependent T cell responses: IgM antibodies are required to elicit contact sensitivity. *J Exp Med* **196**: 1277-1290.

[147] Noonan, F. P., E. C. De Fabo, and H. Morrison. 1988. Cis-urocanic acid, a product formed by ultraviolet B irradiation of the skin, initiates an antigen presentation defect in splenic dendritic cells in vivo. *J Invest Dermatol* **90**: 92-99.

[148] Bastien, Y., and B. D. Mazer. 1994. Detection of the human platelet-activating factor receptor mRNA in human B lymphocytes by polymerase chain reaction on reverse transcripts (RT-PCR). *Biochem Biophys Res Commun* **202**: 1373-1379.

[149] Choquet, D., and K. H. 1988. Dual effects of serotonin on a voltage-gated conductance in lymphocytes. *Proc Natl Acad Sci USA 85*: 4557-4561.

[150] Bastien, Y., B. J. Toledano, N. Mehio, L. Cameron, B. Lamoukhaid, P. Renzi, Q. Hamid, and B. D. Mazer. 1999. Detection of functional platelet-activating factor receptors on human tonsillar B lymphocytes. *J Immunol* **162**: 5498-5505.

[151] Stafforini, D. M., T. M. McIntyre, M. E. Carter, and S. M. Prescott. 1987. Human plasma platelet-activating factor acetylhydrolase. Association with lipoprotein particles and role in the degradation of platelet-activating factor. *J Biol Chem* **262**: 4215-4222.

[152] Sreevidya, C. S., N. M. Khaskhely, A. Fukunaga, P. Khaskina, and S. E. Ullrich. 2008. Inhibition of photocarcinogenesis by platelet-activating factor or serotonin receptor antagonists. *Cancer Res* **68**: 3978-3984.

[153] Sozzani, S., D. Longoni, R. Bonecchi, W. Luini, L. Bersani, G. D'Amico, A. Borsatti, F. Bussolino, P. Allavena, and A. Mantovani. 1997. Human monocyte-derived and CD34+ cell-derived dendritic cells express functional receptors for platelet activating factor. *FEBS Lett* **418**: 98-100.

[154] Schuler, G., and R. M. Steinman. 1985. Murine epidermal Langerhans cells mature into potent immunostimulatory dendritic cells in vitro. *J Exp Med* **161**: 526-546.

[155] Finkelman, F. D., A. Lees, R. Birnbaum, W. C. Gause, and S. C. Morris. 1996. Dendritic cells can present antigen in vivo in a tolerogenic or immunogenic fashion. *J Immunol* **157**: 1406-1414.

[156] Steinbrink, K., M. Wolfl, H. Jonuleit, J. Knop, and A. H. Enk. 1997. Induction of tolerance by IL-10-treated dendritic cells. *J Immunol* **159**: 4772-4780.

[157] Toews, G. B., P. R. Bergstresser, and J. W. Streilein. 1980. Epidermal Langerhans cell density determines whether contact hypersensitivity or unresponsiveness follows skin painting with DNFB. *J Immunol* **124**: 445-453.

[158] Vink, A. A., F. M. Strickland, C. Bucana, P. A. Cox, L. Roza, D. B. Yarosh, and M. L. Kripke. 1996. Localization of DNA damage and its role in altered antigen-presenting cell function in ultraviolet-irradiated mice. *J Exp Med* **183**: 1491-1500.

[159] Vink, A. A., A. M. Moodycliffe, V. Shreedhar, S. E. Ullrich, L. Roza, D. B. Yarosh, and M. L. Kripke. 1997. The inhibition of antigen-presenting activity of dendritic cells resulting from UV irradiation of murine skin is restored by in vitro photorepair of cyclobutane pyrimidine dimers. *Proc Natl Acad Sci USA* **94**: 5255-5260.

[160] Applegate, L. A., R. D. Ley, J. Alcalay, and M. L. Kripke. 1989. Identification of the molecular target for the suppression of contact hypersensitivity by ultraviolet radiation. *J Exp Med* **170**: 1117-1131.

[161] Morison, W. L., C. Bucana, and M. L. Kripke. 1984. Systemic suppression of contact hypersensitivity by UVB radiation is unrelated to the UVB-induced alterations in the morphology and number of Langerhans cells. *Immunology* **52**: 299-306.

[162] Gorman, S., J. W. Y. Tan, J. A. Thomas, S. L. Townley, P. A. Stumbles, J. J. Finlay-Jones, and P. H. Hart. 2005. Primary defect in UVB-induced systemic immunomodulation does not relate to immature or funtionally impaired APCs in regional lymph nodes. *J Immunol* **174**: 6677-6685.

[163] Wang, HW, N. Tedla, A. R. Lloyd, D. Wakefield, and P. H. McNeil. 1998. Mast cell activation and migration to lymph nodes during induction of an immune response in mice. *J Clin Invest* **102**: 1617-1626.

[164] Tanzola, M. B., M. Robbie-Ryan, C. A. Gutekunst, and M. A. Brown. 2003. Mast cells exert effects outside the central nervous system to influence experimental allergic encephalomyelitis disease course. *J Immunol* **171**: 4385-4391.

[165] Hochegger, K., F. Siebenhaar, V. Vielhauer, D. Heininger, T. N. Mayadas, G. Mayer, M. Maurer, and A. R. Rosenkranz. 2005. Role of mast cells in experimental anti-glomerular basement membrane glomerulonephritis. *Eur J Immunol* **35**: 3074-3082.

[166] Khan, M. M., S. Strober, and K. L. Melmon. 1986. Regulatory effects of mast cells on lymphoid cells: the role of histamine type 1 receptors in the interaction between mast cells, helper T cells and natural suppressor cells. *Cell Immunol* **103**: 41-53.

[167] Frandji, P., C. Oskéritzian, F. Cacaraci, J. Lapeyre, R. Peronet, B. David, J. G. Guillet, and S. Mécheri. 1993. Antigen-dependent stimulation by bone marrow-derived mast cells of MHC class II-restricted T cell hybridoma. *J Immunol* **151**: 6318-6328.

[168] Lu, L., E. F. Lind, D. C. Gondek, K. A. Bennett, M. W. Gleeson, K. Pino-Lagos, Z. A. Scott, A. J. Coyle, J. L. Reed, J. Van Snick, T. B. Strom, X. X. Zheng, and R. J. Noelle. 2006. Mast cells are essential intermediaries in regulatory T-cell tolerance. *Nature* **442**: 997-1002.

[169] Gauchat, J. F., S. Henchoz, G. Mazzei, J. P. Aubry, T. Brunner, H. Blasey, P. Life, D. Talabot, L. Flores-Romo, J. Thompson, and et al. 1993. Induction of human IgE synthesis in B cells by mast cells and basophils. *Nature* **365**: 340-343.

[170] Tkaczyk, C., P. Frandji, H. G. Botros, P. Poncet, J. Lapeyre, R. Peronet, B. David, and S. Mecheri. 1996. Mouse bone marrow-derived mast cells and mast cell lines constitutively produce B cell growth and differentiation activities. *J Immunol* **157**: 1720-1728.

[171] Pawankar, R., M. Okuda, H. Yssel, K. Okumura, and C. Ra. 1997. Nasal mast cells in perennial allergic rhinitics exhibit increased expression of the Fc epsilonRI, CD40L, IL-4, and IL-13, and can induce IgE synthesis in B cells. *J Clin Invest* **99**: 1492-1499.

[172] Kawabe, T., T. Naka, K. Yoshida, T. Tanaka, H. Fujiwara, S. Suematsu, N. Yoshida, T. Kishimoto, and H. Kikutani. 1994. The immune responses in CD40-deficient mice: impaired immunoglobulin class switching and germinal center formation. *Immunity* **1**: 167-178.

[173] Xu, J., T. M. Foy, J. D. Laman, E. A. Elliott, J. J. Dunn, T. J. Waldschmidt, J. Elsemore, R. J. Noelle, and R. A. Flavell. 1994. Mice deficient for the CD40 ligand. *Immunity* **1:** 423-431.

[174] Renshaw, B. R., W. C. 3. Fanslow, R. J. Armitage, K. A. Campbell, D. Liggitt, B. Wright, B. L. Davison, and C. R. Maliszewski. 1994. Humoral immune responses in CD40 ligand-deficient mice. *J Exp Med* **180**: 1889-1900.

[175] Herrick, C. A., L. Xu, A. N. McKenzie, R. E. Tigelaar, and K. Bottomly. 2003. IL-13 is necessary, not simply sufficient, for epicutaneously induced Th2 responses to soluble protein antigen. *J Immunol* **170**: 2488-2495.

[176] Defrance, T., P. Carayon, G. Billian, J. C. Guillemot, A. Minty, D. Caput, and P. Ferrara. 1994. Interleukin 13 is a B cell stimulating factor. *J Exp Med* **179**: 135-143.

[177] McKenzie, G. J., C. L. Emson, S. E. Bell, S. Anderson, P. Fallon, G. Zurawski, R. Murray, R. Grencis, and A. N. McKenzie. 1998. Impaired development of Th2 cells in IL-13-deficient mice. *Immunity* **9**: 423-432

In: Immunosuppression: New Research
Editor: Charles B. Taylor, pp. 209-221

ISBN: 978-1-60692-102-9

Chapter 9

Immunosuppressive Therapy in Adult to Adult Living-Related Liver Transplantation

S. Gruttadauria[1,*], J. Viganò[1,2], J.W. Marsh[1], A. Marcos[1] and B. Gridelli[1]

[1]ISMETT, Istituto Mediterraneo per i Trapianti e Terapie ad Alta Specializzazione, UPMC Italy, Palermo, Italy

[2]Scuola di Specializzazione Chirurgia Generale II, Università degli Studi di Pavia, Pavia, Italy

Abstract

Liver transplantation has become the standard treatment for both chronic and acute end-stage liver disease. Because of a progressive increase in the number of patients on waiting list for liver transplant, a number of strategies have been developed in the last few years to increase the donor pool; one of these strategies is adult to adult living-related liver transplantation that showed overall survival similar to deceased donor liver transplantation.

Since adult living-related liver transplantation first became a valuable therapeutic option, the immunosuppressive protocols available to reduce the risk of acute cellular rejection have been continuously changing. Transplanted liver is generally considered immunologically privileged, regardless of the source of donation. Nevertheless, and despite more potential immunological compatibility in living-related transplantation when transplantations are performed between relatives with genetic relationships, acute cellular rejection remains an important risk factor for graft's and patient's loss.

An efficient immunosuppressive protocol, aimed at minimizing potential pharmaceutical side effects and at trying to induce a potential mechanism of tolerance, remains an essential factor for patient's outcome in both deceased donor liver transplantation and living related liver transplantation.

* E-mail address: sgruttadauria@ismett.edu. Telephone: +39-91-2192111. Fax: +39-91-2192400. Correspondence to: Salvatore Gruttadauria, MD, Department of Abdominal Transplant Surgery, Istituto Mediterraneo Trapianti e Terapie ad Alta Specializzazione, Palermo 90127, Italy.

Immunosuppressive therapy based on use of monoclonal antibodies as induction therapy, in combination with calcineurin inhibitor and steroids, or in triple regimen with the addition of azathioprine or mycophenolic acid, results in lower mean acute cellular rejection rates.
In our experience, we report that the use of basiliximab, a monoclonal antibody against interleukin-2 receptor, as induction agent in combination with a steroid-and tacrolimus-based regimen in adult to adult living-related liver transplantation, seems to be an efficient immunosuppressive protocol, with low incidence of cellular rejection, side effects, opportunistic infections or malignancies.

Introduction

Liver transplant outcomes have improved progressively over the last decade, with survivals rates reported to be approximately 82,1% and 67,8% after 1 and 5 years follow up respectively [1].

Improves in surgical technique, post operative management and advances in immunosuppression therapy have contributed significantly to increase long-term survival.

From the immunosuppression standpoint, the immunological barrier to transplantation between unrelated individuals and the subsequent rejection reaction, were the first obstacles surgeons dealing with transplantation have to eliminate. The first success in controlling rejection was reported by Starlz [2] in the early 60s, when a combination of azathioprina and prednisone was used in kidney transplantation. The introduction of cyclosporine into clinical practice at the end of the 70s [3], was the most significant advance in immunosuppressive therapy that marked the beginning of modern era of organ transplantation.

In liver transplantation field, a striking improvement in the clinical results was made when cyclosporine and steroid based immunosoppressive protocols were introduced by Calne [4], with or without azathioprine association. The following step was the introduction of tacrolimus in clinical studies in 1989 [5], that showed better results with significantly fewer episodes of acute, corticosteroid-resistant or refractory rejection in comparison to cyclosporine based protocol, that permits FK506 to become the primary immunosuppressor agent in liver transplantation [6].

In the last 20 years, the majority of liver transplantation centers worldwide applied protocols calcineurin inhibitors and corticosteroids-based. However, both cyclosporine/tacrolimus and corticosteroids chronic therapies are associated with well-known side effects that result in significant morbidities, including nephrotoxicity, neurotoxicity, hypertension, diabetes, infectious complication. Referred to this evidence, by the end on the previous millennium, new several immunosuppressor agents have been introduced in clinical practice to reduce corticosteroids and calcineurin inhibitors dosage and subsequently drug related side effects.

Modern immunosuppressive protocol is aimed at achieving early corticosteroid weaning , maintenance therapy with low dose calcineurin inhibitor, trying to obtain a potential mechanism of tolerance with few drug-related side effects. Antibody induction is a means of reducing the risk of acute cellular rejection in the early post transplant period, with better chances to avoid adverse effects such as nephrotoxicity, compared to calcineurin inhibitor and steroids.

Living Related Liver Transplantation

Since liver transplantation became the standard treatment for both acute and chronic end-stage liver disease, despite immunosuppresion therapy remains a critical point because of graft loss related to acute or chronic rejection, the major pitfalls is the increasing disparity between the number of patients waiting for transplantation and the number of cadaveric liver donors, resulting in a high mortality among on candidates in waiting list for liver transplant [7].

Because of organ shortage, a number of strategies have been developed in the last few years to increase the donor pool.

Living-related liver transplantation (LRLT) was first described by Raia in 1989 [8], then performed successfully in the pediatric population [9], and then proposed as one of the most effective measures to counteract organ-donor shortage for adults. LRLT evolved naturally from other surgical procedures, namely reduced-size liver transplantation and split-liver transplantation [10], based on the segmental anatomy of the liver and on its peculiar capacity to regenerate.

LRLT provides several advantages to the recipient because the transplant operation can be scheduled before the candidate develops life-threatening complication, and lower incidence of post operative primary non function can be expected because donor is always healthy, hemodynamically stable, and preservation time is usually minimized.

However, there has been ongoing debate over the ethics of posing a potential risk to the donor [11], and some uncertainty as to recipient outcomes [12].

Generally the risk of the donor is balanced by the great benefits to the recipient, as well as to donor self-esteem [13].

Since adult to adult living-related liver transplantation (ALRLT) first became a valuable therapeutic option for end-stage liver diseases, the immunosuppressive protocols available to reduce the risk of acute cellular rejection (ACR) have been continually changing.

With the advent of newer immunosuppressive agents, including mycophenolate mofetil, interleukin-2 receptor antibody and sirolimus, experience gained in immunosuppression for deceased donor liver transplantation population, has been applied in ALRLT. Moreover, the particular graft's origin from healthy individual and the risk related to the donor's surgical procedure, urge transplant surgeon to put more thoroughness on immunosuppressive therapy managemet and to abhor graft's loss.

Immunosuppression in Living Related Liver Transplantation

Even when living related transplantation is performed between relatives with genetic relationships, despite more potential immunological compatibility, acute cellular rejection remains an important risk factor for graft's and patient's loss, as well as when donor to recipient biologically relationship is absent.

For this reason, immunosuppressive therapy applied in living related population is often the same one applied in deceased donor population, with a parallel evolution in cyclosporine use first [14] and tacrolimus and other new immunosuppressor agents after [15, 16].

Exception to this rule is when transplantation is performed between identical twins; many authors showed that in solid organ transplanation from a syngenic donor, including liver, kidney, small bowel and pancreas, allografts can be transplanted without immunosuppressive therapy; also in LRLT some authors reported few cases [17].

In the last decades, mainly in deceased donor liver transplantation, among the different new immunosuppresion protocols, several trials have investigated the role of induction therapy with antibody as primary factor to reduce graft and patient loss secondary to immunological complication.

Antibodies may by either polyclonal or monoclonal; polyclonal antibodies have been associated with numerous drug related side effects like leucopenia, infection, increased risk of malignancy, serum sickness [18]; to reduce these adverse effects, monoclonal antibodies have been developped. Particullary monoclonal antibodies specifically targeting the interleukin-2 receptor, were developed to be applied in protocols with early steroid reduction/withdrawal and lower dosage of calcineurin inhibitors [19].

IL-2 receptor antibodies include the chimeric IL-2R antibody basiliximab (Simulect) and the humanized IL-2R antibody daclzumab (Zenapax); both are directed against the alfa chain (CD-25), which is expressed on activated T cells. As inhibitors of IL-2 binding, they prevent ACR by inhibiting IL-2 driven T-cell proliferation.

Randomized trials of basiliximab in kidney transplantation have shown its safety and effectiveness as an induction agent; patients in these studies have a reduction in ACR when compared with patients receiving placebo [20].

In liver transplantation, experience with monoclonal antibodies is less extensive, but several trials have investigated basiliximab in combination with calcineurin inhibitor and steroids, or in triple regimen with the addition of azathioprine, evaluating risk of ACR and the overall incidence of infection, including cytomegalovirus (CMV), mortality and risk of malignancy. These trials noted lower mean ACR rates in the basiliximab group compared with the standard therapy (23% vs 41%) [21,22].

A large multicenter randomized study investigating basiliximab versus placebo in liver transplant recipients showed a lower incidence of ACR (35% Vs 44%) in the basiliximab Group [23].

Following those results, the natural evolution of the immunosuppressive treatment option in LRLT has been the introduction on monoclonal antibody as induction agent [24].

The gold standard in immunosuppressive therapy remains a protocol allowing withdrawal or minimization of immunosuppressive drugs by promoting graft acceptance and the subsequent tolerance.

Many strategies have been developed over years, but nowadays, no one has reached a clinical value. One of this strategies, studied prevalently in kidney transplantation, is infusion of donor-derived hematopoietic cell after recipient myeloconditioning in the peritransplant period [25, 26]. This strategy has been primary applied in patient with renal failure and concomitant hematological malignancies requiring combined bone marrow and kidney transplantation; despite encouraging result, recipient conditioning, usually performed with irradiation or cytotoxic drugs, can be associated with considerable morbidity and mortality and consequently can't be safely applied in the absence of hematological malignancies. With the advent of conditioning protocol with lower toxicity profile, based primary on high dose antithymocite globulin infusion, Donckier et al [27] proposed in 2006 combined living donor liver transplanation and donor stem cell infusion with early immunosuppresion withdrawal, in recipient with no hematological need of bone marrow transplantation. This short series (3 cases) showed good clinical results with immunosuppression withdrawal achived in all patients without evidence of rejection or graft versus host disease; moreover non myeloablative conditioning with antithymocite globulin infusion was toxicity related free. Those results promote more investigation with 2-arm studies, using a control group receiving the same conditioning and immunosuppressive regimen, but without donor stem cell infusion, as suggested by the Author himself.

The Ismett, UPMC Italy Experience

From January 2002 to October 2007 we performed in our institute 77 ALRLT; the immunosuppressive protocol used in the living related population is based on our previous experience with patients who received cadaveric liver donation, both adults and pediatrics [21, 28].

We performed a retrospective analysis with the purpose to evaluate potential different outcome in terms of patient and graft survival, ACR incidence, infectious incidence/recurrence and malignancies, comparing living related transplanted patients and deceased donor transplanted patients submitted to the same immunosuppressive protocol based on basiliximab in combination with tacrolimus and early steroids weaning.

Material and Methods

Since liver transplantation program was started in out institute, until October 2007, we performed 349 liver transplantation in 321 adult patients.

The number of cases has been progressively increasing per year because of extensive use of living donor liver transplantation, split liver transplantation and extended criteria donor whole liver transplantation, with a peak reached in 2006, when we performed 102 liver transplants of witch 24 ALRLT.

In this study we divided the liver transplantation recipients in 2 groups: group 1: 77 ALRLT patients and group 2: 244 deceased donor live transplantation (DDLT) patients.

In both groups, the most common indications for transplantation were hepatocellular carcinoma on C viral cirrhosis (31.17% and 30.88% in group 1 and 2 respectively), and liver cirrhosis secondary to viral etiology (42.86% and 27.93% respectively). Indication for transplantation and MELD score of both groups are summarized in table 1 and 2.

Table 1. Primary indication to transplantation in LRLT; MELD score

Characteristics		N°.	Percent
Diagnosis			
	HCC+HCV	24	31.17%
	HCV	23	29.87%
	HBV	6	7.79%
	PBC	2	2.60%
	Cistic Phibrosis	2	2.60%

Table 1. Continued

Characteristics		N°.	Percent
	HCC+ alcohol	2	2.60%
	HBV-HCV	2	2.60%
	HCC+HBV	2	2.60%
	Carcinoid mets	1	1.30%
	HCC+HCV+HBV	1	1.30%
	Alcohol	1	1.30%
	HBV-HDV	1	1.30%
	HCC+NASH	1	1.30%
	PSC	2	2.60%
	Criptogenic	2	2.60%
	OTC Deficiency	1	1.30%
	Biliary Atresia	1	1.30%
	HCV-HBV-HDV	1	1.30%
	Emangioma	1	1.30%
	HCV+Alcohol	1	1.30%
MELD Score			
	8-10	7	9.09%
	11-20	38	49.35%
	21-30	30	38.96%
	31-40	1	1.30%
	Missing	1	1.30%

Table 2. Primary indication to transplantation in DDLT; MELD score

Characteristics		N°.	Percent
Diagnosis	HCC+HCV	84	30.88%
	HCV	55	20.22%
	REDO OLTx	29	10.66%
	HCC+HBV	21	7.72%
	FHF	19	6.98%
	HBV	8	2.94%
	HBV+HDV	8	2.94%
	HCC+HBV+HDV	7	2.57%
	CRIPTO	6	2.20%
	HCC+ALCOOL	5	1.83%
	HCV+ALCOHOL	5	1.83%
	CBP	4	1.47%
	Colangite Sclerosante	4	1.47%
	ALCOOL	3	1.10%
	Wilson	3	1.10%
	AUTOIMMUNE	2	0.73%
	HBV (Epatite acuta su cronica)	1	0.36%
	EPATITE ACUTA SU CRONICA B	1	0.36%

Table 2. Continued

Characteristics		N°.	Percent
	Fegato policisitico	1	0.36%
	HBV+ALCOOL	1	0.36%
	HCC	1	0.36%
	HCC+EMOCROMATOSI	1	0.36%
	HCC+HCV+EMOCROMATOSI	1	0.36%
	HCV+AUTOIMMUNE	1	0.36%
	HCV+HBV+ESRD	1	0.36%
	HCV+Multiorgan failure	1	0.36%
	Metastasi epatiche da carcinoide	1	0.36%
MELD Score			
	8_10	2	0.74%
	11_20	29	10.66%
	21-30	147	54.04%
	31-40	12	4.41%
	>40	3	1.10%
	Missing	79	29.04%

In ALRLT population, the donors (mean age 32.25 years +/- SD 9.17 years) always had genetic or emotional relationships with the recipients; 43 couples were ABO identical, and 34 compatible; 10 couples were not biological related. Donor liver resections resulted in 75 right hepatectomies and 2 left hepatectomies; graft implantation was performed with the preservation of the recipient inferior vena cava and, in 67 cases, with the use of veno-venous bypass. Donor evaluation and surgical technique have been previously described [11, 29].

In the DDLTs population (donor mean age 45.27 years +/- SD 19.63 years) we performed 119 whole liver transplants, 118 extended criteria donor whole liver transplants and 35 split liver transplants. Demographic characteristics of living and deceased donor and recipient are summarized in table 3 and 4.

The immunosuppressive protocol was identical in both groups, and included 20 mg basiliximab (Simulect®) in association with 500 mg methylprednisolone at the time of liver reperfusion; both were given as IV bolus. An additional 20 mg dose of basiliximab was administered by IV bolus on day 4 after transplantation. Tacrolimus (Prograf®) was administered at 0.15 mg/kg/d by mouth or through the nasogastric tube within 24 hours after the transplant, and adjusted to achieve trough levels in the range of 8 to 10 ng/mL. At 30 days posttransplantation, the target trough level was reduced to 5 to 7 ng/mL. Corticosteroids were administered in a standard rapid taper regimen for the first month: methylprednisolone at 50 mg IV every 6 hours on day 1; 40 mg IV every 6 hours on day 2; 30 mg IV every 6 hours on day 3; 20 mg IV every 6 hours on day 4; and 20 mg IV every 12 hours on day 5; and 20 mg prednisone by mouth or through the nasogastric tube on days 6 to 15; then 10 mg/d for 1 week; and 5 mg/d for 1 additional week. After the first year of activity, we prescribed only methylprednisone 20 mg IV for the first 2 to 3 days and then 20 mg prednisone by mouth, slowly decreasing and weaning from corticosteroids within 1 to 2 months.

Table 3. Demographic characteristics of 77 Living Donors and Recipients.

Characteristics		n°.	Mean+- SD or Percent	n°.	Mean+- SD or Percent
		DONOR		RECIPIENT	
AGE			32.25 ± 9.17		52.71 ± 11.53
	Range		[18;54]		[18;67]
	Classes				
	0-20	6	7.79%	2	2.60%
	21-40	55	71.43%	8	10.39%
	41-60	16	20.78%	50	64.94%
	61-80	6	7.79%	17	22.08%
SEX					
	Male	37	48.05%	29	37.66%
	Female	40	51.95%	48	62.34%
Height (cm)			169.03 ± 8.75		167.45 ± 9.20
Weight (Kg)			68.10 ± 11.65		70.40 ± 12.38
Donor to recipient relationship					
Biologically related		67	87.01%		
	Sibling	10	12.99%		
	Child	53	68.83%		
	Parent	4	5.19%		
Not biologically related		10	12.99%		
	Spouse	5	6.49%		
	other nonbiological	5	6.49%		

Table 4. Demographic characteristics of 244 Cadaveric Donors and Recipients.

Characteristics		n°.	Mean+- SD or Percent	n°.	Mean+- SD or Percent
		DONOR		RECIPIENT	
AGE			45.27 ± 19.63		53.64 ± 10.77
	Range		[8;93]		[18;69]
	Classes				
	0-20	42	15.44%	3	1.23
	21-40	71	26.10%	24	9.84
	41-60	91	33.46%	141	57.79
	61-80	68	25.00%	76	31.15
SEX					
	Male	66	27.05%	106	38.83%
	Female	178	72.95%	167	61.17%

Follow-up ranged from 4 to 1972 days after transplantation in group 1 (mean 558.17 days, SD± 465.45; median 470 days) and from 1 to 2741 days in group 2 (mean 887.16 days, SD± 722.12; median 794 days).

Primary outcomes of this study were: patients and graft survival, incidence of ACR, CMV infection, de novo malignancy, HCV recurrence, and chronic rejection.

In the case of ACR, depending on the gravity of the rejection, the protocol comprised a bolus administration of 500 mg methylprednisolone, to be repeated 3 times; simultaneously, the tacrolimus target level was increased to 8 to 10 ng/mL. The diagnosis of ACR was always biopsy proven.

For CMV prophylaxis, antigenemia-guided pre emptive therapy was applied with pp65 monitoring performed at weeks 2,4,6,8,12 and 16 after transplantation; if positive, oral ganciclovir was used for 6 weeks [30].

Statistical Analysis

Continuous variables are presented as the mean values ± SD, and categorical variables as rates. For survival, the Kaplan-Meier method was used. Patient survival/death, ACR-free time, and infection rate also were measured. The analyses were performed using SPSS (SPSS Inc., Chicago, Ill, United States).

Results

The overall patient survival at 3 yrs in group 1 and group 2 were 84.49% and 89.96%, respectively (p=0.95), while graft survival rates were 79.04% and 79.37% (p=0.58). In the general transplanted population (ALRLT +DDLT), 86.92% of patients were ACR free during the follow-up period, with a rejection-free probability of 93.15% within 3 months. In group 1 and 2, 89.32% and 86.07% of patients were rejection-free respectively during the follow up, with an actuarial rejection-free probability within 3 months of 93.04% (group 1) and 93.51% (group 2). Forty-two patients had episodes of biopsy-proven ACR, 8 cases in group 1 and 34 cases in group 2. In all cases, ACR protocol teatment was sufficient to treat rejection, and OKT3 or other antibody therapy was never required. No patients or grafts were lost due to acute or chronic rejection.

Retransplantation were necessary in 6 cases (7,8%) in group 1, primary for hepatic artery thrombosis, and in 29 cases (11,88%) in group 2 mainly for primary non function and hepatic artery thrombosisis.

We observed 14 cases of HCV recurrence in group 1 (prevalence of 26.92%) and 80 cases in group 2 (prevalence of 54.05%) (p=0.05), with an incidence of HCV recurrence in the first 3 months after transplantation of 3.84% and 14.86%, respectively.

Incidences of HCV recurrence in the first 12 months were 19.23% in group 1 and 41.89% in group 2. In group 1 we observed a higher HCC recurrence compared to group 2 (21,42% vs 2,5%). Eighteen patients developed a CMV infection, 4 in group 1 and 14 in group 2, with CMV infection incidence in the first 3 months after transplantation of 3.89% and 4.5%, respectively. De novo maligancies incidence has been of 6 cases during the follow up: 1 case in group 1 and 5 in group 2. Basiliximab was well tolerated by all patients. No acute side effects were noted, including acute infusion reactions; no cases of tacrolimus related toxicity was observed durino follow up. Table 5 and 6 summarizes primary outcome in both recipient populations.

Table 5. Morbidity and mortality in the ALRLT recipients.

		90d 0-90	1y 91-365	After 1 Year	Total
All deaths (15%)		3	6	3	12
Cause of death	Recurrence of Neoplastic Disease (5,19%)	0	1	3	4
	Sepsis (3.89%)	2	1	0	3
	Multifactorial (6,49%)	1	4	0	5
Retransplants (7.79%)		6	0	0	6
Cause of Retransplant					
	Hepatic Artery Thrombosis (6,49%)	5	0	0	5
	Other (1,29%)	1	0	0	1
ACR (10,38%)		5 (6,49%)	2 (2,58%)	1 (1,29%)	8
CMV infection (5.19%)		3	1	0	4
HCV Recurence (14/52 26.92%)		2	8	4	14
HCC recurrence (6/28 21,42%)		0	2	4	6
Neoplasie De Novo (1,35%)		1	0	0	1
Chronic Rejection		0	0	0	0

Table 6. Morbidity and mortality in the OLTx recipients.

		90d 0-90	1y 91-365	After 1 Year	Total
All deaths (13,52%)		13	11	9	33
Cause of death	Recurrence of Neoplastic Disease (1,22%)	0	1	2	3
	Sepsis (4,5%)	4	4	3	11
	Neoplasia de Novo (0,8%)		1	1	2
	Multifactorial (6,9%)	9	5	3	17
Retransplants (11.88%)		22	3	4	29
Cause of Retransplant	PNF (4,09%)	9	1	0	10
	Hepatic Artery Thrombosis (4,09%)	9	0	1	10
	DGF (1,22%)	3	0	0	3
	Other (2,45%)	1	2	3	6
ACR (13,93%)		17 (50%)	11 (32,35%)	6 (17,64%)	34
CMV infection (5,73%)		11	2	1	14
HCV Reccurence (80/148 54.05%)		22	40	18	80
HCC recurrence (3/120 2.5%)		0	2	1	3
Neoplasie De Novo (2,04%)		0	1	4	5
Chronic Rejection (2,04%)		0	0	0	5

Conclusion

Our single center experience confirm that immunosuppression in living related liver transplantation can be safely based on protocol previous applied on deceased donor liver transplantation. The advent of new immunosuppressor agents like monoclonal antibodies has improuved significantly patient's and graft's outcomes; the introduction of the same agent in LRLT are expected to have the same result as shown preliminary by our results and other authors.

Regarding the use of monoclonal antibodies, basiliximab is the most commonly used (7% of the all liver transplant recipients) because of such advantages as: 1) evidence of reduced overall cost demonstrated by pharmacoeconomic analysis; 2) ease of administration; 3) short term use; 4) no need for blood-level monitoring; 5) lack of major toxicity [31].

Basiliximab induction exhibited no difference in its action in both recipient populations reported in this retrospective comparative analysis.

On the other hand, the data concerning the rate of HCV recurrence in the two different groups of recipients are particularly interesting. In fact our series shows a lower rate of HCV after living related liver transplantation.

References

[1] Waki K.UNOS Liver Registry: ten year survivals. *Clin Transpl.* 2006;:29-39

[2] Starzl TE, Marchioro TL, Waddel WR: The reversal of rejection in human renal homografts with subsequent developement of homografts tolerancerates. *Surg Gynecol Obstet.* 1963 Oct; 117:385-95

[3] Borel JF, Feurer C, Gubler HU, Stähelin H. Biological effects of cyclosporin A: a new antilymphocytic agent. *Agents Actions.* 1976 Jul;6(4):468-75.

[4] Calne RY, Rolles K, White DJ, Thiru S, Evans DB, McMaster P, Dunn DC, Craddock GN, Henderson RG, Aziz S, Lewis P. Cyclosporin A initially as the only immunosuppressant in 34 recipients of cadaveric organs: 32 kidneys, 2 pancreases, and 2 livers. *Lancet.* 1979 Nov 17;2(8151):1033-6.

[5] Starzl TE, Todo S, Fung J, Demetris AJ, Venkataramman R, Jain A. FK 506 for liver, kidney, and pancreas transplantation. *Lancet.* 1989 Oct 28;2(8670):1000-4

[6] 6-A comparison of tacrolimus (FK 506) and cyclosporine for immunosuppression in liver transplantation. The U.S. Multicenter FK506 Liver Study Group. *N Engl J Med.* 1994 Oct 27;331(17):1110-5

[7] Wiesner RH. Patient selection in an era of donor liver shortage: current US policy. *Nat Clin Pract Gastroenterol Hepatol.* 2005 Jan;2(1):24-30

[8] Raia S, Nery JR, Mies S. Liver transplantation from live donors. *Lancet.* 1989 Aug 26;2(8661):497

[9] Otte JB. History of pediatric liver transplantation. Where are we coming from? Where do we stand? *Pediatr Transplant.* 2002 Oct;6(5):378-87.

[10] Heffron TG, Gruttadauria S, Campi O, et al. Surgical innovation in pediatric liver transplantation reduced-size, split, and living related transplantation. *Prob Gen Surg* 1998; 37:2611-3205

[11] Marcos A. Right lobe living donor liver transplantation a review. *Liver Transpl* 2000; 6:3-20.

[12] Gruttadauria S, Mandalà L, Vasta F, Cintorino D, Musumeci A, Marsh W, MarcosA, Gridelli B. Improvements in hepatic parenchymal transection for living related liver donor. *Transplant Proc.* 2005 Jul-Aug;37(6):2589-91.

[13] American Society of Transplant Surgeons' position paper on adult-to-adult living donor liver transplantation. *Liver Transplant* 2000; 6:815

[14] Broelsch CE, Whitington PF, Emond JC, Heffron TG, Thistlethwaite JR, Stevens L, Piper J, Whitington SH, Lichtor JL. Liver transplantation in children from living related donors. Surgical technique and results. *Ann Surg.* 1991 Oct;214(4):428-37

[15] Gruttadauria S, Cintorino D, Piazza T, Mandala L, Doffria E, Musumeci A, Di Trapani G, Arcadipane A, Scianna G, Spada M, Verzaro R, Volpes R, Vizzini G, Palazzo U, Minervini M, Marsh JW, Marcos A, Gridelli B. A safe immunosuppressive protocol in adult-to-adult living related liver transplantation. *Transplant Proc.* 2006 May;38(4):1106-8.

[16] Ringe B, Moritz M, Zeldin G, Soriano H.What is the best immunosuppression in living donor liver transplantation? *Transplant Proc.* 2005 Jun;37(5):2169-71

[17] Yoshizawa A, Takada Y, Fujimoto Y, Koshiba T, Haga H, Nabeshima S, Uemoto S.Liver transplantation from an identical twin without immunosuppression, with early recurrence of hepatitis C. *Am J Transplant.* 2006 Nov;6(11):2812-6.

[18] 18-Brennan DC. Action, efficacy and toxicities: polyclonal antilymphocyte antibodies. In: Norman DJ, Turka LA, eds. Primer on transplantation [ed 2]. Mt. Laurel, NJ, *American Society of Transplantation* 2001, p. 152.

[19] Moser MAJ. Options for induction immunosuppression in liver transplant recipients. *Drugs* 2003; 62: 995.

[20] Adu D, Cockwell P, Ives NJ, et al. Interleukin-2 receptor monoclonal antibodies in renal transplantation: meta-analysis of randomised trials. *BMJ* 2003; 326: 789

[21] Marino IR, Doria C, Scott V.L. Scotti Foglieni C, Lauro A, Piazza T, Cintorino D, Gruttadauria S, Efficacy and safety of basiliximab with a tacrolimus-based regimen in liver transplant recipients, *Transplantation* 2004, 78(6) : 886-891;

[22] Calmus Y, Scheele JR, Gonzalez-Pinto I, Jaurrieta EJ, Klar E, Pageaux GP,Scudamore CH, Cuervas-Mons V, Metselaar HJ, Prestele H, Girault D. Immunoprophylaxis with basiliximab, a chimeric anti-interleukin-2 receptormonoclonal antibody, in combination with azathioprine-containing triple therapy in liver transplant recipients. *Liver Transpl.* 2002 Feb;8(2):123-31.

[23] Neuhaus P, Clavien PA, Kittur D, Salizzoni M, Rimola A, Abeywickrama K, Ortmann E, Chodoff L, Hall M, Korn A, Nashan B; CHIC 304 International Liver Study Group. Improved treatment response with basiliximab immunoprophylaxis after liver transplantation: results from a double-blind randomized placebo-controlled trial. *Liver Transpl.* 2002 Feb;8(2):132-42.

[24] Gruttadauria S et al. Role of basiliximab in the prevention of acute cellular rejection in adult to adult living-related liver transplantation: a single center experience. *Biologics: Targets and Therapy* 2007; 1(1): 69-73

[25] Spitzer TR, Delmonico F, Tolkoff-Rubin N, McAfee S, Sackstein R, Saidman S,Colby C, Sykes M, Sachs DH, Cosimi AB. Combined histocompatibility leukocyte antigen-matched donor bone marrow and renal transplantation for multiple myeloma with end

stage renal disease: the induction of allograft tolerance through mixed lymphohematopoietic chimerism. Transplantation. 1999 Aug 27;68(4):480-4.

[26] Wekerle T, Sykes M.Induction of tolerance. *Surgery*. 2004 Apr;135(4):359-64.

[27] Donckier V, Troisi R, Le Moine A, Toungouz M, Ricciardi S, Colle I, Van Vlierberghe H, Craciun L, Libin M, Praet M, Noens L, Stordeur P, Andrien M,Lambermont M, Gelin M, Bourgeois N, Adler M, de Hemptinne B, Goldman M. Early immunosuppression withdrawal after living donor liver transplantation and donor stem cell infusion. *Liver Transpl*. 2006 Oct;12(10):1523-8.

[28] Cintorino D, Riva S, Spada M, Minervini M, Sonzogni A, Foglieni CS, Gruttadauria S, Verzaro R, Henderson K, Aricò M, Gridelli B. Corticosteroid-free immunosuppression in pediatric liver transplantation: safety and efficacy after a short-term follow-up. *Transplant Proc*. 2006 May;38(4):1099-100.

[29] Salvatore Gruttadauria , J. Wallis Marsh , Davide Cintorino, Domenico Biondo, Angelo Luca , Antonio Arcadipane, Giovanni Vizzini, Riccardo Volpes, Amadeo Marcos, Bruno Gridelli. Adult to Adult Living-related Liver Transplantation: Report on an Initial Experience in Italy.. *Digestive and Liver Disease* 2007 Apr;39(4):342-50.

[30] Singh N, Paterson DL, Gayowski T, Wagener MM, Marino IR.Cytomegalovirus antigenemia directed pre-emptive prophylaxis with oral versus I.V. ganciclovir for the prevention of cytomegalovirus disease in liver transplant recipients: a randomized, controlled trial. *Transplantation*. 2000 Sep 15;70(5):717-22.

[31] Ramirez CB, Marino IR. The role of basiliximab induction therapy in organ transplantation. *Expert Opin Biol Ther*. 2007 Jan;7(1):137-48. Review.

In: Immunosuppression: New Research
Editor: Charles B. Taylor, pp. 223-238

ISBN: 978-1-60692-102-9

Chapter 10

High-Dose Immunosuppression with Autologous Stem Cell Transplantation in Severe Refractory Systemic Lupus Erythematosus

Igor A. Lisukov*, Vera V. Sergeevicheva, Svetlana A. Sizikova, Alexander D. Kulagin[1], Irina V. Kruchkova, Andrey V. Gilevich, Alexey E. Sizikov, Ludmila P. Konenkova, Elena R. Chernykh, Olga Y. Leplina and Vladimir A. Kozlov

Institute of Clinical Immunology RAMS SB, Novosibirsk, Russia
[1]Novosibirsk State Medical University

Abstract

Prolonged studies were carried out to elucidate the role of high dose immunosuppression therapy (HDIST) with autologous hematopoietic stem cell transplantation (SCT) in the treatment of severe and refractory autoimmune disease. In this study, we analyzed single center experience of HDIST followed by SCT for refractory SLE.

The 13 patients with SLE, who had disease progression despite previous treatment with pulse Cy intravenous, prednisolone (standard doses and pulse therapy), oral Cy, azathioprine or metotrexate, were enrolled in the clinic of our institution from 1998 to 2007. All patients were seriously ill, with SLE disease activity indices (SLEDAI) of 6-30, including cases with central nervous system lupus, lung vasculitis, carditis, nephritis with nephrotic syndrome and cytopenia. Autologous hematopoietic stem cells were collected from bone marrow (n=4) or mobilized from peripheral blood with Cy (3g/m2/once) and granulocyte colony-stimulating factor (G-CSF) (n=9). Pretransplant conditioning regimens included BEAM ± ATG (n=2), Melphalan 140 mg/m^2 + Etoposid 1600 mg/m^2 (n=2), Cy 200 mg/kg ± ATG (n=2) and

* E-mail address: depsct@online.nsk.su. Telephone 3832-28-59-56, fax 3832-25-05-22; address correspondence to: Prof. Igor A. Lisukov, Institute of Clinical Immunology RAMS, Yadrintsevskaya str. 14, Novosibirsk 630099, Russia.

Melphalan 120 mg/m^2 (n=1), Cy 140 mg/kg (n=6). Transplanted CD34+ MNC were more than 2x106/kg. Median time to an absolute neutrophil count (ANC) greater than 0.5x10^9 /l and platelet count greater than 50x10^9/l was 11 and 15 days, respectively. Three patients died on days 11, 22 and 63 due to transplant-related complications. All of the patients who died due to transplant-related complications had a long history of corticosteroids treatment, multiple and severe episodes of infections pre-SCT and received more then one anticytostatic drugs or ATG as conditioning regimen. All of the live transplanted patients, who recovered hematopoiesis, showed improvement in disease activity: 8 (CR) and 2 (PR). The median follow up is now 14 months. One patient died due to lung vasculitis progression 8 years after SCT. We conclude that HDIST followed by SCT for refractory SLE is feasible and effective, and achievement of prolonged, corticosteroid-free remissions is a reality.

Keywords: stem cell transplantation, systemic lupus erythematosus

Introduction

Some of the patients with SLE are damaged severely or fatally from uncontrolled disease progression, and conventional treatments are not effective. High-dose immunosuppression and SCT have been proposed as an investigational therapy for patients with severe refractory autoimmune diseases including SLE [1-5]. This approach is supported by hematopoietic SCT in animal autoimmune disorders [7-10] and in patients undergoing transplantation for hematologic disease who also have a coincidental autoimmune disease [11-12]. The rationale for using SCT to treat autoimmune disease is to maximally suppress or ablate the immune system and then rescue the patient from prolonged cytopenia by infusing autologous stem cells. Eradication of autoreactive cells by the conditioning regimen, redistribution of an altered cellular and humoral immunological network or thymic re-education are discussed as potential mechanisms for response ("reprogramming of the immune system") [13-17]. The EBMT/EULAR Registry has collected retrospective data on autoSCT from more than 460 patients with autoimmune diseases [18]. Transplantation-related mortality (TRM) for all autoimmune disease has been reported to be 8.6% [17-19]. TRM was 12% for 51 patients undergoing transplantation for SLE [18]. Remission of disease activity was seen in 33/50 (66%) evaluable patients by six months, of which 10/31 (32%) subsequently relapsed after six months [18].

We describe 13 patients with primary severe SLE who received HDIST and auto-SCT in our institution from 1998 to 2007 (Table 1). Six patients were registered in the EBMT/EULAR database.

Table 1. Results of autologous SCT in patients with SLE

	Sex/Age	Duration of SLE, years	Previous treatment	Organ involvement	Regimen	Number of infused cells	Results	Follow-up
Patient 1	F/21	3	oral corticosteroids, azathioprine, Cy pulse (1)	Lung, Renal	BEAM+ATG	$2.4x10^8$/kg (BM)	Complete remission	5 years
Patient 2	F/29	14	oral corticosteroids, azathioprine, Cy pulse (7), oral Cy (7g)	Renal, Serositis	BEAM	$1.2x10^8$/kg (BM)	Died on day 11 (sepsis)	
Patient 3	F/21	7	oral corticosteroids, azathioprine, Cy pulse (6)	CNS, Renal	Melphalan 120 mg/m^2 + etoposide 1600 mg/m^2	$1.3x10^8$/kg (BM)	Partial response	3.3 years
Patient 4	F/15	5	oral corticosteroids, azathioprine, Cy pulse (3), oral Cy (20,8g)	Renal	Melphalan 140 mg/m^2 + etoposide 1600 mg/m^2	$1.3x10^8$/kg (BM)	Died on day 22 (sepsis)	
Patient 5	F/19	9	oral corticosteroids, Cy pulse (9)	Renal, Cytopenia	Cy 200 mg/kg + ATG	$20.6x10^6$/kg (PBSC)	Died on day 63 (CMV)	
Patient 6	F/25	4	oral corticosteroids, azathioprine, Cy pulse (7)	Renal, CNS, Cytopenia	Cy 200 mg/kg	$18x10^6$/kg (PBSC)	Complete remission	3 years
Patient 7	F/42	7	oral corticosteroids, azathioprine, Cy pulse (9)	Lung, Heart (carditis) Renal	Cy 120 mg/kg	$7x10^6$/kg (CD34+ PBSC)	Complete remission	2.5 years

Table 1. Continued

	Sex/Age	Duration of SLE, years	Previous treatment	Organ involvement	Regimen	Number of infused cells	Results	Follow-up
Patient 8	F/34	8	oral corticosteroids, azathioprine, Cy+methylprednisolone pulse (6).	Renal, CNS	Melphalan 120 mg/m^2	$3.8x10^6$/kg (CD34+ PBSC)	Partial remission	1 year
Patient 9	F/24	1	oral corticosteroids, azathioprine, Cy+methylprednisolone pulse (6)	Renal	Cy 120 mg/kg	$4.3x10^8$/kg (CD34+ PBSC)	Complete remission	1 year
Patient 10	F/15	8	oral corticosteroids, Cy pulse (4), oral Cy (24g)	Renal, Lung, Heart (coronariitis)	Cy 120 mg/kg	$4.3x10^6$/kg (CD34+ PBSC)	Complete remission	6 months
Patient 11	F/25	2.5	oral corticosteroids, mtx, Cy+ methylprednisolone pulse pulse (4), cyclosporin A.	Renal, Lung, Heart (carditis)	Cy 130mg/kg	$5.9x10^6$/kg (CD34+ PBSC)	Complete remission	4 months
Patient 12	F/36	3	oral corticosteroids, Cy pulse (4), cyclosporin A	Renal cytopenia	Cy 120 mg/kg	$2.6x10^6$/kg (CD34+ PBSC)	Complete remission	3 months
Patient 13	F/34	4.5	oral corticosteroids, Cy pulse (9)	Renal, CNS	Cy 120 mg/kg	$3.6x10^6$/kg (PBSC)	Complete remission	3 months

Patient Selection

From April 1998 through February 2007, 13 females aged 15 to 41 years and suffering from SLE were enrolled in a high-dose immunosuppression (HDIST) with autologous hematopoietic stem cell transplantation (SCT) study at a single medical center.

Patient eligibility depended on a refractory to standard immunosuppression therapies and either organ- or life-threatening visceral involvment. The inclusion criteria were: not controlled with pulse therapy Cy glomerulonephritis (World Health Organization [WHO] class III-IV), central nervous system (CNS) lupus, vasculitis involving the lung or heart, or transfusion-dependent autoimmune cytopenias. Evaluation of eligible patients by two independent rheumatologists and transplant physicians, informed consent and approval by the ethical committee were part of the protocol [13, 16].

Hematopoietic Stem Cell Procurement

Autologous hematopoietic stem cells were collected from bone marrow only for the first four patients (n=4) under general anaesthesia, and all subsequent patients underwent peripheral blood hematopoietic stem cell collection (n=9). Three patients, on whom bone marrow harvests was performed, achieved suboptimal MNC count ($<2x10^8$). PBSC mobilized from peripheral blood with Cy 4g/m^2 and granulocyte colony-stimulating factor (G-CSF) (filgrastim) at 10 μg/kg subcutaneous daily with leukapheresis initiated when the white blood cells count reached $1x10^9$/l (n=9). Apheresis was continued daily until the number of harvested progenitor cells reached a minimum of $2x10^6$ CD34+ cells/kg body weight. Successful collection from all of the patients was achieved after two to three leukapheresis sessions. The harvests were not manipulated. Stem cell products were cryopreserved at –80°C for at least two weeks after collection.

Conditioning Regimen

The conditioning regimen was not started until at least 14 days after PBSC apheresis. Pretransplant conditioning regimens included BEAM (BCNU 300 mg/m^2 on day -7; Etoposid 800 mg/m^2 and Ara-C 800 mg/m^2 on days -6, -5, -4, -3; Melphalan 120 mg/m^2 on day -2) with antithimocyte globulin (ATG) at a dose of 30mg/kg infused over 10 hours on day 0 (n=1), BEAM (n=1); Etoposid 1600 mg/m^2 on day -2 with Melphalan 140 mg/m^2 on day -1 (n=2); Cy 200 mg/kg in divided doses of 50 mg/kg/day intravenously on days -6, -5, -4, -3 with ATG (total doses 60 mg/kg) infused over 10 hours in divided doses of 30 mg/kg/day on days +1, +2 (n=2); Melphalan 120 mg/m^2 (n=1); and Cy 200-140 mg/kg intravenously in divided doses for four days -6, -5, -4, -3 (n=6).

Supportive Care

Before, during and for 24 hours after treatment with high dose cyclophosphamide, patients received hyperhydratation with forced diuresis and urometexan (Mesna) infusion for the prevention of haemorrhagic cystitis. Patients were treated in a single room without air filtration. All patients followed a standardized supportive care protocol including antiemetic therapy, analgesia for mucositis, transfusion support, and venoocclusive disease prophylaxis. A low microbial diet, oral daily fluoroquinolone (1 g/d) changed to intravenouse cefepime upon presentation of neutropenic fever, fluconazole (400 mg/d) and acyclovir (10 mg/kg/d) and aerosolized amphotericin B (10 mg daily twice) were started upon admission and discontinued when the ANC rebounded to $0.5x10^9$/l. All patients continued to receive prednisolone 15-30 mg/d. Methylprednisolone (1g) was administered intravenously 30 minutes before each dose of ATG. All patients underwent BMT, received subcutaneous G-CSF (filgrastim) 5 μg/kg started the day of hematopoietic stem cell infusion and continued until the ANC was greater than $1x10^9$ /l for three consecutive days. Platelets irradiated with 25 Gy and red blood cells were given to maintain platelet count greater than 20,000/μL and hemoglobin level greater than 8.0 g/dL. For the first six months after transplantation, patients were treated with daily oral fluconazole and trimethoprim/sulfamethoxazole orally three times a week.

Table 2. Characteristics of the patients before SCT

	Anti-dsDNA, IU/ml[c]	C3 / C4, g/l[d]	ESR, mm/hr[e]	SLEDAI score
P1	580	0.42 / 0.1	58	18
P2	160	0.7 / 0.1	25	14
P3	740	0.74 /<0.1	65	30
P4	860	0.4 / 0.16	46	22
P5	107	0.66 /0.11	40	6
P6	1084	0.48 /<0.1	40	15
P7	13	0.3 / 0.1	27	2
P8	34	0.7 / 0.12	50	26
P9	260	0.7 /<0.1	29	12
P10	170	0.4 / 0.2	25	5
P11	50	0.55 /0.1	23	21
P12	18	0.9 /0.2	6	18
P13	98	0.72 /<0.1	25	14

Anti-dsDNA, antibodies to double stranded DNA were determined according to the manufacturer`s instructions (IMMCO Diagnostics Inc., USA) by enzyme linked immunosorbent assay (ELISA). Results were expressed in IU/ml, using Wo/80 as ultimate standard (negative result <50 IU/ml, positive result >60 IU/ml);

C3/C4, levels of the 3rd and 4th complement components were determined in immunoassay (BECKMAN Array[R] 360 system). The normal ranges were 0.8-2.0 g/l for C3 and 0.16-0.47 g/l for C4;

ESR, erythrocyte sedimentation rate, mm/hr

Assessment of Disease Status [18-22]

Patients returned for scheduled follow-up at 1, 3, 6 and 12 months and then yearly thereafter. If a patient was not able to return for follow-up, medical records and laboratory blood testing results were collected from the local hospital.

Outcome was based on assessments before SCT (Table 2) and at 1, 3, and 6 months and yearly after transplantation. Early clinical response was evaluated using local interphysician vignettes, according the American College of Rheumatology Response criteria for SLE clinical trail: responder index for lupus erythematosis (RIFLE) criteria and improvement was revealed after mobilization regimen, including Cy [20].

Outcome was based on physical examination, serology (antibodies to double stranded DNA, antinuclear antibodies [ANA], anticardiolipin antibodies, C3 component level and lupus anticoagulant), lupus disease activity index (SLEDAI) [21], and response of pretransplant abnormalities in involved organ systems (e.g., serum creatinine, 24-hour urine protein and creatinine clearance in nephritis, chest radiograph, and necessary imaging status, and pulmonary function tests in pneumonitis, and evaluation of neurologic deficits in CNS lupus). Antibodies to double stranded DNA (anti-dsDNA) were determined according to the manufacturer`s instructions (IMMCO Diagnostics Inc., USA) by enzyme linked immunosorbent assay (ELISA). Results were expressed in IU/ml, using Wo/80 as ultimate standard (negative result <50 IU/ml, positive result >60 IU/ml). The presence of ANA was determined by the HEp-2000 indirect fluorescent antibody test system in accordance with the manufacturer`s instructions (IMMCO Diagnostics Inc., USA). Improvement was defined as a 50% improvement in any baseline parameter with no deterioration in any objective parameter. Criteria for complete remission requires SLEDAI ≤ 3, prednisolone dose <10 mg daily and absence of other immunosuppressive therapy.

Results

Patient data before SCT are summarized in Table 1. All patients had been treated unsuccessfully with Cy (intravenous pulse and oral) and other immunosupressive drugs. The reinfused bone marrow (n=4) contained median nucleated cell counts of $1.55x10^8$/kg (range 1.2-$2.4x10^8$/kg). The reinfused peripheral blood stem cell harvest (n=9) contained median $4.34x10^6$/kg (range 2.6-$20x10^6$/kg) CD34+ cells. Median time to an absolute neutrophil count (ANC) greater than $0.5x10^9$ /l and platelet count greater than $50x10^9$/l was 11 and 15 days, respectively. Three patients died on days 11, 22 and 63 due to transplant-related complications. All of the live transplanted patients, who recovered hematopoiesis, showed improvement in disease activity: 8 (CR) and 2 (PR). The median follow-up is now 15 months. One patient died due to SLE relapse: lung vasculitis progression 8 years after SCT.

Transplant-Related Mortality (Toxity)

Main causes of death in patients with transplant-related mortality before engraftment were infections (mucositis, pneumonia, sepsis) and hemorrhage (gastrointestinal bleeding) during the severe postchemotherapy cytopenia. All of the patients who died due to transplant-related complications had a long history of corticosteroid treatment, multiple and severe episodes of infections pre-SCT, and received more than one anticytostatic drug or ATG as conditioning regimen. One patient developed secondary cytopenia due to virus-induced engraftment failure after hematopoiesis recovery. We present lethal cases in detail below.

Patient 1. The 29-year-old woman had a 14-year history of SLE, including arthritis, pericarditis, WHO class III glomerulonephritis, and elevated titers of ANA. The symptoms responded to corticosteroids, azathioprine and Cy. In November 1994 the patient developed nephrotic syndrome with proteinuria 3.3 g/l, acute renal failure (ARF), abdominal syndrome, ascite, anasarca and high titers of ANA (1:320). Pulse Cy intravenous (3 g in one month) in combination with pulse methylprednisolone intravenous was given with improvement. The disease was controlled by continuous therapy of oral prednisolone (minimum dose 20 mg daily) and azathioprine 150 mg/d and was complicated by frequent infections, including bacterial pneumonia, pyelonephritis, varicella zoster virus infection. In May 1998, relapse of the nephrotic syndrome with ARF was diagnosed, and the remission of SLE was not achieved despite treatment with pulse Cy and methylprednisolone. The patient was not on dialysis. In November 1998 the patient underwent HDC (BEAM) followed by unmanipulated auto-BMT (1.2×10^8/kg of nucleated cells). Treatment was managed according to a standard supportive care protocol. The patient developed severe mucositis (grade 4), sepsis followed by multiorgan failure, severe hemorrhage (gastric bleeding) and died on day +11.

Patient 2. The 15-year-old female patient had suffered from SLE since 1995. SLE symptoms were arthritis, discoid rash, malar rash, photosensitivity, fever, elevated titers of ANA (1:160) and elevated titers of anticardiolipin antibodies. The treatment with 1 mg/kg/d prednisolone and 400 mg Cy weekly was started but did not induce complete response. Discoid rash, arthralgias and serological symptoms were uncontrolled. Eight months later, prednisolone was reduced to 20 mg/d because of side effects. In January 1998, lupus nephritis was diagnosed. The treatment with oral Cy (in May 1998 total dose was 20.8g) with addition of penicillamine, azathioprine and increased corticosteroids was continued without significant improvement. Therefore, three pulses of 1g Cy intravenous were given at monthly intervals. However, the patient's condition deteriorated, lupus nephritis progressed, and disease activity remained high (SLEDAI 22). The option of HDC was discussed with the patient's parents and performed after approval by the ethics committee. In April 2000, unmanipulated non-cryopreserved autologous marrow (1.32×10^8/kg of nucleated cells) was reinfused after conditioning of the recipient with a combination of etoposide 1600 mg/m^2 on day -2 and melphalan 140 mg/m^2 on day -1. In the posttransplantation period, the patient developed severe mucositis and enteropathy (day +5), sepsis followed by multiorgan failure (day +10), severe hemorrhage (gastrointestinal bleeding), pneumonia (day +12) and died on day +22. ANC reached 0.5×10^9/l on day +15.

Patient 3. The 19-year-old woman had suffered from SLE (arthritis, malar rash, carditis, pneumonitis, and immunologic disorder) since 1993. The treatment with 1 mg/kg/d prednisolone induced complete response that lasted until 1999. Relapse of SLE with lupus erythema and elevated titers of ANA was diagnosed in January 1999. In August 2000, the patient presented with severe cutaneous vasculitis, cytopenia (platelets 45×10^9/l, leukocytes 1.2×10^9/l), fever, and nephritis despite treatment with oral prednisolone 0.5 mg/kg/d. There was no sustained improvement with pulse intravenous Cy (7.4 g in 9 months) in combination with oral prednisolone (60-25 mg daily) and pulse intravenous methylprednisolone (total dose 5 g). The disease activity decreased, but cutaneous vasculitis, cytopenia and serological symptoms were uncontrolled. The functions of major organs were adequate. She was selected for high-dose immunosuppression and autologous SCT. Priming was done with Cy 4 g/m^2 followed by G-CSF 480 μg/d subcutaneously. Significant regress of symptoms of cutaneous vasculitis and absence of cytopenia were achieved. Prednisolone was reduced to 10 mg/d. Two months later, conditioning with Cy 50 mg/kg daily for 4 days with ATG 30 mg/kg daily for 3 days was given. Transplantation of 20.8×10^6/kg CD34+ autologous stem cells was performed on October 2002. Engraftment occurred on day 10 (leukocytes 9.0×10^9/l, platelets 80×10^9/l). On day 20 the patient developed fever, abnormal liver function (ALT 4.1 mmol/l [normal<0.68], AST 2.0 mmol/l [normal<0.68], total bilirubin level 6.08 mg/dl [normal<1.2]) and severe pancytopenia (leukocytes 0.2×10^9/l, platelets 30×10^9/l, haemoglobin 7 g/dl), and on day 30 severe enteropathy. On the basis of clinical signs, positive results in polymerase chain reaction assay, detection of cytomegalovirus (CMV) inclusions in bone marrow, CMV disease was diagnosed. We started treatment with intravenous ganciclovir 10 mg/kg daily in combination with intravenous immunoglobulin 0.5 g/kg for five consecutive days, and thereafter once weekly maintenance was given. After two weeks, the liver function returned to normal and the symptoms of enterocolitis regressed. Unfortunately, the patient remained pancytopenic (despite the administration of G-CSF), developed sepsis and pneumonia, and died on day 63 from multiorgan failure.

Overall and Disease-Free Survival

All of the transplanted patients who recovered stabile hematopoiesis showed rapid improvement in clinical disease activity. The median follow-up is now 15 months. The probability of disease-free survival or complete remission is defined as requiring no SLE-activity and immunosuppressive medication, except physiologic doses of prednisolone (<10 mg/day); however the time of entering remission was several months, often because of long-term high-dose pre-SCT corticosteroid therapy that had to be withdrawn gradually to avoid abstinence syndrome. Improvement or normalization of serology achieved after a long time (ANA, anti-ds DNA) occurred in patients entering clinical remission (mean six months). We not exclude the possibility that this owes to cyclophosphomaide-resistant specific memory B-cells with prolonged persistence.

The partial remission was defined in two patients who suffered from CNS-lupus and mild symptoms remained after SCT. One patient, admitted to our hospital in November 1999, was severely disabled (lower paraplegia and failure of pelvic function due to myelitis) with SLEDAI 30. The total observation time after transplantation is now 74 months. The functions of bladder and bowel returned to normal, but mild lower paraplegia and serology activity remain which require prolonged immunosuppression therapy with steroids. The second SLE patient presented with organic encephaloneuropathies: abnormalities in neurocognitive function, such as memory and intellect; reflectory tetraplegia; and sensitive ataxia in pretrasplantation period, presenting with mild neurological symptoms now (one year after SCT): headache, depression and transitory psychosis. Patient need in symptomatic, antipsychotic treatment. Immunosupression by sreroid and cyclosporin is continuing.

The longest continuous duration of SLE remission has been eight years. Disease progression-related mortality despite initial response occurred once after long-term stable clinical and immunological remission. The case report follows.

Patient. The 21-year-old woman with SLE developed lung vasculitis in 1995. She was treated with corticosteroids 0.5 mg/kg over 10 weeks with some clinical improvement. Prednisolone was reduced to 10 mg/d. In 1997, lupus nephritis was diagnosed, and pulse Cy intravenous was given but withdrawn because of allergic dermatitis. The treatment with prednisolone 1 mg/kg and azathioprine was started but did not produce any effect. In March 1998 the patient was admitted to our hospital with dyspnea, progressive pulmonary hypertension (Doppler echo showed estimated systolic pulmonary artery pressure [sPAP] of 49 mm Hg), arthritis, proteinuria (5.3 g/24 hour), renal failure (creatinine clearance 50 ml/min), and elevated titres of ANA (1:160). In April 1998, HDC according to the BEAM protocol followed by unmanipulated autologous bone marrow transplantation (BMT) was applied. On day 0, ATG ("ATGAM" 30 mg/kg) was given for in vivo T cell depletion. The patient developed moderate mucositis and enteropathy (grade 2), neutropenic fever (FUO) with response to the ceftriaxone 4 g/d + tobramycin 240 mg/d, and genital herpes infection with response to the famciclovir 750 mg/d. Haemorrhage was mild. The time to achieve an ANC exceeding $0.5x10^9/l$ and platelet count exceeding $50x10^9/l$ was respectively 16 and 19 days. After 6 months, complete remission of SLE was established. The SLEDAI decreased from 18 to 0, pulmonary and renal function recovered, and ANA titres were negative. The oral prednisolone was withdrawn after 10 months of BMT. The follow up at this time was over five years. The patient was in stable clinical and immunologic remission and returned to work. In November 2006, the patient was admitted to the hospital with symptoms of respiratory insufficiency. Physical and laboratory examination revealed progression of lung vasculitis (Doppler echo showed high sPAP, CT scanning revealed bullous pneumonitis) and pregnancy of 8 weeks gestation. After therapeutic abortion, treatment with cyclosporine 150 mg and prednisolone 30 mg daily once was started with transitory clinical improvement, but the patient died due to repeating spontaneous pneumothorax after 8 years after SCT.

The aim of high-dose immunosupression is to destroy self-reactive lymphocytes. We evaluate the efficacy and toxicity of ASCT with specific attention to long-term immune reconstitution. Immunological features were assessed before ASCT and at 1, 3, and 6 months and yearly after transplantation. HDIT induced profound lymphocytopenia. Mean absolute lymphocyte counts were back to baseline level at 6 months. The CD4/CD8 ratio significantly decreased at 1 month after ASCT due to reduced proportions of CD4 T-cells and remained stable for 6 months. There were no significant changes from pretherapy in the proportions of CD4+DR+ and CD8+DR+ lymphocytes. At 1 month posttransplant, the number of naïve CD4+45RA+ cells was reduced significantly as well as CD8+45RA+ cells, but these subpopulations recovered completely at 6 months after ASCT. CD8+45RO+ cells decreased steadily during the posttransplant follow-up. Before conditioning, in vitro T-cell mitogenic responses were decreased in most patients with a trend toward a baseline level at 3 months after ASCT.

Conclusion

Patients with refractory and active lupus involving multiple organ systems despite a relatively young age traditionally have a high disease-related mortality rate. Continuing failing therapy for such patients is problematic, but necessary to confirm that the increased risk HDIST with auto-SCT would be offset by better disease control, and induced long-term remission or partial response with clinical improvement in all refractory live SLE patients who underwent SCT in our center.

Three patients died due to serious infections in the early posttransplantation period. Among them, the nucleated cell counts in the reinfused graft product in the two fatal cases (case 1 and case 2) were less than $2x10^8$/kg recipient body weight, and this was probably not enough for stable hematopoiesis recovery. Although there is no universal agreement, recommended optimal CD 34+ cell dose ($2-5x10^8$ /kg) for successful engraftment after autologous myeloablative SCT for patient with malignancies has been accepted by most clinicians [23]. Non-myeloablative conditioning regimen used in most our patient carries virtually no risk of non-engraftment after SCT. However, our results (data not shown) demonstrated a correlation between infused CD34+ cell dose and faster WBC and platelet engraftment supporting the role of autologous SC in shortening the period of neutropenia and critical trombocytopenia. Thus, for all patients in whom HSC collection was unsuccessful in achieving an adequate number of CD 34+ cells, repeat bone marrow harvest or mobilization should be performed [23, 24]. In our study, G-CSF in combination with Cy did not cause a disease flare-up [25]. Most patients showed an improvement in disease activity after high dose Cy and G-CSF for PBSC mobilization before pretransplant conditioning [5]. Only one patient, receiving Cy-mobilization, experienced severe complications and developed pneumonia and skin infection during the pretransplantation period.

Culture-negative neutropenic fever, although common during early posttransplantation regimen, was transient and easily controlled with empiric antibiotic therapy.

All of the patients who died due to transplant-related complications received more than one anticytostatic drug in myeloablative doses or ATG as conditioning regimen. The conditioning regimen for autoimmune disease used to eliminate self-reactivity lymphocytes within the patient was designed depending on whether the investigator wanted to either specifically target lymphocytes (lymphoablative, i.e., non-myeloablative regimen) or to destroy the entire hematopoietic bone marrow compartment (myeloablative regimen). In cancers, autologous HSCT regimens are designed to be myeloablative, as the rationale is to destroy leukemic cancer-causing stem cells. [1]. The goal of autologous HSCT for autoimmune diseases is to generate new self-tolerant lymphocytes after elimination of self- or auto-reactive lymphocytes (i.e., lymphoablation), rather than ablate and reconstitute the entire hematopoietic compartment (myeloablation). Non-myeloablative regimens are often considered safer owing to lower organ toxicity, the more rapid engraftment following non-myeloablative HSCT demonstrated herein also supports of non-myeloablative regimens compared to myeloablative regimens. Therefore, in SLE, there are no reports comparing engraftment and responses after non-myeloablative compared to myeloablative regimens for autologous HSCT [1, 4].

Consistent with previous reports, we think that intensification of the chemotherapy is not a justified risk for SLE patients, and we stopped using myeloablative conditioning regimens specific for malignant disease. Now we used a dose-escalated Cy for conditioning, a standard lupus medication [4, 5]

One of the most important complications was cardiotoxicity, possibly related to direct Cy toxicity and hyperhydration. The patient selection is important to reduce TRM and complete cardiological assessment before transplantation is highly recommended [26]. Careful patient selection, especially cardiac function evaluation, which is often underestimated in SLE-patient, may avoid mortality [26].

A few patients developed CMV disease after AutoSCT [27]. We did not routinely monitor this or CMV viremia. One patient, who was severely immunosuppressed owing to chronic use of high-dose steroids for more than 9 years, was found to have fatal CMV-disease after ATG-including regimen, which was more characteristic of a postallotransplant complication. It may be cause for a recommendation to use standard CMV pretrasplant prophylaxis and CMV-monitoring for SLE patients with a long-term history of immunosuppessive therapy. Positive CMV surveillance assay are the grounds for prompt treatment with ganciclovir [28]. Also, compared with patients with cancer, patients with lupus have a long history of chronic immunosuppression and appear unusually prone to infections during mobilization and after transplantation, mandating aggressive preemptive antimicrobial (i.e., antifungal and antiviral) prophylaxis [29].

Addition of ATG for SCT for SLE treatment further maximizes immunosuppression, because of specific target T-cells [30]. Equine ATG caused acute toxicities that mimicked active SLE flare-ups and did not target memory B cells [27,30]. Because we obtained significant clinical response and low rate of severe infection, when treating with Cy alone, ATG seemed not to be necessary for the conditioning [5].

We did not find differences in T-cell recovery between patients with complete and partial response or between patients treated with different regimens. But we noted more rapid, numerous and functional T-cell recovery in SLE patients treated with ASCT compared with lymphoma patients (data not shown).

Other method of immunoablation, such as anti-CD20 monoclonal antibody (Rituximab), may be an important therapeutic approach for the treatment of patients intolerant to HDIST with auto-SCT. Because Rituximab is generally well tolerated and selectively depletes B cells, its role in immune-mediated diseases is now also being explored [31-34]. Future SLE transplant protocol should consider substituting ATG with rituximab or alemtuzumab, which target both T and B-cells [35,36]. We did not incorporate ATG into the conditioning regimen from 2003 on.

Thus, the complication of autologous SCT is connected with patient selection, the choice of conditioning regimen, and supportive care during and after transplantation.

There are two among our groups of patients who developed symptoms of SLE during pregnancy (one patient during fatal progression of the disease and one patient at the onset of the disease). Patients with SLE have normal fertility and should not be discouraged from having children. However, given the high frequency of SLE flare-ups during pregnancy, SLE pregnancies should be regarded as high risk and close monitoring for disease activity is mandatory throughout the pregnancy [37,38].

The involvement of the central nervous system (CNS) is one of the major causes of morbidity and mortality in systemic lupus erythematosus (SLE) patients [3,39]. Among the neurologic manifestations of SLE, the most common are the organic encephalopathies, which basically comprise all potential variations of acute confusion, lethargy, or coma; chronic dementias; depression, mania, or other affective disturbances; psychosis; cranial nerve abnormalities (most prominently, optic neuritis); stroke; peripheral neuropathy; etc. Acute or subacute mental status changes may be secondary to diffuse cerebritis but should be differentiated from focal cortical dysfunction resulting from thromboembolic cerebrovascular accident (CVA) or from diffuse changes resulting from electrolyte or metabolic derangements (accentuated by concomitant renal failure) [39].

Spinal cord involvement in SLE patient is rare but devastating. Transverse myelitis, and subacute-to-chronic demyelinating syndromes may cause severe invalidity [40,41]. Management of central nervous system (CNS) involvement still remains one of the most challenging, and using HDIST does not solve problems completely. Our two patients with CNS involvment did not achieve Cr after SCT but dramatically improved. Recently, the use of intrathecal methotrexate and dexamethasone have been reported in a small series of patients, with a good outcome in patients with severe CNS manifestations.

It should be mentioned that all of our patients had experienced multiple and severe episodes of infections pre-SCT, and long-term history of corticosteroid therapy (3-14 years). The remissions were achieved despite a previous history of refractory or relapsing disease, indicating the potential efficacy of this procedure. It was anticipated that control of clinical lupus activity was reflected by marked falls of anti-ds DNA antibodies, normalization of complement levels and reduction or withdrawal of corticosteroids.

In concert with the consensus report from EULAR and EBMT [16], patients should be selected for autoSCT who have severe disease and are refractory to conventional therapy. In selecting patients, consideration should be given to the balance between disease severity and organ damage. For patients with SLE, in contrast with malignancies, since organ compromise is due to lupus, impaired visceral organ function is not ultimately a contraindication, but is one of the major indications for SCT. While this makes the transplant procedure more complicated, marked organ improvement—particularly of the lung, the kidney and the central nervous system—has occurred following Cy-contained mobilization and SCT. Thus preexisting dysfunction of kidneys, liver, and lung are associated with increased mortality from transplant regimens. Treatment of such patients remains a difficult clinical problem. The presence of poor prognostic indicators would provide additional support in patient selection for future SCT studies. Recently, prognostic indicators suggesting a poor outcome in SLE have been proposed [43]. These are renal dysfunction, hypertension, anemia, low C3, central nervous system involvement and thrombocytopenia. Patients with these prognostic features have a considerably shortened life span. Thus, the 10-year survival of patients without features is estimated to be 86% compared with 60% of patients with these features. The quality of response to conventional therapy may be a useful criterion in selection of patients earlier in disease. Pulse Cy (500-1000 mg/m^2) is generally considered the standard of care. Eligibility for SCT patients with nonrenal visceral involvement need only fail corticosteroids and 3 months of pulse Cy. For patients in whom the indication is nephritis, active disease must be present despite at least 6 cycles of monthly pulse Cy [17].

Judicious selection of patients earlier in disease or in remission, but with a high risk of relapse or further progression, will improve the results of treatment and transplantation-related complication.

References

[1] Burt R., Marmont A, Oyama Y, Slavin S. Randomized Controlled Trials of Autologous Hematopoietic Stem Cell Transplantation for Autoimmune Diseases The Evolution From Myeloablative to Lymphoablative Transplant Regimens. *ARTHRITIS and RHEUMATISM* 2006; Vol. 54, No. 12: pp 3750–3760.

[2] Marmont A, van Lint M, Gualandi F, Bacigalupo A. Autologous marrow stem cell transplantation for severe systemic lupus erythematosus of long duration. *Lupus* 1997; 6: 545-548.

[3] Trysberg E, Lindgren I, Tarkowski A. Autologous stem cell transplantation in case of treatment resistant central nervous system lupus. *Ann. Rheum. Dis.* 2000; 59: 236-238.

[4] Burt R and E Traynor A Hematopoietic stem cell transplantation for systemic erythematosus *Arthritis Res. Ther.* 2003, 5:207-209.

[5] Tsukamoto H, Nagafuji K, Horiuchi T, A phase I-II trial of autologous peripheral blood stem cell transplantation in the treatment of refractory autoimmune disease *Ann Rheum Dis* 2006; 65;508-514.

[6] Lisukov IA, Sizikova SA, Kulagin AD. High-dose Immunosuppression with Autologous Stem Cell Transplantation in Severe Refractory Systemic Lupus Erythematosus *Lupus* 2004; Vol 13: 89-94.

[7] Ikehara S. Bone marrow transplantation for autoimmune diseases. *Acta Haematol.* 1998; 99: 116-132.

[8] Van Bekkum D.W. Review: BMT in experimental autoimmune diseases. *Bone Marrow Transplant* 1993; 11: 183 –187.

[9] Knaan-Shanzer S., Houben P., Van Bekkum D.W. Remission induction of adjuvant arthritis in rats by total body irradiation and autologous bone marrow transplantation. *Bone Marrow Transplant* 1992; 8: 333-338.

[10] Van Bekkum D.W. Experimental basis for treating autoimmune diseases with bone marrow transplants. *Stem cells* 1996; 14: 463-465.

[11] Liu Yin J, Jowitt S. Resolution of immune-mediated diseases following allogeneic bone marrow transplantation for leukemia. *Bone Marrow Transplant* 1992; 9:31.

[12] Salzman P, Tami J, Jackson C, Clinical remission of myasthenia gravis after high dose chemotherapy and autologous transplantation with CD34+ stem cells. *Blood* 1994; 84 (abstract 206a).

[13] Tyndall A., Fassas A., Passweg J. et al. Autologous haematopoietic stem cell transplants for autoimmune diseases – feasibility and transplant-related mortality. *Bone Marrow Transplant* 1999; 24: 729–734.

[14] Tyndall A., Gratwohl A. Haematopoietic stem and progenitor cells in the treatment of severe autoimmune diseases. *Ann. Rheum. Dis.* 1996; 35: 149–151.

[15] Marmont A. Stem cell transplantation for severe autoimmune diseases: progress and problems. *Haematologica* 1998; 83: 733 – 743.

[16] Tyndall A, Gratwohl A. Blood and marrow stem cell transplants in autoimmune disease: a consensus report written on behalf of the European League Against Rheumatism (EULAR) and the European Group for Blood and Marrow Transplantation (EBMT). *British Journal of Rheumatology* 1997; 36: 390–392.

[17] Burt R, Slavin S, Burns W, Marmont A. Induction of tolerance in autoimmune diseases by hematopoietic stem cell transplantation: getting closer to a cure? *Blood* 2002; 99: 768-784.

[18] Jayne D, Passweg J, Marmont A et al. Autologous stem cell transplantation for systemic lupus erythematosus. *Lupus*; 2004;13 (3):168-76.

[19] Openshaw H, Nash R, McSweeney P. High-dose immunosupression and hematopoietic stem cell transplantation in autoimmune disease: clinical review. *Biol Blood Marrow Transplant* 2002; 8: 233-248.

[20] American College of Rheumatology, *The American College of Rheumatology Response Criteria for Systemic Lupus Erythematosus Clinical Trials ARTHRITIS and RHEUMATISM* 2004, Vol. 50, No. 11, pp 3418–3426.

[21] Bombardier C, Gladman D. Derivation of the SLEDAI. A disease activity index for lupus patients. The committee on prognosis studies in SLE. *Arthritis Rheum.* 1992; 35: 630-640.
[22] Isenberg D, Ramsey-Goldman R. Assessing patients with lupus: towards a drug responder index. *Rheumatology* 1999; 38: 1045-1049.
[23] Ketterer N, Salles G,. High CD34+ cell counts decrease hematologic toxicity of autologous peripheral blood progenitor cell transplantation. *Blood* 1998; 91: 3148–3155.
[24] Statkutel L, Verda L Mobilization, harvesting and selection of peripheral blood stem cells in patients with autoimmune diseases undergoing autologous hematopoietic stem cell transplantation. *Bone Marrow Transplantation* 2007, 00, pp 1–13.
[25] Gottenberg JE, Roux S, Desmoulins F, ClercD, Mariette X. Granulocyte colony-stimulating factor therapy resulting in a flare of systemic lupus erythematosus: comment on the articleby Yang and Hamilton. *Arthr. Rheum.* 2001; 44: 2458–2460.
[26] Loberiza FR Jr, Zhang MJ, Lee SJ, et al. Association of transplant center and physician factors on mortality after hematopoietic stem cell transplantation in the United States. *Blood.* 2005;105:2979-2987.
[27] Burt R, Traynor A, Statkute L Nonmyeloablative Hematopoietic Stem Cell Transplantation for Systemic Lupus Erythematosus, *JAMA*, 2006, Vol 295, No. 5 527-535.
[28] Salzberger B, Bowden RA, Neutropenia in allogeneic marrow transplant recipients receiving ganciclovir for prevention of cytomegalovirus disease: risk factors and outcome. *Blood.* 1997;90:2502-2508.
[29] Kang I, Park SH. Infectious complications in SLE after immunosuppressive therapies. *Curr. Opin. Rheumatol.* 2003;15:528-534.
[30] Young N, Speck B. Antithymocyte and antilymphocyte globulins: clinical trials and mechanism of action. *Prog. Clin. Biol. Res.* 1984;148:221-226.
[31] Arzoo K, Sadeghi S, Liebman H. Treatment of refractory antibody mediated autoimmune disorders with an anti-CD20 monoclonal antibody (rituximab). *Ann. Rheum. Dis.* 2000; 61: 922-924.
[32] Looney R.J. Treating human autoimmune disease by depleting B cells. *Ann. Rheum Dis.* 2002; 61: 863-866.
[33] Eisenberg R. SLE: rituximab in lupus. *Arthritis. Res. Ther.* 2003;5:157-159.
[34] Anolik JH, Barnard J, Cappione A, et al. Rituximab improves peripheral B cell abnormalities in human systemic lupus erythematosus. *Arthritis. Rheum.* 2004;50:3580-3590.
[35] Willis F, Marsh JC, Bevan DH, et al. The effect of treatment with Campath-1H in patients with autoimmune cytopenias. *Br. J. Haematol.* 2001; 114:891-898.
[36] Cohen Y, Polliack A, Nagler A. Treatment of refractoryautoimmune diseases with ablative immunotherapy using monoclonal antibodies and/or high dose chemotherapy with hematopoietic stem cell support. *Curr. Pharm. Des.* 2003;9:279-288.
[37] Georgiou P.E., Politi E.N. et al. Outcome of lupus pregnancy: a controlled study *Rheumatology* 2000;39:1014-1019.
[38] Mok CC, Wong R W S Pregnancy in systemic lupus erythematosus *Postgrad Med. J.* 2001; Vol:77:157-165.
[39] Sannal G, Bertolaccini ML, Mathieu A Central nervous system lupus: a clinical approach to therapy. *Lupus* (2003) 12, 935–942.

[40] Schantz V, Oestergaard LL, Junker P. Shrinking spinal cord following transverse myelopathy in a patient with systemic lupus erythematosus and the phospholipid antibody syndrome. *J. Rheumatol.* 1998; 25: 1425–1428.
[41] Yazawa S, Kawasaki S, Ohi T *et al.* Development of severe longitudinal atrophy of thoracic spinal cord following lupus-related myelitis. *Intern. Med.* 2001; 40: 353–357.
[42] Dong Y, Zhang X, Tang F, Tian X, Zhao Y, Zhang F. Intrathecal injection with methotrexate plus dexamethasone in the treatment of central nervous system involvement in systemic lupus erythematosus. *Chin. Med. J. (Engl)* 2001; 114: 764–766.
[43] Hahn B.H. The potential role of autologous stem cell transplantation in patients with SLE. *J. Rheumatol.* 1997; 24 (Suppl 48): 89-93.

In: Immunosuppression: New Research
Editor: Charles B. Taylor, pp. 239-269
ISBN: 978-1-60692-102-9

Chapter 11

Experimental Approaches for Transplantation of Islets in the Absence of Immunosuppression

Bart J. de Haan, Marijke M. Faas, Albert F. Hamel and Paul de Vos*

Transplantation biology and Immunoendocrinology, Department of Pathology and Laboratory Medicine, section of Medical Biology, University of Groningen, Hanzeplein 1, 9700 RB Groningen, The Netherlands.

Abstract

Transplantation of insulin producing cells in diabetic patients requires technologies to transplant tissues in the absence of immunosuppression since the side effect of immunosuppression can never be an acceptable alternative for insulin therapy. Much effort has been put into the development of immunomodulating technologies to transplant genetically or otherwise modified islet tissue in order to decrease the immunogenicity of the islet tissue. A number of these approaches have been shown to be effective in small rodents and to allow for life-long survival of islet grafts[1,2]. In spite of some successes it has not yet come to clinical application. Another approach is immunoisolation of tissue by encapsulation of pancreatic islets to protect the tissue from the host immune system by an artificial membrane. Basically, there are three major approaches of encapsulation. These include intravascular macrocapsules, which are anastomosed to the vascular system as AV shunt, extravascular macrocapsules, which are mostly diffusion chambers transplanted at different sites, and extravascular microcapsules transplanted in the peritoneal cavity. All systems have been shown to be successful in preclinical studies. These studies also showed that not all approaches meet the technical or physiological requirements for application in men. The extravascular approach provides advantages over the intravascular systems since it is associated with fewer complications such as thrombosis and infection. Microcapsules, due to their spatial characteristics, offer better diffusion capacity than macrocapsules. Recent

* E-mail address: B.J.DE.HAAN@MED.RUG.NL. Phone: (31) (50) 3611045, Fax: (31) (50) 3619911, Address correspondence to:. De Vos, Ph.D.Pathology and Laboratory Medicine, Section of Medical Biology, University of Groningen, Hanzeplein 19700 RB Groningen, The Netherlands.

progress in biocompatibility of microcapsules has brought this technology near clinical application. Critical issues such as limitations in the functional performance and survival are being discussed. The latest results show that both issues can be solved by transplantation of microencapsulated islets near blood vessels in prevascularized solid supports. Also, latest insights will be presented into the composition of the membranes for immuoisolating devices and the associated biocompatibility.

Introduction

The general goal in the treatment of insulin dependent diabetes mellitus (IDDM) is the prevention of late complications, and thereby improvement of the quality of patient life. There is no dispute that euglycemia is of essential importance to reach that goal. Euglycemia may be achieved by intensified insulin treatment, and the results of the Diabetes Control and Complications trial clearly demonstrate that this approach is effective since it delays the onset and reduces the progression of diabetic complications [3]. Intensified treatment, however, is not a simple achievement since it requires multiple daily injections, frequent monitoring, dosage adaptations and, thus, patient compliance. Also, it is associated with frequent episodes of severe hypoglycemia and with glycemic unawareness. A principally different approach to achieve euglycemia is to provide the diabetic patient with an endogenous rather than an exogenous source of insulin by the transplantation of endocrine pancreatic tissue. Pancreatic organ transplantation is now an established mode of treatment with a worldwide experience of more than 15.000 cases [4,5]. Results have substantially improved during the past two decades and present patient and one-year graft survival rates almost equal to those of kidney transplantation (respectively 98% and 85%). A successful pancreas transplant provides almost normal glucose homeostasis, but it requires life-long immunosuppressive medication. Since it is still unclear whether the advantage of a pancreas transplant over continued insulin treatment outweighs the disadvantage of obligatory immunosuppression, most transplant centers still restrict themselves to combined pancreas and kidney transplantation in diabetic patients with end-stage renal failure [4,6].

Islet transplantation, in contrast to pancreas transplantation, requires no major surgery.

Recent improvements in the technology are the administration of non-glucocorticoid immunosuppression (sirolimus, tacrlimus, daclizumab) by the Edmonton-group which is associated with one-year graft survival of 100% of the transplanted diabetic patients [7]. These advances have led to a tremendous growth in the number of research groups involved in human islet transplantation. Unfortunately, not all these groups have achieved the same level of success, which is usually attributed to different degrees in ‘experiences’ in efficacious isolation of functional islets. However, in spite of the inability of many groups to fully reproduce the Edmonton results, the general impression is that recent advances of the Edmonton group have brought islet-transplantation close to widespread clinical application.

Another pertinent advantage of islet transplantation over whole pancreas transplantation is that successful islet transplantation without immunosuppression might be achieved by relatively simple methods such as immunomodulation, genetic engineering of islets and immunoisolation. These experimental approaches will be discussed in the present paper in view of future clinical applications.

Immunomodulation

An attractive feature of free isolated islets is the ability to immunomodulate the tissue before transplantation in order to reduce the immunogenicity. During the past two decades various technical approaches have been tested to delete antigen-presenting cells in islets and to reduce the presentation of immunogenic peptides on islet cells. These approaches include culture at low temperatures[8] or under ultraviolet light [9,10], pretreatment with neutralizing or deleting antibodies [11], immunosuppressive drug pretreatment such as cyclophosphamide or deoxyguanosine pretreatment [12], cryopreservation [13,14], or irradiation [15]. All these technologies have proven successful in small rodents with graft survival rates for periods up to a year. Unfortunately, however, when applied in large animal models only temporary instead of prolonged survival of islet tissue was observed. Although the reasons for the difference in success of immunomodulation between rodents and large mammals remain to be studied it has been suggested that a plausible difference is the more complex and still not well understood biochemistry of human islets.

A very promising approach of immunomodulation is targeting the donor-derived costimulatory activity. It has been shown that coating of murine islet allografts with antibodies against co-stimulatory molecules CTLA4-Ig facilitates engraftment and induces permanent tolerance in 50% of the recipients [16]. This blockade of co-stimulatory molecules is also the basis of many genetic approaches to overcome graft rejection and will be discussed in more detail in the next section.

Genetic Engineering of Islets

In the past decade, islets have been genetically modified in order to block costimulatory molecules, to induce expression of Fas ligand (FasL) or immunosuppressive cytokines, and to inhibit gene transcription of regulatory proteins, such as nuclear factor-B [17-19]. However, the majority of present experimental strategies to reduce rejection of islet allografts by genetic engineering are aiming on blockade of the costimulatory pathway. This approach will be discussed in more detail in the next sections.

After transplantation of 'foreign' islets T-cell activation occurs which causes the upregulation of at least two essential co-stimulatory molecules. One of the molecules, CTLA4, binds B7 with a high affinity and provides a negative signal to the T cell. The other molecule, ICOS, binds B7H/B7RP-1, and is required for an adequate humoral immune response and induction of cytokine production such as interleukin 4. Many groups involved in genetic engineering of islet-tissue have focussed in the past decade on the potential application of CTLA4-Ig for blockade of the costimulatory pathway. The main reason for that is the observation that T cells involved in rejection and in autoimmunity express high levels of CD80 (B7.1) and CD86 (B7.2) antigens both in rodent and humans. CTLA4-lg is a genetically engineered fusion protein of human CTLA4 and the IgG 1 Fc region, and prevents T-cell activation by binding with high affinity to human B7.

There are several successful approaches for delivery of CTLA4-Ig in the vicinity of transplanted islets. Chahine et al. [20] observed that cotransplantation of myoblasts transfected with CTLA4-Ig cDNA and syngenic to the host, significantly prolonged murine islet allograft survival. This approach, however, did only induce permanent survival when CTLA4-Ig was combined with blockade of the leukocyte function-associated-1 pathway by applying an additional monoclonal antibody (Fig. 1). Gainer et al [21,22] transfected CTLA4-Ig cDNA directly into islets rather than cells in the vicinity of the tissue and showed prolonged allograft survival in 50% of the recipients. Unfortunately, this method did not provide full protection since the islets showed peri-insulitis. The reason for this peri-insulitis is probably related to the fact that transfection is not permanent: the level of CTLA4-Ig obtained in transfected islets does vary ninefold, and the constructs disappear after 21-28 days [22].

The success of genetic engineering of islet cells in large mammals and humans remains to be proven but an optimistic view is realistic since a single CTLA4-Ig bolus improved renal allograft survival in a series of five Cynomolgus monkeys for periods longer than 50 days [23]. This suggest that similar mechanism of co-stimulation occur in large mammals and plausibly also in humans.

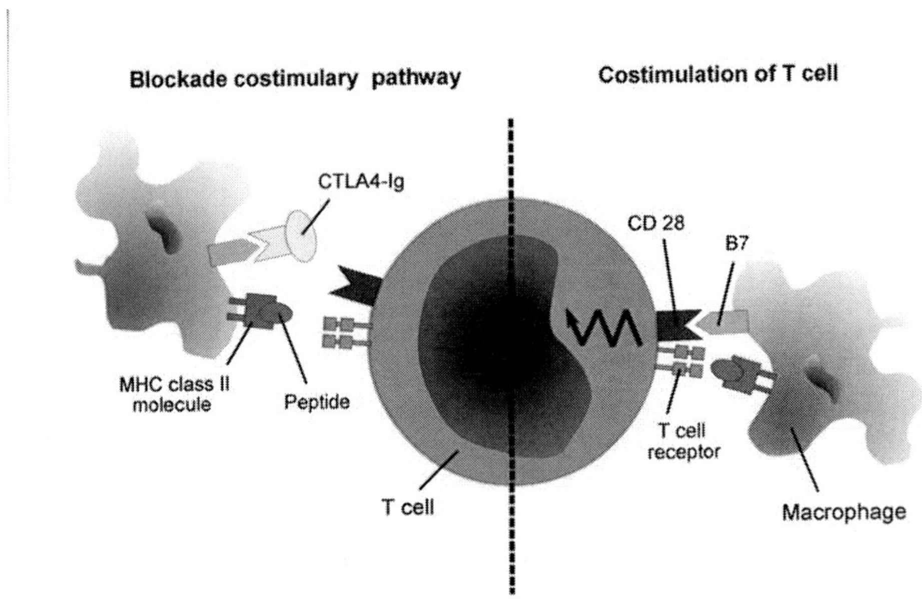

Figure 1. Schematic representation of T-cell stimulation after the presentation of a peptide by a macrophage. The macrophage presents the peptide to the T-cell receptor in context of MHC class 2. Simultaneously the CD28 receptor binds the macrophage co-stimulatory molecule B7 (right panel). Blocking the co-stimulatory pathway with CTLA4-Ig occurs by high affinity binding of this antibody to the B7 molecule thus preventing low affinity binding to CD28. As a result the peptide will not be presented to the T cell (left panel).

Immunoisolation

The possibility of transplanting cells in immunoprotective membranes for organ replacement dates back to 1933. At that time, Bisceglie [24] replaced the endogenous pancreas by transplanting insulin producing tissue encapsulated in a semipermeable but immunoprotective membrane to study the effects of absence of vascularization on the survival of tissues. It took, however, until 1943 before the concept of immunoisolation was established by Algire [25] who recognized that graft failure was delayed by encapsulating allo- and xenogenic tissues before transplantation. The group of Algire was also the first to illustrate the importance of biocompatibility since they found that graft failure was always accompanied by cellular overgrowth of the membranes. At present, transplantation of cells in immunoisolating devices is under study for the treatment of a wide variety of diseases, including Hemophilia B [26], anemia [27], dwarfism [28], kidney [29] and liver failure[30] pituitary [31] and central nervous system insufficiencies [32], and diabetes mellitus [33]. For diabetes mellitus research there are two major encapsulaton systems: macro- and microencapsulation (Fig. 2). The macrocapsules contain groups of islets enveloped together in one immunoisolating membrane that can be implanted as extravascular and intravascular device. With microencapsulation the islets are individually enveloped by their own capsule. These two approaches will be discussed in the next section.

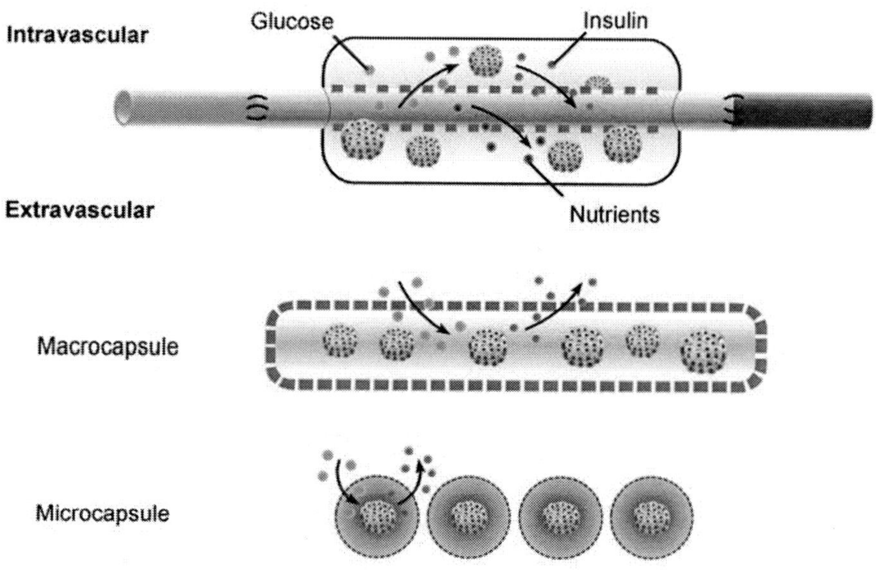

Figure 2. Immunoisolation in intravasculair and extravasculair devices.In immunoisolation with intravascular macrocapsule devices, islets are seeded on the outside of artificial capillaries, in close contact with the bloodstream. The extravascular capsules have a higher diffusion distance to the bloodstream due to the lack of vascularisation. Immunoisolation in extravascular macrocapsules there are several islets encapsulated in one capsule, while immunoisolation in extravascular microcapsules involves individual encapsulated islets.

Macrocapsules

Extravascular Macrocapsules

The extravascular macrocapsules can be implanted with minimal surgery in different sites such as the peritoneal cavity [34-37], the subcutaneous site [38-44], or the renal capsule [45]. The concept of extravascular devices does not require vascular anastomoses, since it is based on the principle of diffusion chambers [46]. The geometry may be planar in the form of a flat, circular double layer or tube-like as a so-called hollow fiber [46]. The surgical risks are much lower with extravascular than with the intravascular devices. Also, they can be readily retrieved, and they can be produced in a relatively simple way.

Many different biomaterials have been applied for the production of extravascular macrocapsules (Table 1). The hollow fiber geometry is usually preferred over the planar membranes for their smaller foreign body response [47]. Most studies on hollow fibers use fibers made of polyacrylonitrile and polyvinylchloride copolymer (PAN-PVC) [48,49]. They have been produced with a smooth or fenestrated outer skin with the same spongy matrix as applied in the intravascular. The design with the smooth outer skin proved to be the most successful since it provokes much less fibrosis than the rough fenestrated surface which allows host tissue to grow into the spongy matrix. Many modifications of this concept have been proposed in order to further improve the biocompatibility. One of those was the coating of the membranes with poly-ethyleenoxide to reduce protein adsorption [50]. Biocompatibility problems with extravascular macrocapsules are usually deleterious only to the function of the encapsulated tissue and have no or only minimal risk for the recipient. These biocompatibility problems are usually related to toxicity and activation of non-specific foreign body reactions resulting in fibrotic overgrowth with subsequent necrosis of the encapsulated tissue.

Table I. Main components of capsules proposed for macroencapsulation of pancreatic islets

Membrane Geometry Proposed by	Geometry	Proposed by
nitro-cellulose acetate	Planar	Algire 1943 [25]
polycarbonate	Planar	Strautz 1970 [187]
2-hydroxyethyl methacrylate (HEMA)	Planar	Klomp et al 1979 [57]
polytetrafluoroethylene	Planar	Rafael et al 1999
polyacrylonitrile and polyvinylchloride	Tubular	Archer et al 1980 [34] Zekorn
cellulose	Tubular	et al 1989
polyamide	Tubular	[188] Zekorn et al 1989 [188] Kessler
acrylonitrile and sodium-methallyl sulfonate(AN69)	Tubular	et al 1991 (59)
alginate-based		
polyvinyl alcohol (PVA)	Tubular	Lanza et al 1995 [189]
polyisobutylene	Tubular	Gamian et al 1999 [190]
	Tubular	Isayeva et al 2003 [191]

During the past few years, an interesting trend has been the growing number of groups applying hydrogels for extravascular macrocapsules. Hydrogels provide a number of features which are advantageous for the biocompatibility of the membranes. Firstly, as a consequence of the hydrophilic nature of the material, there is almost no interfacial tension with surrounding fluids and tissues, which minimizes the protein adsorption and cell adhesion. Furthermore, the soft and pliable features of the gel reduce the mechanical or frictional irritations to surrounding tissue. And, finally, they provide a high degree of permeability for low molecular weight nutrients and metabolites, which is required for the optimal functioning of living cells[51,52].

Many hydrogels have been applied, such as gels prepared of alginate [53-55], agarose [37,56], 2-hydroxyethyl methacrylate HEMA [57,58] and a copolymer of acrylonitrile and sodium-methallyl sulfonate, AN69 [59]. Primary attention has been focussed on the hydrogel membrane AN69, which induced only minimal fibrosis in the peritoneal cavity of rats [60,61] but had low permeability for insulin [60,61]. Kessler et al [60,61] have introduced corona discharge to obtain a membrane with a more hydrophobic surface. Less molecules adhered to the surface of such membranes, which improved not only the permeability for insulin but also its long-term biocompatibility. One year after implantation in rats, only few macrophages were found on the membrane's surface. Moreover, encouraging results were reported by Jain et al who demonstrated functional porcine islets transplanted in agarose macrobeads almost 200 days after intraperitoneal transplantation into BB rats [37].

Intravascular Macrocapsules

The intravascular device is usually composed of a microporous tube with blood flow through its lumen and with a housing on its outside containing the implanted tissue [62,63]. The device is implanted by vascular anastomoses to the vessels of the host. The most intensively studied intravascular device is the modified diffusion chamber of Chick et al [64]. It is technically advanced and has been tested extensively in small [65] as well as in large animals [65,66] The original device was composed of a number of small diameter artificial capillaries contained by one large diameter tube. The artificial capillaries were composed of fibers of polyacrylonitrile and polyvinylchloride copolymer (PAN-PVC) similar to those used in extravascular devices [48][49]. This PAN-PVC ultrafiltration capillary design [31] has a lumen loaded with islets at the outside of the artificial capillaries. The design permits for close contact between the islets and blood, separated only by the microporous walls of the capillaries. These devices were found to induce normoglycemia in diabetic rats [65], dogs [66] and monkeys [65] but required systemic anticoagulation. The duration of this normoglycemia was usually restricted to several hours and successes of a somewhat longer duration were exceptional. Clotting of the blood in the lumen of these small diameter artificial capillaries proved to be a major obstacle, in spite of anticoagulant medication in massive doses. This thrombus formation was an early sign of insufficient biocompatibility, and has led to the use of tubular membranes with larger diameters in the hope of minimizing or eliminating clot formation in the absence of systemic anticoagulation.

The latter large lumen device is composed of a single, coiled, and tubular membrane with an internal diameter of 5-6 mm. The membrane is somewhat modified but still composed of PAN-PVC with a nominal molecular weight cutoff of 50 kDa. This membrane was found to be rather successful, since these devices implanted as high flow arteriovenous fistulas could remain patent for periods of seven weeks in the absence of systemic anticoagulant therapy

[67]. This success is in part explained by the high flow rates through the device which prevents adhesion of cells to the membranes or collection of those cells in the immediate vicinity [48].

Allo- and xenogenic islets in the high flow devices were successfully transplanted to diabetic dogs [68-73] but the efforts to improve the blood-compatibility have probably interfered with the efficacy of the device as an implantation site for islets. This view is derived from the following observations. First, two devices per recipient instead of one were required to achieve adequate secretion capacity while maintaining the same numbers of islets per device [74]. Furthermore, it has not been possible to load the space between the membranes and the housing with an islet-tissue density higher than 5-10% of the volume [31], in spite of the fact that the large lumen is exposed to arterial blood with optimal concentrations of nutrients and oxygen. It is quite plausible that the high flow rates through the device, which are required to keep the device patent, do not allow sufficient exchange of glucose, insulin and nutrients to permit long term survival and adequate function of the islets.

There are also indications that the materials applied in this kind of devices are not only thrombogenic but also insufficiently compatible with long term functional survival of the islets. For example, the PTFE as used for vascular anastomosis of the device has been shown to induce IL-1β production by macrophages [75], which cytokine is lethal for islets [76,77]. It is quite plausible that IL-1β causes loss of high numbers of islets during the period between implantation and complete integration of the prothesis since macrophages are usually the first cells to invade the implant [78-80]. This is another explanation for the fact that so many islets divided over two devices are required for maintaining normoglycemia in dogs.

Although the intravascular devices have shown some degree of success, the problems mentioned above should be solved if clinical application is considered. Even then, the complications associated with any type of vascular prosthetic surgery remain a serious threat, such as thrombosis, either primary or secondary to intimal hyperplasia at the venous anastomosis, defects of the device, or infection. This is a major drawback for wide application in large numbers of diabetic patients since any alternative to conventional insulin treatment should preferably carry no additional risk.

Microcapsules

Microencapsulation is the technique by which each islet is enveloped in its own, spherical semipermeable membrane. Several arguments favor microcapsules over macrocapsules. Their spherical shape offers better diffusion capacity because of a better surface/volume ratio. Microcapsules cannot be easily disrupted, they are mechanically stable, they do not require complex or expensive manufacturing procedure, and they can be implanted into the patient by a simple injection procedure.

Reportedly, the clinical experience is still restricted to one recipient [81], but several research groups are concentrating on transplantation of microencapsulated islets in the experimental setting [42,43,82,83,83-104]. Although successful encapsulated islet grafts do induce normoglycemia in streptozotocin diabetic rodents recipients, some authors have reported reduced functional performance in response to glucose challenge [51,95,105-107].

For several years, we have been concentrating on microencapsulation and we have directed our efforts to a step-wise analysis of the factors influencing performance of the microencapsulated grafts. To this end, we have been using only one technique of alginate-polylysine microencapsulation as initially introduced by Lim and Sun [33], instead of testing other materials in a trial and error approach. Our aim is to define the conditions, which must be met for successful transplantation of microencapsulated islets as a feasible treatment of insulin dependent diabetes mellitus.

The Principle of Microencapsulation

The vast majority of groups apply hydrogels for production of microcapsules since these hydrogels are associated with optimal survival of the enveloped cells. Table 2 lists the most commonly applied biomaterials for this technique. A major distinction exists between water-soluble polymers such as alginates and water insoluble polymers such as HEMA-MMA. Water insoluble polymers are preferred by a number of groups [58,108-110] since it is assumed that after implantation they are more stable than water soluble polymers. However, a major obstacle in using water insoluble polymers for encapsulation of cells is the use of an organic solvent, which usually interferes with cellular function [58,111].

Table 2. Main components of capsules proposed for microencapsulation of pancreatic islets

Main component of the capsule	Source	Initially proposed by
Alginate	Alga	Lim and Sun 1980 (33) Zielinski 1994
Chitosan	Alga	(192)
Agarose	Alga	Iwata et al 1989 (96) Dawson et al 1987
Poly(hydroxyethylmetacrylate-methyl	Synthetic	(193)
methacrylate)(HEMA-MMA)	Synthetic	Kessler et al 1991 (59)
Copolymers of acrylonitrile (AN69)	Synthetic	Shimizu et al 1996 (194)
Protamine-heparine	Synthetic	Tatarkiewicz 1994 (195)
N-isopropylacrylamide	Synthetic	Sefton et al 1997 (196)
Polyacryates	Synthetic	Cruise et al 1999 (84)
Polyethyleneglycol (PEG)	Synthetic	Boninsegna 2003 (197)
Silica		

We, like others [98,103,104,112-114], have concentrated on alginate based capsules since they have repeatedly been found not to interfere with cellular function. Despite of their solubility in aqueous solutions, they have been shown to be stable for years in small and large animals and recently also in men [72,81,115]. The encapsulation technique is based on entrapment of individual islets in an alginate droplet, which is transformed into a rigid bead by gelification in a divalent cation solution, mostly rich in Ca^{2+}. The droplets are formed by forcing an alginate/cell mixture through a needle, which is installed in a droplet generator. In principle we can distinguish three techniques of droplet generation (Fig. 3). The first and most commonly applied approach, is the air-driven droplet generator [116].

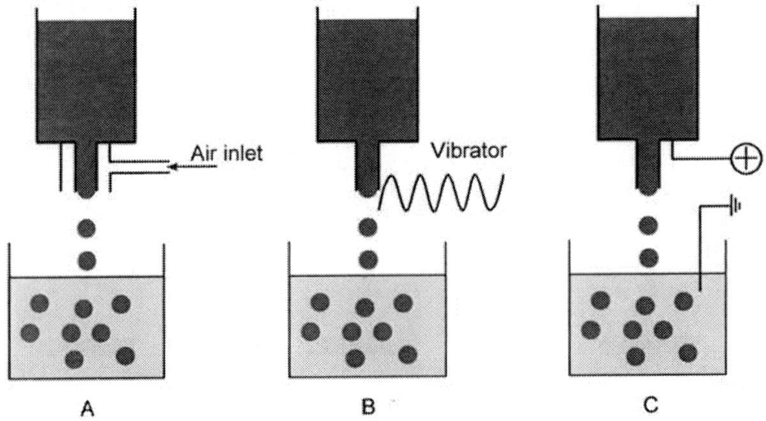

Figure 3. The basic principle of encapsulation is the formation of droplets by forcing an alginate/cell mixture through a needle, which is installed in a droplet generator. We can distinguish three techniques of droplet generation. The air-driven droplet generator (A) where droplets are formed by a co-axial airstream around the tip of a needle, which forces droplets of alginate to detach from the needle-tip. The size of the droplets can be decreased by increasing the airflow rate. With the vibration technique (B) detachment of the droplets from the needle is forced by substituting the airstream for vibration. With the latest technique, the voltage driven dropletgenerator (C), the dropletsize is controlled by a voltage difference between needle and gelification solution.

In these devices droplets are formed by a co-axial airstream around the tip of a needle which forces droplets of alginate to detach from the needle-tip. The size of the droplets can be decreased by increasing the airflow rate. In order to increase the production rate of droplets some groups have introduced a new approach by substituting the needle in de droplet generator for a vibration [117]. These devices do not need an airstream and by increasing the vibration frequency, the production rate can be increased while the droplet size decreases. Both the air-driven dropletgenerator and the vibration device have one major disadvantage, they do not allow for reproducible production of droplets with a size smaller than 500 μm [118]. Devices that produce capsules smaller than 500 μm may be mandatory since it has repeatedly been shown that small capsules are needed for optimal exchange of nutrients and metabolics as well as for adequate function of the enveloped cells. Therefore, a third category of devices has been introduced. These are the so-called voltage driven dropletgenerators. The technique of this device is based on administration of electrostatic forces to pull droplets off a needle-tip. The bead size can be varied by increasing the electrostatic potential between the gelling bath and the needle. Reportedly, this technique allows for reproducible production of droplets of 300 μm [103] but in our hands even smaller droplets of 175 μm can be readily obtained. Although the smallest capsule possible is prefered, it should be noted that the size of the capsules is not only limited by the technology applied but also by the size of the tissue to be encapsulated. With islet-encapsulation the size will be limited by the diameter of the islets which vary between 50 and 350 μm.

The next step in the encapsulation process is the gelification. Alginate-molecules are composed of mannuronic (M) and guluronic acids (G). The alginate-molecules are connected by Ca^{2+} through binding of consecutive blocks of G-molecules on each of both molecules.

The most commonly applied alginate-based capsule is the alginate-polylysine system. The beads are coated with a polylysine membrane by suspending the beads in a poly-L-lysine (PLL) solution. During this step PLL binds to mixed sequences of G and M in the alginate molecules [119,120]. This induces the formation of complexes at the capsule surface consisting of α-helical PLL surrounded by superhelically orientated polysaccharide chains [120]. The presence of these complexes decreases the porosity of the membrane. By varying the molecular weight, the concentration of the polylysine, and the incubation time one can modulate the porosity of the capsule membrane [94,121-126]. Usually, ten-minute incubation in 0.1 % polylysine with a molecular weight of 22 kDa is sufficient to form an immunoprotective membrane. However, it should be emphasized that the binding of polylysine does not only depend upon the incubation time and the molecular weight of the polylysine but also on the type and concentration of alginate [125,127] as well as on the incubation temperature [124,125,127]. In a final step, to provide biocompatibility, the capsules are suspended in a solution of alginate or other negatively charged molecules [124,127] to bind all positively charged polylysine residues still present at the capsule surface. We do not apply EGTA or citrate [111] to liquify the inner core of the capsule. The reason for this modification of the original Lim and Sun method [33] was, that we have observed many capsules loosing their integrity during the treatment.

A very important aspect of adequate biocompayibility, is a smooth and mechanically stable microcapsule. In our laboratory we have observed that high- rather than low-G alginates produce smooth beads with no obvious tails or strains. Moreover, we have found that after implantation, alginates with low-G concentrations had a tendency to swell with subsequent breakage of the PLL membrane followed by cellular overgrowth of the capsules. Therefore, for our studies we have chosen the alginate with an intermediate G-concentration.

The stability of the capsule is determined by stability of a membrane and stability of an alginate core. The stability of the membrane can be controlled by the PLL-step since shorter incubation time, lower PLL concentrations, and lower PLL molecular weight than described above, were associated with an increase of the number of capsules with broken membranes. Additionally, incubation at 4°C instead of room temperature led to less stable microcapsules. In spite of all the improvements in the stability of the capsules, tissue reactions still continued to interfere with longevity of the graft survival. We have found that other factors, not directly related to the production procedure per se, were responsible for the tissue reaction as a sign of insufficient biocompatibility of microcapsules.

Present Insights in Tissue Reponses Against Microcapsules

A major obstacle in the application of immunoisolation has been insufficient biocompatibility of the capsules which induced overgrowth of the capsules by inflammatory cells with necrosis of the enveloped therapeutic cells as a consequence [52,128]. It was shown that this insufficient biocompatibility of capsules is influenced by many factors. We found that the number of capsules that will be affected by cellular overgrowth is dependent on the chemical characteristics of the capsule-materials applied. We have shown that pure alginate rather than commercially available crude alginates should be applied for encapsulation [52].

Crude alginates are contaminated with several inflammatory substances such as polyphenols, which are associated with severe inflammatory reactions after implantation. When pure alginates are applied with an intermediate-G content we were able to reduce the overgrowth from 80-100% of the capsules to a portion of only 2-10% of the capsules. Also, it is important that there are no unbound PLL residues on the capsule surface. When PLL is not adequately bound by alginate it provokes a strong inflammatory response after implantation. The adequacy of binding of PLL depends on the composition of the alginate applied. Alginates are composed of blocks of guluronic acid (G-blocks), blocks of mannuronic acid (M-blocks), and alternating blocks of guluronic acid and mannuronic acid (G-M blocks). Adequate binding of PLL mainly depends on the amount of G-M blocks in the alginate. Small lower variations in the G-M content results in less efficient binding of PLL with overgrowth of the capsule surface as a consequence [119,120,129,130]. For adequate binding of PLL and neutralising the majority of its proinflammatory effects we have to apply a so-called intermediate-G alginate with 45% G and 30 % G-M blocks. Recently, our group has shown that, when adequately produced, empty capsules for cell-immunoisolation can survive for two years in the peritoneal cavity of rats [115].

It was found that the 2-10% overgrowth was caused by individual imperfections on a portion of the capsules such as protruding cells (Fig. 4) and incomplete bound PLL on the surface.

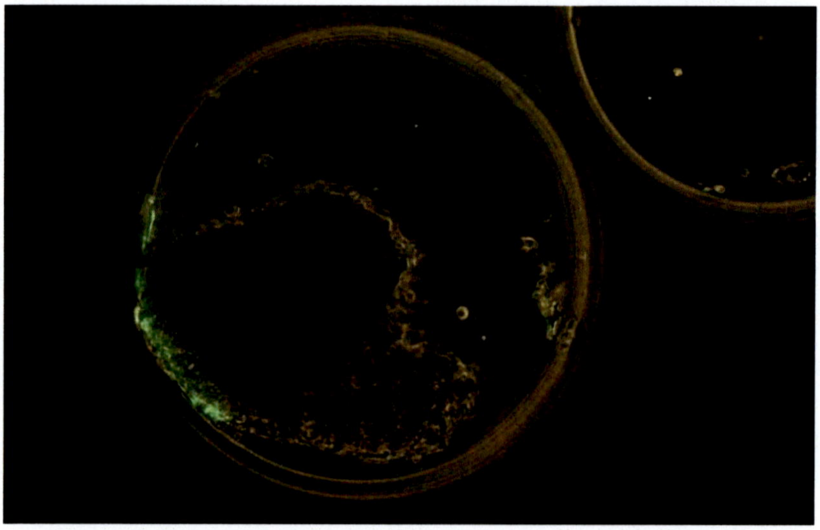

Figure 4. Inadequate encapsulation of pancreatic islets. The islet is incompletely encapsulated. Islet cells protruding from the capsule are specifically labeled by the FITC-labeled lectin RCA-I . (original magnification x 100).

These imperfections are difficult to avoid in the current technological approach since we apply flexible alginates (with intermediate-G content) which is associated with some capsules with protruding cells. Also, the present technology is susceptible for small variations in G-M content in the alginate sources which cause tissue responses as the consequence of insufficient neutralisation of the proinflammatory PLL on the capsule surface [129,131-134]. In an attempt to solve the cell protrusion problem we have tested the biocompatibility of alginate-PLL capsules prepared of high-G alginates since from our *in vitro* studies follows that alginate with a high guluronic acid content (> 53%) provides stronger capsules with less protruding cells than capsules prepared of alginate with an intermediate guluronic acid content [52]. Unfortunately, these high-G alginates could not be applied for cell encapsulation since they were associated with severe tissue responses *in vivo* due to inefficacious binding of the proinflammatory polylysine.

In order to provide more insight in the structure of alginate-PLL capsules we have performed an physico-chemical analysis of the capsules by applying X-ray photoelectron spectroscopy [129,130,135]. This technique allows for identification of the chemical groups on the surface of the capsule on an atomic level. Up to now the capsule was assumed to be composed of a core of Ca-alginate which is enveloped by a membrane composed of two layers, *i.e.* an inner layer of alginate-PLL and an outer layer of Ca-alginate [33,136,137]. The data, which have lead to this model, were almost exclusively obtained by studying the chemical interactions of PLL with solved, non-Ca^{2+} bound and often individual components of alginate (*i.e* guluronic (G)-acid and mannuronic (M)-acid monomers) and not by studying the chemical structure of the capsules as such. In our studies on true capsules, we never observed Ca^{2+} in the membrane of the capsules, which has the following implications for the assumed structure of the capsules. First, the alginate-PLL layer is not composed of the combination of alginate-PLL and Ca^{2+}-alginate but of the alginate-PLL only. The absence of Ca^{2+} also implies that the outer Ca-alginate layer does not exist and, consequently, that the membrane is not composed of two but of one layer only. Finally, we found sodium in the membrane, which is bound by carboxyl groups on consecutive blocks of G- and M-molecules, which remain unbound between the complexes of PLL and mixed sequences of G and M. Figure 5 shows the actual structure of alginate-PLL capsules.

These findings have serious implications for biocompatibility issues associated with microcapsules since it implies that the proinflammatory PLL is always on the surface of the capsules in direct contact with the inflammatory cells. It suggests that, for optimal biocompatibility, we have to focus on understanding and improving the interaction of the inflammatory polycations with alginate rather than improving the second coating step with alginate. Alternatively, we can perform an additional envelopment step of the capsules to prevent direct contact between the polycation with the surrounding tissues in the implantation site.

Purified intermediate-alginates reduced the overgrowth from 80-100% to a portion of only 2-10% of the capsules. When tested with encapsulated rat pancreatic islet allografts we found that this reduction in overgrowth did bring about an increase in graft survival time from 3 to 6 months. This illustrated that improving the quality of the capsules is a successful strategy in order to increase the longevity of the grafts. At this point it was unclear what caused failure of the cells since it was generally assumed that the loss of 2-10% of capsules could not explain the failure of the remaining 90-98% of the capsules [138]. In search of factors contributing to graft failure we analysed in subsequent investigations the inflammatory responses against the grafts. This was done at various time points between implantation and graft failure. The first new finding was that the responses against the grafts were not static as generally assumed [132,139-142] but dynamic [135] with involvement of different cell types as will be discussed in detail in the following section.

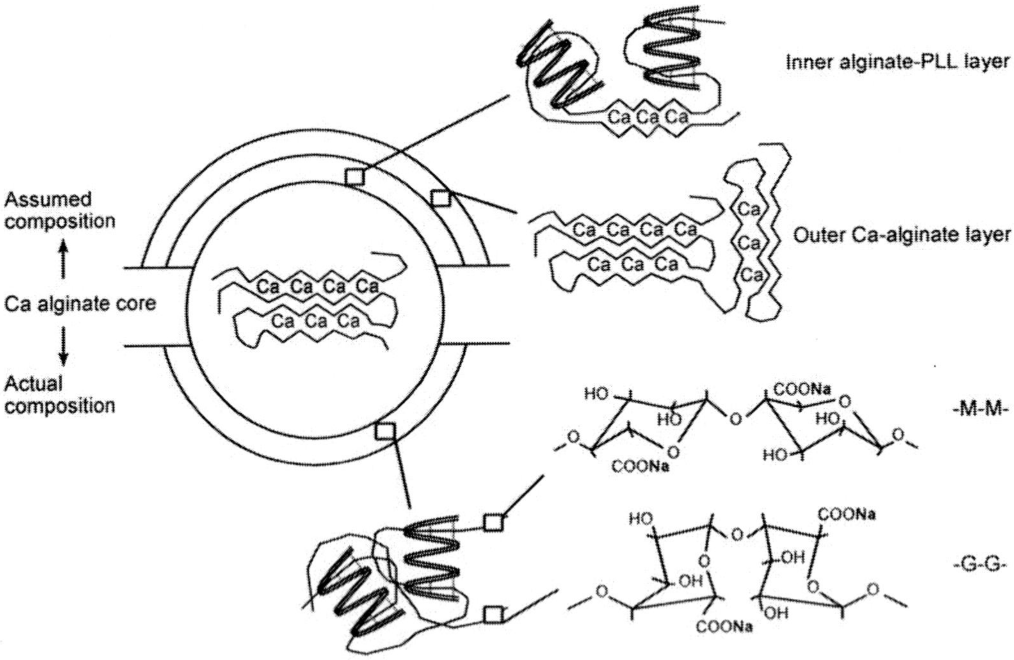

Figure 5. Schematic representation of the composition of the alginate-PLL membranes. In the assumed model the alginate core is surrounded with two layers. The inner layer of alginate-PLL is considered to be formed by two types of interactions. The first type is that of the interaction between the PLL and mixed sequences of guluronic acid (G) and manuronic acid (M) in the alginate molecules. This interaction reduces the permeability of the capsules by inducing the formation of complexes at the surface of α-helical PLL surrounded by superhelically orientated polysaccharide molecules. The other interaction is that between Ca^{2+} and alginate which is already formed in the gelation step in 100 mM $CaCl_2$. In the actual model the outer layer is composed of only one alginate-PLL layer containing PLL and Na^+ without the Ca-alginate. The Na^+ ions are bound by carboxyl groups present in the alginate.

The very first step in the tissue response is probably not related to the implantation of the 'foreign' capsules but to the required surgical procedure for implantation. Although it is only minor surgery, the procedure is associated with tissue damage as illustrated by the observation of erythrocytes in the peritoneal cavity at the first day after implantation. The bleedings and subsequent tissue repair is associated with the introduction of serum factors in the peritoneal cavity and release of bioactive proteins such as fibrinogen, trombin, and fibronectin[143]. These factors will have chemotactic effects on inflammatory cells which cells will subsequently migrate to the peritoneal site [144-147]. The bioactive proteins are adsorbed by the foreign polymers as of day 5 [135] resulting in adherence of cells at a portion of the capsules. These adherent cells were found to produce the cytokines IL-1β, TNF-α, and TGF-β, which further activate inflammatory cells in the vicinity of the foreign materials [143,147-149]. The observation of high numbers of basophils in the cellular infiltrate suggests that basophils play an important role in the host response against immunoisolated cells. Basophiles are strong producers of bioactive proteins and cytokines such as histamine [150-154], monocyte and macrophage chemoattractant proteins (MIP and MCP) [151,155], IL-4 [154,156,157], and IL-13 [154,158-160]. These cytokines are well known to have chemotactic and activating effects on inflammatory cells such as granulocytes, macrophages and fibroblasts. The above-described response is most severe during the first two weeks after implantation. In these two weeks, basophils and granulocytes gradually disappear from the graft site while macrophages and fibroblasts remain attached to a portion of 2-10% the capsules [135].

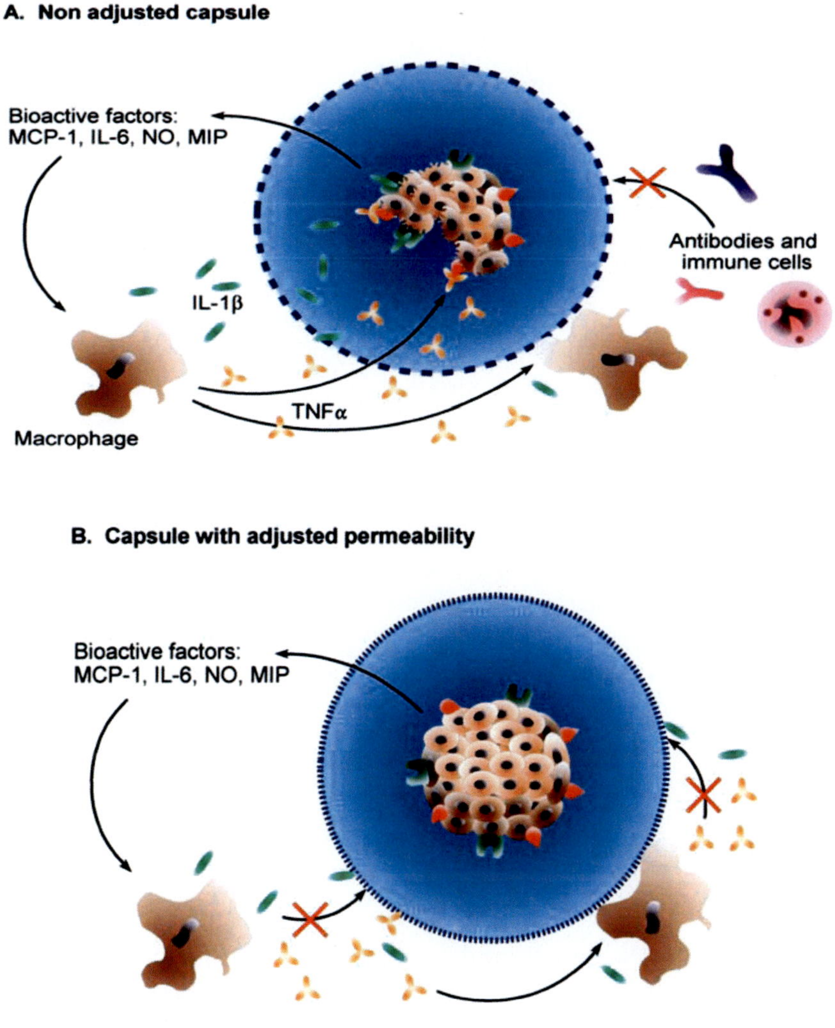

Figure 6. **A.** Schematic representation that a small amount of overgrowth on capsules can have a pronounced effect on the functional survival of the encapsulated grafts. The macrophages on the 2-10% overgrown capsules stay activated and the release of cytokines results in elevated apoptosis in the engrafted cells and release of graft-derived cytokines such as MCP-1 in the 90-98% nonovergrown capsules. The effect of this is a continuing circle of activation and loss of 40-80% of the cells in the graft [161]. **B**. Decreasing the permeability by chemical modification of the capsules prevents diffusion of large and multimeric cytokines such as TNF-α as well as small (e.g. IL-1β) cytokines, produced by the activated macrophages, into the capsules. The mechanism is that the chemical modifications for decreasing the permeability increased the negative charges of the alginate in the capsules, which induces repulsion of the negative charges on the tested cytokines-molecules.

Recently, by performing both *in vitro* and *ex vivo* studies, we showed that even this small amount of overgrown capsules can have a pronounced effect on the functional survival of the encapsulated grafts. The macrophages on the 2-10% overgrown capsules stay activated (as indicated by upregulation of IL-1β and TNF-α mRNA) as of the moment of implantation until at least day 28 after implantation. This results in elevated apoptosis in the engrafted cells and release of graft-derived cytokines such as MCP-1 in the 90-98% nonovergrown capsules. The effect of this is a continuing circle of activation and loss of 40-80% of the cells in the graft (Fig. 6A) [161]. Therefore, we now consider this latter response and consequently the overgrowth on 2-10% of the capsules an important deleterious factor for adequate graft survival.

Permeability of Capsules for Cytokines

As discussed in the preceding sections diffusion of graft-derived and inflammatory cell-derived cytokines is a major threat for the longevity of the encapsulated grafts. The permeability of the capsules for cytokines has always been a subject of debate. Scepticists have always assumed that the membranes of capsules can not adequately protect against deleterious cytokines with an approximate molecular weight of insulin or essential nutrients (5-15 kDa). Therefore, diffusion of cytokines into the capsules has always been the Achilles heel of immunoisolation. Recently, combined efforts of our group and that of Prof. Marchetti in Pisa have shown that this is not an insurmountable problem. It has been shown that the final effect of cytokines is dependent on the combined presence of different cytokines and on the concentration of cytokines [162]. We found *in vitro* that decreasing the permeability by chemical modification of the capsules prevents diffusion into the capsules of large and multimeric cytokines such as TNF-α. Also, diffusion of small cytokines (e.g. IL-1β) was reduced by changing the permeability of the membrane which was unexpected as the molecular weight of small cytokines such as IL-1β (17 kDa) was far below the molecular cut-off of the applied capsules (100 kDa) (Fig.6B). The mechanism is that the chemical modifications for decreasing the permeability increased the negative charges of the alginate in the capsules which induces repulsion of the negative charges on the tested cytokines-molecules. The observation that capsules can be selectively made impermeable for cytokines is very important since this can overcome the problem of the continuing circle of activation of cells in the overgrowth due the release of graft derived cytokines [163]

Also, we found evidence that cytokines may not interfere with islet function in case of xenografting of encapsulated islets in humans. We have observed that following exposure to a combination of human cytotoxic cytokines, a marked decrease in functional survival and a high percentage of apoptotic cells could be found in human islets but not in bovine islets [164]. Preliminary data show that this is due, at least in part, to the fact that xenogenic islet cells are less capable to bind and to take up human cytokines. This implies that, at least in some combinations, even when capsules are applied which are permeable for cytokines, the function and survival of xenogenic islet-sources will be less affected.

Metabolic Function of Encapsulated Islet Grafts

Adequate regulation of glucose levels by an encapsulated pancreatic islet graft requires a minute to minute regulation of blood glucose. In order to design such a transplant, it is mandatory to have sufficient insight in factors influencing the kinetics of insulin secretion by encapsulated islets. Functional performance of encapsulated grafts has mainly been studied with microencapsulated grafts. Therefore, in the next section we will mainly concentrate on the graft function of recipients of microencapsulated islets.

Insulin responses of encapsulated islets are influenced by the permeability of the capsule membrane and not by the islet-diameters or capsule diameter in the routinely applied 500-800 μm range. During our comparison of the glucose induced insulin responses of islets with different sizes, we surprisingly found no size-dependent differences in insulin secretion. This lack of effect of islet-size on insulin-secretion should probably be explained by the fact that in isolated islets the glucose is penetrating the islets by passive diffusion instead of by active transport to each, individual islet-cell by the bloodstream. This passive diffusion of glucose is predictably less efficient than active transport in normal, vascularized islets in the native pancreas [165,166]. Consequently, the glucose around large isolated islets will only stimulate islet-cells in the periphery rather than the more centrally located islet-cells.

The observation that encapsulated small, 90-120 μm islets show similar instead of lower glucose induced insulin responses than 150-180 and 210-300 μm islets suggests that the inclusion of only small islets in encapsulated grafts will have no consequences for the functional performance of the grafts. This is a pertinent consideration since small islets are associated with less protrusion [94,127,167] and, therefore, a lower rate of failing encapsulated islets. Another advantage of application of small islets is the reduction of problems associated with insufficient nutrition and central necrosis of the encapsulated islets with sizes larger than 150 μm [138]. This necrosis has been shown to be a major cause of failure of encapsulated grafts [52,138]. However, the effects of application of only the small rather than the large islets on longevity of encapsulated islet grafts requires some further research considerations since longevity of the graft is determined by the size of the graft volume [168,169] which volume is mainly determined by the number of large islets in the transplant [168,170,171].

Intraperitoneal transplantation of a microencapsulated islet graft restored normoglycemia in streptozotocin diabetic rat recipients within one week after transplantation. This normalization of blood glucose levels was associated with an evident metabolic improvement as illustrated by a normalization of body weight, normal HBAc1 levels and by a dramatic reduction in daily urine production. When functioning grafts were tested by oral or intravenous glucose challenge, glucose tolerance was found to be rather adequate as indicated by maximum glucose levels of 8.3 mM after the consumption of a glucose-rich meal but a rise in systemic insulin levels was never observed.

We have further substantiated this observation experimentally by assessing portal and systemic insulin responses and glucose levels after gradual infusion of low amounts of insulin into the peritoneal cavity, thereby mimicking the gradual release of insulin from the capsules of intraperitoneal graft. We found that the dose-dependent rise of insulin and decrease of glucose levels with intraperitoneal insulin infusion were strongly delayed and reduced as well as prolonged in comparison to intraportal insulin infusion [172][106]

The fact that the peritoneal cavity is not an optimal site for islet transplantation is also shown by the fact that the C-peptide level (which is released from islets in an equimolar concentration but not absorbed by abdominal organs and does not undergo hepatic extraction) is increased in the systemic circulation of an transplanted diabetic mice after an meal. However, this increase is delayed and decreased compared to normal mice[107]. The reason for the peritoneal cavity being less accommodating for transplanted islets is the lack of neovascularisation which also results in a relative hypoxia [31,173].

The absence of revascularization of the encapsulated islets interferes with both the functional performance and the longevity of the grafts [52,162,174]. Apparently, it is obligatory for clinical applications to find a site where encapsulated islets are in close contact with the blood stream. Unfortunately, it is difficult to find such a site since it should combine the capacity to bear a large graft volume in the immediate vicinity of blood vessels. Reported sites allowing for successful islet transplantation in mammals such as the liver [168,175-177], the spleen [168,178-180], and the renal capsule [40,169,181] do not meet these requirements since they can never carry the volumes of more than 100 ml of capsules required for transplantation in man [81,116,125]. To overcome this obstacle, we have recently introduced the concept of an intraperitoneally implanted solid support system for pancreatic islets [174]. This site allows for implantation of high numbers of islets, which can readily be retrieved and, theoretically, can be designed as such that it is highly vascularized.

This solid support system was developed of expanded polytetrafluoroethylene (ePTFE) since ePTFE have been shown to be biocompatible and to become neovascularized after implantation in the peritoneal cavity. Initially, we applied the concept of Thompson et al [182,183] in which solid supports are coated with collagen type IV (*i.e.* the collagen type predominantly present in the basal membrane) and acidic-fibroblast growth factors (a-FGF) to facilitate the ingrowth of blood vessels [174,182,183]. This solid support was shown to be very efficacious since normoglycemia was induced in all diabetic rats with islet transplants in the solid supports while this was only the case in 40% of the diabetic rats transplanted with islets in the unmodified peritoneal cavity without the solid support [174].

In our subsequent studies on vascularization of solid supports, we have focused on VEGF–165 [184-186], which is considered to have the greatest potential as angiogenic stimulus when compared to other angiogenic growth factors like acidic-fibroblast growth factor, basic-fibroblast growth factor, platelet derived growth factor, epidermal growth factor, epidermal growth factor, transforming growth factor alpha and beta, interleukines (IL-8 and TNF) or prostaglandines. Our present experimental approach is to stimulate vascularization of the solid supports applicable for encapsulated islets. These supports were prepared of flat sheet of ePTFE which were coated with collagen type IV and subsequently implanted in the peritoneal cavity in the immediate vicinity of the liver in order to promote portal drainage of insulin.

Concluding Remarks

It is clear that tremendous advances have been made in immunoisolation of pancreatic islets during the last few decades. It was shown that insufficient biocompatibility of capsules is influenced by many factors. When pure alginates are applied with an intermediate-G content we were able to reduce the overgrowth to a portion of only 2-10% of the capsules.

This overgrowth in vivo on this small portion of the capsules is caused by individual imperfections on the capsule surface such as inadequate islet encapsulation, incomplete covering of the inflammatory PLL and the effect of the surgical procedure. Recent new insight has shown that these imperfections on the small portions of capsules are not without consequences. The imperfections attract inflammatory cells such as macrophages. These macrophages stay activated for prolonged periods of time since they remain activated by bioactive factors released by the islet-tissue in the capsules [161]. This is an important observation since it implies that for successful transplantation we should not only focus on finding adequate biomaterials but also delete the effects of the enveloped cells in sustaining the inflammatory response.

Another obstacle on the route to successful transplantation of encapsulated islets is the absence of an adequate islet source. Irrespective of the species (i.e. rat or human) we require multiple donors for a single transplantation. It is mandatory to gain sufficient insight in which factors determine success or failure of an islet isolation procedure. For islet-encapsulation it is of an additional importance that the islets are sufficiently 'clean', i.e. not contaminated with exocrine tissue since this holds the risk of protrusion of cells[94,167] and death of the encapsulated islets as a consequence.

Furthermore, the encapsulated islets should closely follow the kinetics of insulin release of a free, nonencapsulated islet. Therefore, we require the smallest capsule possible. However, decreasing the capsule diameter holds the risk of protrusion of cells. It has been shown that protrusion can be minimized by application of only the small islets in the graft rather than the larger islets. Whether application of only small islets has consequences for the functional performance of the grafts remains to be determined.

We have shown that lowering the permeability of the capsules by increasing the PLL incubation time can provide a mean to overcome the obstacle of diffusion of cytokines into the capsules. The efficacy of this approach for the blockade of the inflammatory responses induced by the islet in the capsules *in vivo* remains to be confirmed but it shows that obstacles which seem to be insurmountable can be solved by a step-wise analysis of factors determine success and failure of encapsulated grafts.

References

[1] Laumonier T, Potiron N, Boeffard F, Chagneau C, Brouard S, Guillot C, Soulillou JP, Anegon I, Le Mauff B: CTLA4Ig Adenoviral` Gene Transfer Induces Long-Term Islet Rat Allograft Survival, Without Tolerance, After Systemic but Not Local Intragraft Expression. *Hum.Gene Ther.* **14**:561-575, 2003

[2] Demeterco C, Levine F: Gene therapy for diabetes. *Front Biosci.* **6**:D175-D1912001

[3] The effect of intensive treatment of diabetes on the development and progression of long-term complications in insulin-dependent diabetes mellitus. The Diabetes Control and Complications Trial Research Group. *N.Engl.J.Med.* **329**:977-986, 1993

[4] Robertson RP, Davis C, Larsen J, Stratta R, Sutherland DE: Pancreas and islet transplantation for patients with diabetes. *Diabetes Care* **23**:112-116, 2000

[5] Sutherland DE, Gruessner AC, Gruessner RW: Pancreas transplantation: a review. *Transplant.Proc.* **30**:1940-1943, 1998

[6] Kronson JW, Gillingham KJ, Sutherland DE, Matas AJ: Renal transplantation for type II diabetic patients compared with type I diabetic patients and patients over 50 years old: a single-center experience. *Clin.Transplant.* **14**:226-234, 2000

[7] Shapiro AM, Lakey JR, Ryan EA, Korbutt GS, Toth E, Warnock GL, Kneteman NM, Rajotte RV: Islet transplantation in seven patients with type 1 diabetes mellitus using a glucocorticoid-free immunosuppressive regimen. *N.Engl.J.Med.* **343**:230-238, 2000

[8] Faustman D, Lacy PE, Davie JM: Transplantation without immunosuppression. *Diabetes* **31** Suppl 4:11-16, 1982

[9] Hardy MA, Lau H, Weber C, Reemtsma K: Pancreatic islet transplantation. Induction of graft acceptance by ultraviolet irradiation of donor tissue. *Ann.Surg.* **200**:441-450, 1984

[10] Lau H, Reemtsma K, Hardy MA: The use of direct ultraviolet irradiation and cyclosporine in facilitating indefinite pancreatic islet allograft acceptance. *Transplantation* **38**:566-569, 1984

[11] Faustman DL, Steinman RM, Gebel HM, Hauptfeld V, Davie JM, Lacy PE: Prevention of rejection of murine islet allografts by pretreatment with anti-dendritic cell antibody. *Proc.Natl.Acad.Sci.U.S.A* **81**:3864-3868, 1984

[12] Morris PJ, Finch DR, Garvey JF, Poole MD, Millard PR: Suppression of rejection of allogeneic islet tissue in the rat. *Diabetes* **29** Suppl 1:107-112, 1980

[13] Bowen KM, Andrus L, Lafferty KJ: Successful allotransplantation of mouse pancreatic islets to nonimmunosuppressed recipients. *Diabetes* **29** Suppl 1:98-104, 1980

[14] Zeng Y, Peterson L, Levisetti M, Torres M, Montag A, Thistlethwaite J-RJ: Immunomodulation of human islets results in prolonged in vivo islet graft survival. *Transplant.Proc.* **27**:611-612, 1995

[15] Bhalla RK, Rich SJ, James RF, Bell PR, London NJ: The immunomodulation of cryopreserved pancreatic islets by gamma irradiation. A feasibility study. *Transplantation* **56**:1045-1047, 1993

[16] Steurer W, Nickerson PW, Steele AW, Steiger J, Zheng XX, Strom TB: Ex vivo coating of islet cell allografts with murine CTLA4/Fc promotes graft tolerance. *J.Immunol.* **155**:1165-1174, 1995

[17] Hsu PN, Lin HH, Tu CF, Chen NJ, Wu KM, Tsai HF, Hsieh SL: Expression of human Fas ligand on mouse beta islet cells does not induce insulitis but is insufficient to confer immune privilege for islet grafts. *J.Biomed.Sci.* **8**:262-269, 2001

[18] Turvey SE, Gonzalez-Nicolini V, Kingsley CI, Larregina AT, Morris PJ, Castro MG, Lowenstein PR, Wood KJ: Fas ligand-transfected myoblasts and islet cell transplantation. *Transplantation* **69**:1972-1976, 2000

[19] Takeda Y, Gotoh M, Dono K, Grochowiecki TR, Kimura F, Okuyama M, Shimizu J, Nagano H, Umeshita K, Sakon M, Miyasaka M, Monden M: Acceptance of islet allografts transplanted with Fas ligand expressing testicular allografts. *Transplant.Proc.* **31**:624, 1999

[20] Chahine AA, Yu M, McKernan MM, Stoeckert C, Lau HT: Immunomodulation of pancreatic islet allografts in mice with CTLA4Ig secreting muscle cells. *Transplantation* **59**:1313-1318, 1995

[21] Gainer AL, Suarez-Pinzon WL, Min WP, Swiston JR, Hancock-Friesen C, Korbutt GS, Rajotte RV, Warnock GL, Elliott JF: Improved survival of biolistically transfected

mouse islet allografts expressing CTLA4-Ig or soluble Fas ligand. *Transplantation* **66**:194-199, 1998

[22] Gainer AL, Korbutt GS, Rajotte RV, Warnock GL, Elliott JF: Expression of CTLA4-Ig by biolistically transfected mouse islets promotes islet allograft survival. *Transplantation* **63**:1017-1021, 1997

[23] Kirk AD, Harlan DM, Armstrong NN, Davis TA, Dong Y, Gray GS, Hong X, Thomas D, Fechner J-HJ, Knechtle SJ: CTLA4-Ig and anti-CD40 ligand prevent renal allograft rejection in primates. *Proc.Natl.Acad.Sci.U.S.A* **94**:8789-8794, 1997

[24] Bisceglie VV: Uber die antineoplastische Immunitat. *Krebsforsch* **40**:141-158, 1933

[25] Algire GH: An adaption of the transparant chamber technique to the mouse. *J.Natl.Cancer Inst.* **4**:1-11, 1943

[26] Liu HW, Ofosu FA, Chang PL: Expression of human factor IX by microencapsulated recombinant fibroblasts. *Hum.Gene.Ther.* **4**:291-301, 1993

[27] Koo J, Chang TSM: Secretion of erythropoietin from microencapsulated rat kidney cells. *Int J Artif Organs* **16**:557-560, 1993

[28] Chang PL, Shen N, Westcott AJ: Delivery of recombinant gene products with microencapsulated cells in vivo. *Hum.Gene.Ther.* **4**:433-440, 1993

[29] Cieslinski DA, Humes HD: Tissue engineering of a bioartificial kidney. *Biotechnol.Bioeng.* **43**:678-681, 1994

[30] Uludag H, Sefton MV: Metabolic activity and proliferation of CHO cells in hydroxyethyl methacrylate-methyl methacrylate (HEMA-MMA) microcapsules. *Cell Transplant.* **2**:175-182, 1993

[31] Colton CK: Implantable biohybrid artificial organs. *Cell Transplantation* **4**:415-436, 1995

[32] Aebischer P, Goddard M, Signore AP, Timpson RL: Functional recovery in hemiparkinsonian primates transplanted with polymer-encapsulated PC12 cells. *Exp.Neurol.* **126**:151-158, 1994

[33] Lim F, Sun AM: Microencapsulated islets as bioartificial endocrine pancreas. *Science* **210**:908-910, 1980

[34] Archer J, Kaye R, Mutter G: Control of streptozotocin diabetes in Chinese hamsters by cultured mouse islet cells without immunosuppression: a preliminary report. *J.Surg.Res.* **28**:77-85, 1980

[35] Loudovaris T, Jacobs S, Young S, Maryanov D, Brauker J, Johnson RC: Correction of diabetic nod mice with insulinomas implanted within Baxter immunoisolation devices. *J.Mol.Med.* **77**:219-222, 1999

[36] Lanza RP, Beyer AM, Chick WL: Xenogeneic humoral responses to islets transplanted in biohybrid diffusion chambers. *Transplantation* **57**:1371-1375, 1994

[37] Jain K, Asina S, Yang H, Blount ED, Smith BH, Diehl CH, Rubin AL: Glucose control and long-term survival in biobreeding/Worcester rats after intraperitoneal implantation of hydrophilic macrobeads containing porcine islets without immunosuppression. *Transplantation* **68**:1693-1700, 1999

[38] Lacy PE, Hegre OD, Gerasimidi Vazeou A, Gentile FT, Dionne KE: Maintenance of normoglycemia in diabetic mice by subcutaneous xenografts of encapsulated islets. *Science* **254**:1782-1784, 1991

[39] Juang JH, Bonner-Weir S, Vacanti JP, Weir GC: Outcome of subcutaneous islet transplantation improved by a polymer device. *Transplant.Proc.* **27**:3215-3216, 1995

[40] Juang JH, Bonner-Weir S, Wu YJ, Weir GC: Beneficial influence of glycemic control upon the growth and function of transplanted islets. *Diabetes* **43**:1334-1339, 1994

[41] Scharp DW, Swanson CJ, Olack BJ, Latta PP, Hegre OD, Doherty EJ, Gentile FT, Flavin KS, Ansara MF, Lacy PE: Protection of encapsulated human islets implanted without immunosuppression in patients with type I or type II diabetes and in nondiabetic control subjects. *Diabetes* **43**:1167-1170, 1994

[42] Suzuki K, Bonner-Weir S, Trivedi N, Yoon KH, Hollister-Lock J, Colton CK, Weir GC: Function and survival of macroencapsulated syngeneic islets transplanted into streptozocin-diabetic mice. *Transplantation* **66**:21-28, 1998

[43] Suzuki K, Bonner-Weir S, Hollister-Lock J, Colton CK, Weir GC: Number and volume of islets transplanted in immunobarrier devices. *Cell Transplant.* **7**:47-52, 1998

[44] Tatarkiewicz K, Hollister-Lock J, Quickel RR, Colton CK, Bonner-Weir S, Weir GC: Reversal of hyperglycemia in mice after subcutaneous transplantation of macroencapsulated islets. *Transplantation* **67**:665-671, 1999

[45] Siebers U, Zekorn T, Bretzel RG, Planck H, Renardy M, Zschocke P, Federlin K: Histocompatibility of semipermeable membranes for implantable diffusion devices (bioartificial pancreas). *Transplant.Proc.* **22**:834-835, 1990

[46] Scharp DW, Mason NS, Sparks RE: Islet immuno-isolation: the use of hybrid artificial organs to prevent islet tissue rejection. *World J.Surg.* **8**:221-229, 1984

[47] Woodward SC: How fibroblasts and giant cells encapsulate implants: considerations in design of glucose sensors. *Diabetes Care* **5**:278-281, 1982

[48] Colton CK, Avgoustiniatos ES: Bioengineering in development of the hybrid artificial pancreas. *J.Biomech.Eng.* **113**:152-170, 1991

[49] Lanza RP, Borland KM, Lodge P, Carretta M, Sullivan SJ, Muller TE, Solomon BA, Maki T, Monaco AP, Chick WL: Pancreatic islet transplantation using membrane diffusion chambers. *Transplant.Proc.* **24**:2935-2936, 1992

[50] Shoichet MS, Winn SR, Athavale S, Harris JM, Gentile FT: Poly(ethylene oxide)-grafted thermoplastic membranes for use as cellular hybrid bio-artificial organs in the central nervous system. *Biotech.Bioeng.* **43**:563-572, 1994

[51] De Vos P, Van Schilfgaarde R. Biocompatibility Issues. In Kühtreiber WM, Lanza RP, Chick WL., eds. Cell encapsulation technology and therapeutics. Boston: Birkhäuser, 1999; 63-79.

[52] De Vos P, Tatarkiewicz K: Considerations for successful transplantation of encapsulated pancreatic islets. *Diabetologia* **45**:159-173, 2002

[53] Lanza RP, Chick WL: Encapsulated Cell Therapy. *Scientific American Science and Medicine* **4**:16-25, 1995

[54] Lanza RP, Hayes JL, Chick WL: Encapsulated cell technology. *BioTechnology* **14**:1107-1111, 1996

[55] Lanza RP, Kuhtreiber WM, Ecker DM, Marsh JP, Staruk JE, Chick WL: A simple method for xenotransplanting cells and tissues into rats using uncoated alginate microreactors. *Transplant.Proc.* **28**:8351996

[56] Iwata H, Takagi T, Amemiya H: Agarose microcapsule applied in islet xenografts (hamster to mouse). *Transplant.Proc.* **24**:9521992

[57] Klomp GF, Ronel SH, Hashiguchi H, D'Andrea M, Dobelle WH: Hydrogels for encapsulation of pancreatic islet cells. *Trans.Am.Soc.Artif.Intern.Organs* **25**:74-76, 1979

[58] Sefton MV: The good, the bd and the obvious: 1993 Clemson Award for Basic Research-Keynote Lecture. *Biomaterials* **14** (15):1127-1134, 1993
[59] Kessler L, Pinget M, Aprahamian M, Dejardin P, Damge C: In vitro and in vivo studies of the properties of an artificial membrane for pancreatic islet encapsulation. *Horm.metab.Res.* **23**:312-317, 1991
[60] Kessler L, Legeay G, Jesser C, Damgé C, Pinget M: Influence of corona surface treatment on the properties of an artificial membrane used for Langerhans islets encapsulation: Permeability and biocompatibility studies. *Biomaterials* **16**:185-191, 1995
[61] Kessler L, Legeay G, West R, Belcourt A, Pinget M: Physicochemical and biological studies of corona-treated artificial membranes used for pancreatic islets encapsulation: Mechanism of diffusion and interface modification. *J.Biomed.Mater.Res.* **34**:235-245, 1997
[62] Knazek RA, Gullino PM, Kohler PO, Dedrick RL: Cell culture on artificial capillaries: an approach to tissue growth in vitro. *Science* **178**:65-66, 1972
[63] Chick WL, Like AA, Lauris V: Beta cell culture on synthetic capillaries: an artificial endocrine pancreas. *Science* **187**:847-849, 1975
[64] Chick WL, Like AA, Lauris V, Galletti PM, Richardson PD, Panol G, Mix TW, Colton CK: A hybird artifical pancreas. *Trans.Am.Soc.Artif.Intern.Organs* **21**:8-15, 1975
[65] Sun AM, Parisius W, Healy GM, Vacek I, Macmorine HG: The use, in diabetic rats and monkeys, of artificial capillary units containing cultured islets of Langerhans (artificial endocrine pancreas). *Diabetes* **26**:1136-1139, 1977
[66] Maki T, Lodge JP, Carretta M, Ohzato H, Borland KM, Sullivan SJ, Staruk J, Muller TE, Solomon BA, Chick WL, et al: Treatment of severe diabetes mellitus for more than one year using a vascularized hybrid artificial pancreas. *Transplantation* **55**:713-717, 1993
[67] Galletti PM, Trudell LA, Panol G, Richardson PD, Whittemore A: Feasibility of small bore AV shunts for hybrid artificial organs in nonheparinized beagle dogs. *Trans.Am.Soc.Artif.Intern.Organs* **27**:185-187, 1981
[68] Maki T, Mullon CJ, Solomon BA, Monaco AP: Novel delivery of pancreatic islet cells to treat insulin- dependent diabetes mellitus. *Clin.Pharmacokinet.* **28**:471-482, 1995
[69] Maki T, O'Neil JJ, Porter J, Mullon CJP, Solomon BA, Monaco AP: Long-term function of porcine islets in xenogeneic hosts. *Transplant.Proc.* **28**:8071996
[70] Maki T, Otsu I, O'Neil JJ, Dunleavy K, Mullon CJP, Solomon BA, Monaco AP: Treatment of diabetes by xenogeneic islets without immunosuppression - Use of a vascularized bioartificial pancreas. *Diabetes* **45**:342-347, 1996
[71] Lanza RP, Chick WL: Transplantation of encapsulated cells and tissues. *Surgery* **121**:1-9, 1997
[72] Lanza RP, Chick WL: Immunoisolation: At a turning point. *Immunology Today* **18**:135-139, 1997
[73] Lanza RP, Lodge P, Borland KM, Carretta M, Sullivan SJ, Beyer AM, Muller TE, Solomon BA, Maki T, Monaco AP, et al: Transplantation of islet allografts using a diffusion-based biohybrid artificial pancreas: long-term studies in diabetic, pancreatectomized dogs. *Transplant.Proc.* **25**:978-980, 1993
[74] Lanza RP, Sullivan SJ, Chick WL: Perspectives in diabetes. Islet transplantation with immunoisolation. *Diabetes* **41**:1503-1510, 1992

[75] Krause TJ, Robertson FM, Liesch JB, Wasserman AJ, Grecos RS: Differential production of IL-1 on the surface of biomaterials. *Arch.Surg.* **125**:1158-1160, 1990

[76] Sandler S, Eizirik DL, Sternesjo J, Welsh N: Role of cytokines in regulation of pancreatic B-cell function. *Biochem.Soc.Trans.* **22**:26-30, 1994

[77] Cetkovic Cvrlje M, Eizirik DL: TNF-alpha and IFN-gamma potentiate the deleterious effects of IL- 1 beta on mouse pancreatic islets mainly via generation of nitric oxide. *Cytokine.* **6**:399-406, 1994

[78] Remes A, Williams DF: Immune response in biocompatibility. *Biomaterials* **13**:731-743, 1992

[79] Hunt JA, Flanagan BF, McLaughlin PJ, Strickland I, Williams DF: Effect of biomaterial surface charge on the inflammatory response: evaluation of cellular infiltration and TNF alpha production. *J.Biomed.Mater.Res.* **31**:139-144, 1996

[80] Anderson JM, Langone JJ: Issues and perspectives on the biocompatibility and immunotoxicity evaluation of implanted controlled release systems. *J.Controlled Release.* **57**:107-113, 1999

[81] Soon Shiong P, Heintz RE, Merideth N, Yao QX, Yao Z, Zheng T, Murphy M, Moloney MK, Schmehl M, Harris M, et al: Insulin independence in a type 1 diabetic patient after encapsulated islet transplantation. *Lancet* **343**:950-951, 1994

[82] Calafiore R, Basta G, Luca G, Boselli C, Bufalari A, Cassarani MP, Giustozzi GM, Brunetti P: Transplantation of pancreatic islets contained in minimal volume microcapsules in diabetic high mammalians. *Ann.N.Y.Acad.Sci.* **875**:vol1999

[83] Weber CJ, Safley S, Hagler M, Kapp J: Evaluation of graft-host response for various tissue sources and animal models. *Ann.N.Y.Acad.Sci.* **875**:vol1999

[84] Cruise GM, Hegre OD, Lamberti FV, Hager SR, Hill R, Scharp DS, Hubbell JA: In vitro and in vivo performance of porcine islets encapsulated in interfacially photopolymerized poly(ethylene glycol) diacrylate membranes. *Cell Transplant.* **8**:293-306, 1999

[85] Kulseng B, Skjak-Braek G, Ryan L, Andersson A, King A, Faxvaag A, Espevik T: Transplantation of alginate microcapsules: generation of antibodies against alginates and encapsulated porcine islet-like cell clusters. *Transplantation* **67**:978-984, 1999

[86] Calafiore R, Basta G, Osticioli L, Luca G, Tortoioli C, Brunetti P: Coherent microcapsules for pancreatic islet transplantation: A new approach for bioartificial pancreas. *Transplant.Proc.* **28**:812-813, 1996

[87] Grohn P, Klock G, Schmitt J, Zimmermann U, Horcher A, Bretzel RG, Hering BJ, Brandhorst D, Brandhorst H, Zekorn T, et al: Large-scale production of Ba(2+)-alginate-coated islets of Langerhans for immunoisolation. *Exp.Clin.Endocrinol.* **102**:380-387, 1994

[88] Siebers U, Zekorn T, Horcher A, KlÖck G, Houben R, Frank H, Bretzel RG, Zimmermann U, Federlin K: Microencapsulated transplantation of allogeneic islets into specifically presensitized recipients. *Transplant.Proc.* **26**:787-788, 1994

[89] Zimmermann U, KlÖck G, Federlin K, Hannig K, Kowalski M, Bretzel RG, Horcher A, Entenmann H, Sieber U, Zekorn T: Production of mitogen-contamination free alginates with variable ratios of mannuronic acid to guluronic acid by free flow electrophoresis. *Electrophoresis* **13**:269-274, 1992

[90] Ar'Rajab A, Bengmark S, Ahren B: Insulin secretion in streptozotocin-diabetic rats transplanted with immunoisolated islets. *Transplantation* **51**:570-574, 1991

[91] Basic D, Vacek I, Sun AM: Microencapsulation and transplantation of genetically engineered cells: A new approach to somatic gene therapy. *Artif.Cells Blood Substitutes Immobilization Biotechnol.* **24**:219-255, 1996

[92] Chicheportiche D, Reach G: In vitro kinetics of insulin release by microencapsulated rat islets: effect of the size of the microcapsules. *Diabetologia* **31**:54-57, 1988

[93] Crooks CA, Douglas JA, Broughton RL, Sefton MV: Microencapsulation of mammalian cells in a HEMA-MMA copolymer: effects on capsule morphology and permeability. *J.Biomed.Mater.Res.* **24**:1241-1262, 1990

[94] De Vos P, De Haan BJ, Wolters GHJ, Van Schilfgaarde R: Factors influencing the adequacy of microencapsulation of rat pancreatic islets. *Transplantation* **62**:888-893, 1996

[95] De Vos P, De Haan BJ, Wolters GHJ, Strubbe JH, Van Schilfgaarde R: Improved biocompatibility but limited graft survival after purification of alginate for microencapsulation of pancreatic islets. *Diabetologia* **40**:262-270, 1997

[96] Iwata H, Amemiya H, Matsuda T, Takano H, Hayashi R, Akutsu T: Evaluation of microencapsulated islets in agarose gel as bioartificial pancreas by studies of hormone secretion in culture and by xenotransplantation. *Diabetes* **38** Suppl 1:224-225, 1989

[97] Korbutt GS, Elliott JF, Ao Z, Flashner M, Warnock GL, Rajotte RV: Microencapsulation of neonatal porcine islets: Long-term reversal of diabetes in nude mice and in vitro protection from human complement mediated cytolysis. *Transplant.Proc.* **29**:21281997

[98] Sandler S, Andersson A, Eizirik DL, Hellerstrom C, Espevik T, Kulseng B, Thu B, Pipeleers DG, Skjak Braek G: Assessment of insulin secretion in vitro from microencapsulated fetal porcine islet-like cell clusters and rat, mouse, and human pancreatic islets. .*Transplantation* **63**:1712-1718, 1997

[99] Stevenson WT, Sefton MV: Graft copolymer emulsions of sodium alginate with hydroxyalkyl methacrylates for microencapsulation. *Biomaterials* **8**:449-457, 1987

[100] Sun AM: Advantages of microencapsulation as an immunoprotection method in the transplantation of pancreatic islets. *Ann.Transplant.* **2**:55-62, 1997

[101] Yderstroede KB: Pancreatic islet transplantation. Experimental and clinical aspects. *Dan.Med.Bull.* **34**:323-329, 1987

[102] Zhou M, Chen D, Yao Q, Xia Z, Wang C, Zhu H: Microencapsulation of rat islets prolongs xenograft survival in diabetic mice. *Chin.Med.J.Engl.* **111**:394-397, 1998

[103] Halle JP, Leblond FA, Pariseau JF, Jutras P, Brabant MJ, Lepage Y: Studies on small (<300 microns) microcapsules: II--Parameters governing the production of alginate beads by high voltage electrostatic pulses. *Cell Transplant* **3**:365-372, 1994

[104] Duvivier-Kali VF, Omer A, Parent RJ, O'Neil JJ, Weir GC: Complete protection of islets against allorejection and autoimmunity by a simple barium-alginate membrane. *Diabetes* **50**:1698-1705, 2001

[105] De Vos P, Vegter D, Strubbe JH, De Haan BJ, Van Schilfgaarde R: Impaired glucose tolerance in recipients of an intraperitoneally implanted microencapsulated islet allograft is caused by the slow diffusion of insulin through the peritoneal membrane. *Transplant.Proc.* **29**:756-757, 1997

[106] De Vos P, Vegter D, De Haan BJ, Strubbe JH, Bruggink JE, Van Schilfgaarde R: Kinetics of intraperitoneally infused insulin in rats: functional implications for the bioartificial pancreas. *Diabetes* **45**:1102-1107, 1996

[107] Tatarkiewicz K, Garcia M, Omer A, Van Schilfgaarde R, Weir GC, De Vos P: C-peptide responses after meal challenge in mice transplanted with microencapsulated rat islets. *Diabetologia* **44**:646-653, 2001

[108] Wells GD, Fisher MM, Sefton MV: Microencapsulation of viable hepatocytes in HEMA-MMA microcapsules: a preliminary study. *Biomaterials* **14**:615-620, 1993

[109] Bartkowiak A, Canaple L, Ceausoglu I, Nurdin N, Renken A, Rindisbacher L, Wandrey C, Desvergne B, Hunkeler D: New multicomponent capsules for immunoisolation. *Ann.N.Y.Acad.Sci.* **875**:vol1999

[110] Rihova B: Immunocompatibility and biocompatibility of cell delivery systems. *Adv.Drug Deliv.Rev.* **42**:65-80, 2000

[111] Fritschy WM, Wolters GH, Van Schilfgaarde R: Effect of alginate-polylysine-alginate microencapsulation on in vitro insulin release from rat pancreatic islets. *Diabetes* **40**:37-43, 1991

[112] Klock G, Frank H, Houben R, Zekorn T, Horcher A, Siebers U, Wohrle M, Federlin K, Zimmermann U: Production of purified alginates suitable for use in immunoisolated transplantation. *Appl.Microbiol.Biotechnol.* **40**:638-643, 1994

[113] Kulseng B, Thu T, Espevik T, Skjåk-Bræk G: Alginate polylysine microcapsules as immune barrier: permeability of cytokines and immunoglobulins over the capsule membrane. *Cell Transplantation* **6**:387-394, 1997

[114] Sawhney AS, Hubbell JA: Poly(ethylene oxide)-graft-poly(L-lysine)copolymers to enhance the biocompatibility of poly(L-lysine)-alginate micocapsules membranes. *Biomaterials* **13** (12):863-870, 1992

[115] De Vos P, Van Hoogmoed CG, van Zanten J, Netter S, Strubbe JH, Busscher HJ: Long-term biocompatibility, chemistry, and function of microencapsulated pancreatic islets. *Biomaterials* **24**:305-312, 2003

[116] De Vos P, De Haan BJ, Van Schilfgaarde R: Upscaling the production of encapsulated islets. *Biomaterials* **18**:1085-1090, 1997

[117] Serp D, Cantana E, Heinzen C, von Stockar U, Marison IW: Characterization of an encapsulation device for the production of monodisperse alginate beads for cell immobilization. *Biotechnol.Bioeng.* **70**:41-53, 2000

[118] De Haan BJ, Faas MM, De Vos P: Factors influencing insulin secretion from encapsulated islets. *Cell Transplant.* **12**:617-625, 2003

[119] Bystricky S, Malovikova A, Sticzay T: Interaction of acid polysaccharides with polylysine enantiomers, conformation probe in solution. *Carbohydrate Polymers* **15**:299-308, 1991

[120] Bystricky S, Malovikova A, Sticzay T: Interaction of alginate and pectins with cationic polypeptides. *Carbohydr.Res.* **13**:283-294, 1990

[121] King GA, Daugulis AJ, Faulkner P, Goosen MFA: Alginate-Polylysine Microcapsules of Controlled Membrane Molecular Weight Cutoff for Mammalian Cell Culture Engineering. *Biotechnol.Prog.* **3**:231-240, 1987

[122] Vandenbossche GM, Van Oostveldt P, Remon JP: A fluorescence method for the determination of the molecular weight cut-off of alginate-polylysine microcapsules. *J.Pharm.Pharmacol.* **43**:275-277, 1991

[123] Vandenbossche GM, Bracke ME, Cuvelier CA, Bortier HE, Mareel MM, Remon JP: Host reaction against alginate-polylysine microcapsules containing living cells. *J.Pharm.Pharmacol.* **45**:121-125, 1993

[124] Vandenbossche GM, Bracke ME, Cuvelier CA, Bortier HE, Mareel MM, Remon JP: Host reaction against empty alginate-polylysine microcapsules. Influence of preparation procedure. *J.Pharm.Pharmacol.* **45**:115-120, 1993

[125] De Vos P, Wolters GH, Fritschy WM, Van Schilfgaarde R: Obstacles in the application of microencapsulation in islet transplantation. *Int.J.Artif.Organs* **16**:205-212, 1993

[126] Van Schilfgaarde R, De Vos P: Factors influencing the properties and performance of microcapsules for immunoprotection of pancreatic islets. *.J.Mol.Med.* **77**:199-205, 1999

[127] Uludag H, de-Vos P, Tresco PA: Technology of mammalian cell encapsulation. *Adv.Drug Deliv.Rev.* **42**:29-64, 2000

[128] Colton CK: Engineering challenges in cell-encapsulation technology. *Trends Biotechnol.* **14**:158-162, 1996

[129] De Vos P, Van Hoogmoed CG, Busscher HJ: Chemistry and biocompatibility of alginate-PLL capsules for immunoprotection of mammalian cells. *J Biomed Mater Res.* **60**:252-259, 2002

[130] Van Hoogmoed CG, Busscher HJ, De Vos P: Fourier transform infrared spectroscopy studies of alginate-PLL capsules with varying compositions. *J.Biomed.Mater.Res.* **67A**:172-178, 2003

[131] De Vos P, De Haan B, Van Schilfgaarde R: Effect of the alginate composition on the biocompatibility of alginate-polylysine microcapsules. *Biomaterials* **18**:273-278, 1997

[132] Strand BK, Ryan L, In 't Veld P, Kulseng B, Rokstad AM, Skjåk-Braek G, Espevik T: Poly-L-lysine induces fibrosis on alginate microcapsules via the induction of cytokines. *Cell Transplant* **10**:263-277, 2001

[133] King A, Lau J, Nordin A, Sandler S, Andersson A: The effect of capsule composition in the reversal of hyperglycemia in diabetic mice transplanted with microencapsulated allogeneic islets. *Diabetes Technol.Ther.* **5**:653-663, 2003

[134] Koch S, Schwinger C, Kressler J, Heinzen C, Rainov NG: Alginate encapsulation of genetically engineered mammalian cells: comparison of production devices, methods and microcapsule characteristics. *J.Microencapsul.* **20**:303-316, 2003

[135] De Vos P, Van Hoogmoed CG, De Haan BJ, Busscher HJ: Tissue responses against immunoisolating alginate-PLL capsules in the immediate posttransplant period. *J.Biomed.Mater.Res.* **62**:430-437, 2002

[136] Thu B, Bruheim P, Espevik T, Smidrod O, Soon-Shiong P, Skjak-Braek G: Alginate polycation microcapsules. I. Interaction between alginate and polycation. *Biomaterials* **17**:1031-1040, 1996

[137] Dupuy B, Arien A, Perrot Minnot A.: FI-IR of membranes made with alginate-polylysine complexes. Variations with mannuronic or guluronic content of the polysaccharides. *Art.Cells., Blood subs., and Immob.Biotech.* **22**:71-82, 1994

[138] De Vos P, van Straaten JF, Nieuwenhuizen AG, de Groot M, Ploeg RJ, De Haan BJ, Van Schilfgaarde R: Why do microencapsulated islet grafts fail in the absence of fibrotic overgrowth? *.Diabetes* **48**:1381-1388, 1999

[139] Zhou D, Kintsourashvili E, Mamujee S, Vacek I, Sun AM: Bioartificial pancreas: alternative supply of insulin-secreting cells. *Ann.N.Y.Acad.Sci.* **875**:208-218, 1999

[140] King A, Sandler S, Andersson A: The effect of host factors and capsule composition on the cellular overgrowth on implanted alginate capsules. *J. Biomed. Mater. Re.* **57**:374-383, 2001

[141] Horcher A, Zekorn T, Siebers U, KlÖck G, Frank H, Houben R, Bretzel RG, Zimmermann U, Federlin K: Transplantation of microencapsulated islets in rats: Evidence for induction of fibrotic overgrowth by islet alloantigens released from microcapsules. *Transplant.Proc.* **26**:784-786, 1994

[142] Rafael E, Wu GS, Hultenby K, Tibell A, Wernerson A: Improved survival of macroencapsulated islets of Langerhans by preimplantation of the immunoisolating device: a morphometric study. *Cell Transplant.* **12**:407-412, 2003

[143] Tang L, Eaton JW: Natural responses to unnatural materials: A molecular mechanism for foreign body reactions. *Mol.Med.* **5**:351-358, 1999

[144] Tang L, Jennings TA, Eaton JW: Mast cells mediate acute inflammatory responses to implanted biomaterials. *Proc.Natl.Acad.Sci.U.S.A.* **95**:8841-8846, 1998

[145] Hu WJ, Eaton JW, Tang L: Molecular basis of biomaterial-mediated foreign body reactions. *Blood* **98**:1231-1238, 2001

[146] Tang L, Ugarova TP, Plow EF, Eaton JW: Molecular determinants of acute inflammatory responses to biomaterials. *J Clin.Invest.* **97**:1329-1334, 1996

[147] Rihova B: Immunocompatibility and biocompatibility of cell delivery systems. *Adv.Drug Deliv.Rev.* **42**:65-80, 2000

[148] Babensee JE, Anderson JM, McIntire LV, Mikos AG: Host response to tissue engineered devices. *Adv.Drug Deliv.Rev.* **33**:111-139, 1998

[149] Hunt JA, McLaughlin PJ, Flanagan BF: Techniques to investigate cellular and molecular interactions in the host response to implanted biomaterials. *Biomaterials* **18**:1449-1459, 1997

[150] Falcone FH, Haas H, Gibbs BF: The human basophil: a new appreciation of its role in immune responses. *Blood* **96**:4028-4038, 2000

[151] Kobayashi H, Ishizuka T, Okayama Y: Human mast cells and basophils as sources of cytokines. *Clin.Exp.Allergy* **30**:1205-1212, 2000

[152] Huntley JF: Mast cells and basophils: a review of their heterogeneity and function. *J.Comp.Pathol.* **107**:349-372, 1992

[153] Schedle A, Samorapoompichit P, Fureder W, Rausch-Fan XH, Franz A, Sperr WR, Sperr W, Slavicek R, Simak S, Klepetko W, Ellinger A, Ghannadan M, Baghestanian M, Valent P: Metal ion-induced toxic histamine release from human basophils and mast cells. *J.Biomed.Mater.Res.* **39**:560-567, 1998

[154] Schroeder JT, MacGlashan D-WJ, Lichtenstein LM: Human basophils: mediator release and cytokine production. *Adv.Immunol.* **77**:vol 2001

[155] Tang L, Jennings TA, Eaton JW: Mast cells mediate acute inflammatory responses to implanted biomaterials. *Proc.Natl.Acad.Sci.U.S.A.* **95**:8841-8846, 1998

[156] Brunner T, Heusser CH, Dahinden CA: Human peripheral blood basophils primed by interleukin 3 (IL-3) produce IL-4 in response to immunoglobulin E receptor stimulation. *J. Exp.Med.* **177**:605-611, 1993

[157] Arock M, Merle-Beral H, Dugas B, Ouaaz F, Le-Goff L, Vouldoukis I, Mencia-Huerta JM, Schmitt C, Leblond-Missenard V, Debre P: IL-4 release by human leukemic and activated normal basophils. *J. Immunol.* **151**:1441-1447, 1993

[158] Wedemeyer J, Galli SJ: Mast cells and basophils in acquired immunity. *Br.Med.Bull.* **56**:936-955, 2000

[159] Li H, Sim TC, Alam R: IL-13 released by and localized in human basophils. *J Immunol.* **156**:4833-4838, 1996

[160] Falcone FH, Haas H, Gibbs BF: The human basophil: a new appreciation of its role in immune responses. *Blood* **96**:4028-4038, 2000

[161] De Vos P, Smedema I, van Goor H, Moes H, van Zanten J, Netters S, de Leij LF, de Haan A, De Haan BJ: Association between macrophage activation and function of micro-encapsulated rat islets. *Diabetologia* **46**:666-673, 2003

[162] De Vos P, Marchetti P: Encapsulation of pancreatic islets for transplantation in diabetes: the untouchable islets. *Trends Mol.Med.* **8**:363-366, 2002

[163] De Vos P, Smedema I, van Goor H, Moes H, van Zanten J, de Leij LFM, De Haan BJ: Association between macrophages activation and function of microencapsulated islets. *Diabetologia* 2003

[164] Piro S, Lupi R, Dotta F, Patane G, Rabuazzo MA, Marselli L, Santangelo C, Realacci M, Del-Guerra S, Purrello F, Marchetti P: Bovine islets are less susceptible than human islets to damage by human cytokines. *Transplantation* **71**:21-26, 2001

[165] Monta~na E, Bonner-Weir S, Weir GC: Transplanted beta cell response to increased metabolic demand. Changes in beta cell replication and mass. *J.Clin.Invest.* **93**:1577-1582, 1994

[166] Bonner Weir S: Regulation of pancreatic Beta-cell mass in vivo. *Recent Prog. Horm. Res.* **49**:91-104, 1994

[167] De Vos P, De Haan BJ, Pater J, Van Schilfgaarde R: Association between capsule diameter, adequacy of encapsulation, and survival of microencapsulated rat islet allografts. *Transplantation* **62**:893-899, 1996

[168] van Suylichem PT, Strubbe JH, Houwing H, Wolters GH, Van Schilfgaarde R: Rat islet isograft function. Effect of graft volume and transplantation site. *Transplantation* **57**:1010-1017, 1994

[169] van Suylichem PT, Strubbe JH, Houwing H, Wolters GH, Van Schilfgaarde R: Insulin secretion by rat islet isografts of a defined endocrine volume after transplantation to three different sites. *Diabetologia* **35**:917-923, 1992

[170] Wolters GH, van Suylichem PT, Van Deijnen JH, Van Schilfgaarde R: Factors influencing the isolation process of islets of Langerhans. *Horm.Metab.Res.Suppl.* **25**:20-26, 1990

[171] Wolters GH, van Suylichem PT, Van Deijnen JH, Van Schilfgaarde R: Increased islet yield by improved pancreatic tissue dissociation: the effects of bovine serum albumin and calcium. *Transplant.Proc.* **21**:2626-2627, 1989

[172] De Vos P, De Haan BJ, Vegter D, Hillebrands JL, Strubbe JH, Bruggink JE, Van Schilfgaarde R: Insulin levels after portal and systemic insulin infusion differ in a dose-dependent fashion. *.Horm.Metab.Res.* **30**:721-725, 1998

[173] Avgoustiniatos ES, Colton CK: Effect of external oxygen mass transfer resistances on viability of immunoisolated tissue. *Ann NY Acad.Sci.* **31**:145-167, 1997

[174] De Vos P, Hillebrands JL, De Haan BJ, Strubbe JH, Van Schilfgaarde R: Efficacy of a prevascularized expanded polytetrafluoroethylene solid support system as a transplantation site for pancreatic islets. *Transplantation* **63**:824-830, 1997

[175] Gardemann A, Jungermann K, Grosse V, Cossel L, Wohlrab F, Hahn HJ, Blech W, Hildebrandt W: Reinnervation of pancreatic islets and regulation of insulin secretion by hepatic sympathetic nerves after intraportal transplantation of islets into livers of diabetic rats. *Exp.Clin.Endocrinol.Diabetes* **103** Suppl. 2:107-111, 1995

[176] Andersson A, Korsgren O, Jansson L: Intraportally transplanted pancreatic islets revascularized from hepatic arterial system. *Diabetes* **38** Suppl 1:192-195, 1989

[177] Dunger A, Korsgren O, Andersson A: DNA replication in mouse pancreatic islets transplanted subcapsularly into the kidney or intraportally into the liver. Influence of unilateral nephrectomy or partial hepatectomy. *Transplantation* **49**:686-689, 1990

[178] Kneteman NM, Warnock GL, Evans MG, Nason RW, Rajotte RV: Prolonged function of canine pancreatic fragments autotransplanted to the spleen by venous reflux. *Transplantation* **49**:679-681, 1990

[179] Feldman SD, Hirshberg GE, Dodi G, Raizman ME, Scharp DW, Ballinger WF, Lacy PE: Intrasplenic islet isografts. *Surgery* **82**:386-394, 1977

[180] Beattie GM, Hayek A: Islet cell mass and the longevity of islet grafts in diabetic rats. *Cell Transplant.* **2**:119-122, 1993

[181] Ar'Rajab A, Ahren B, Alumets J, Logdberg L, Bengmark S: Islet transplantation to the renal subcapsular space improves late complications in streptozotocin-diabetic rats. *Eur.Surg.Res.* **22**:270-278, 1990

[182] Thompson JA, Haudenschild CC, Anderson KD, DiPietro JM, Anderson WF, Maciag T: Heparin-binding growth factor 1 induces the formation of organoid neovascular structures in vivo. *Proc.Natl.Acad.Sci.U.S.A.* **86**:7928-7932, 1989

[183] Thompson JA, Anderson KD, DiPietro JM, Zwiebel JA, Zametta M, Anderson WF, Maciag T: Site-directed neovessel formation in vivo. *Science* **241**:1349-1352, 1988

[184] Trivedi N, Steil GM, Colton CK, Bonner-Weir S, Weir GC: Improved vascularization of planar membrane diffusion devices following continuous infusion of vascular endothelial growth factor. *Cell Transplant.* **9**:115-124, 2000

[185] Neufeld G, Cohen T, Gengrinovitch S, Poltorak Z: Vascular endothelial growth factor (VEGF) and its receptors. *FASEB J.* **13**:9-22, 1999

[186] Frelin C, Ladoux A, D'angelo G: Vascular endothelial growth factors and angiogenesis. *Ann.Endocrinol.Paris.* **61**:70-74, 2000

[187] Strautz RL: Studies of hereditary-obese mice (obob) after implantation of pancreatic islets in Millipore filter capsules. *Diabetologia* **6**:306-312, 1970

[188] Zekorn T, Siebers U, Filip L, Mauer K, Schmitt U, Bretzel RG, Federlin K: Bioartificial pancreas: the use of different hollow fibers as a diffusion chamber. *Transplant.Proc.* **21**:2748-2750, 1989

[189] Lanza RP, Ecker D, Kühtreiber WM, Staruk JE, Marsh J, Chick WL: A simple method for transplanting discordant islets into rats using alginate gel spheres. *Transplantation* **59**:1485-1487, 1995

[190] Gamian E, Kochman A, Rabczynski J, Burczak K: Badanie biokompatybilnosci i funkcjonowania protezy wewnatrzwydzielniczej czesci trzustki, wykonanej z zasiedlonych zywymi wyspami trzustki makrokapsulek PVA. [Biocompatibility testing and function of a pancreatic prosthesis consisting of viable pancreatic islets encapsulated in PVA macrocapsules]. *Polim.Med.* **29**:3-20, 1999

[191] Isayeva IS, Kasibhatla BT, Rosenthal KS, Kennedy JP: Characterization and performance of membranes designed for macroencapsulation/implantation of pancreatic islet cells. *Biomaterials* **24**:3483-3491, 2003

[192] Zielinski BA, Aebischer P: Chitosan as a matrix for mammalian cell encapsulation. *Biomaterials* **15**:1049-1056, 1994

[193] Dawson RM, Broughton RL, Stevenson WT, Sefton MV: Microencapsulation of CHO cells in a hydroxyethyl methacrylate- methyl methacrylate copolymer. *Biomaterials* **8**:360-366, 1987

[194] Shimizu S, Yamazaki M, Kubota S, Ozasa T, Moriya H, Kobayashi K, Mikami M, Mori Y, Yamaguchi S: In vitro studies on a new method for islet microencapsulation using a thermoreversible gelation polymer, N-isopropylacrylamide-based copolymer. *Artif.Organs* **20**:1232-1237, 1996

[195] Tatarkiewicz K, Sitarek E, Fiedor P, Sabat M, Orlowski T: Protamine-heparin membrane for cell microencapsulation. *Transplant.Proc.* **26**:35091994

[196] Sefton MV, Hwang JR, Babensee JE: Selected aspects of the microencapsulation of mammalian cells in HEMA-MMA. *Ann.N.Y.Acad.Sci.* 831260-70 *LHM:vol1997

[197] Boninsegna S, Bosetti P, Carturan G, Dellagiacoma G, Dal Monte R, Rossi M: Encapsulation of individual pancreatic islets by sol-gel SiO2: a novel procedure for perspective cellular grafts. *J.Biotechnol.* **100**:277-286, 2003

In: Immunosuppression: New Research
Editor: Charles B. Taylor, pp. 271-282

ISBN: 978-1-60692-102-9

Chapter 12

Oxidative Stress Peripheral Markers in Graves' Ophthalmopathy Patients during Combined Immunosuppression

***Janusz Bednarek*[1], *Henryk Wysocki*[2] *and Jerzy Sowiński*[1]**
[1] Department of Endocrinology, Metabolism and Internal Medicine;
[2] Department of Cardiology and Intensive Therapy, Poznań University of Medical Sciences, Poznań, Poland

Abstract

Graves' ophthalmopathy is considered an inflammatory disorder of autoimmune background, and changed reactive oxygen species (ROS) metabolism presumably plays a role in pathogenesis of autoimmune diseases. Corticosteroids and radiotherapy are principal measures of infiltrative ophthalmopathy treatment, and their therapeutic effect is partially connected with influence on ROS generation systems. In this chapter we analyse the both therapeutic methods influence on extracellular oxidative stress markers in Graves' ophthalmopathy patients. Plasma indices of free radical generation and scavenging were determined in 20 euthyroid patients with infiltrative Graves' ophthalmopathy initially, after orbital irradiation combined with intensive corticotherapy and off steroid treatment. 24 healthy volunteers and 25 euthyroid Graves' patients without ophthalmopathy served as controls. The changes suggesting peripheral oxidative stress presence (increased hydrogen peroxide, lipid hydroperoxides and ceruloplasmin levels and superoxide dismutase and catalase activities, reduced glutathione peroxidase and glutathione reductase activities) were still found just after radiotherapy, in spite of concurrent corticosteroid treatment. However, longer follow up revealed the ROS metabolism markers normalization in individuals off the therapy. Changed peripheral oxidative stress markers in Graves' ophthalmopathy patients are corrected by the combined immunosuppressive treatment. This effect presumably depends on regression of the orbital inflammatory lesions.

Keywords: autoimmune thyroid disease, Graves' ophthalmopathy, oxidative stress, radiotherapy, corticosteroids

Introduction

Graves' disease is an autoimmune disorder of the thyroid gland characterized by production of TSH receptor stimulating autoantibodies [1], what results in hyperthyroidism. Infiltrative ophthalmopathy, presented in Graves' patients, is considered an inflammatory disorder of autoimmune background [2]. The autoimmune process is induced presumably due to sharing antigenic epitopes (e.g. TSH receptor [3]) by thyroid and retroocular tissues [4]. Activated T lymphocytes stimulate orbital fibroblasts for proliferation and synthesis of glycosaminoglycans *via* cytokine network [5]. It leads to extraocular muscles enlargement and clinically overt ophthalmopathy development. Later, typical of an active phase inflammatory changes are replaced by fibrotic lesions (an inactive phase) [6].

Reactive oxygen species (ROS) are involved in pathogenesis of various neoplastic, degenerative, metabolic, inflammatory and ischemic diseases [7]. The extent of oxidative damage depends on a balance of ROS production and efficiency of antioxidant system, composed of specific enzymes and non-enzymatic components (distributed in tissues and circulating blood). There is growing evidence that changed ROS metabolism plays an important role in pathogenesis of autoimmune disorders [8]. Experimental data suggest that the presence of oxidative stress and the initiation of the immune response in Graves' disease may be closely related [9].

At present, a few experimental studies document an involvement of ROS in pathogenesis of the infiltrative eye changes in Graves' disease. Burch et al. [10] show anti-TSH receptor antibodies react with orbital fibroblasts superoxide dismutase (SOD), which reveals homologues fragment to TSH receptor. They prove higher prevalence of anti-SOD antibodies in Graves' patients compared to controls. ROS stimulate proliferation of retroocular fibroblasts from patients with Graves' ophthalmopathy, which is inhibited by methimazole [11]. Thyrostatics also inhibit ROS-induced expression of 72 kDa heat shock protein in Graves' retroocular fibroblasts [12]. However, little is known about peripheral ROS metabolism in patients with Graves' ophthalmopathy.

Corticosteroids are widely used for the suppression of inflammation in chronic inflammatory and autoimmune diseases, such as asthma, rheumatoid arthritis or inflammatory bowel disease, all of which are associated with increased expression of inflammatory genes. Systemic corticotherapy is also a mainstay of treatment of infiltrative Graves' ophthalmopathy. Corticosteroids increase anti-inflammatory proteins genes transcription and inhibit inflammatory factors genes expression [13]. *In vitro* studies suggest that the anti-inflammatory action of corticosteroids depends, at least partially, on an interference with the formation of ROS by phagocytes [14]. Corticosteroids produce significant inhibition of superoxide anion release by human monocytes [15,16] and granulocytes [17]. They may also raise leucocyte intracellular levels of ROS scavenging enzymes, as superoxide dismutase, catalase and glutathione peroxidase [18].

Low dose radiotherapy is another principal method of medical treatment employed in infiltrative Graves' ophthalmopathy [4]. Irradiation therapeutic effectiveness in inflammatory diseases may be connected with functional changes of lymphocytes, monocytes and macrophages [19]. It is suggested that ionizing radiation effect is connected with modification of ROS and nitric oxide generation systems [20, 21]. These mechanisms are presumably responsible for immunomodulatory and anti-inflammatory action of low dose irradiation, leading to swelling reduction and pain relief [21].

The aim of the research described in this chapter was a complex estimation of corticosteroids and radiotherapy influence on blood extracellular indices of ROS generation and free radical scavenging in patients with infiltrative Graves' ophthalmopathy.

Patients and Methods

Patients

The study was performed on 3 groups of subjects. A. Twenty euthyroid patients (14 females and 6 males, aged 45.6 ± 9.4, mean ± SD) with Graves' disease, which had manifested untreated, advanced eye changes in class 3b – 5 according to the American Thyroid Association (ATA) classification [22] for no longer than 5 months (*an ophthalmopathy group*). These individuals revealed high values (≥4) of a Clinical Activity Score [23] (5.1 ± 1.1, mean ± SD). B. Twenty five euthyroid patients (17 females and 8 males, aged 41.8 ± 8.9) with Graves' disease and no clinically overt infiltrative ophthalmopathy (ATA class 0 – 1) (*a non-ophthalmopathy group*). C. Twenty four healthy volunteers (15 females and 9 males, aged 44.9 ± 10.2) (*a control group*). Excluding criteria were alcohol drinking, presence of diabetes mellitus, hypertension, liver or kidney disorders, severe vascular diseases, other endocrine, immunological or inflammatory disorders, hyperlipaemia, regular drug ingestion or antioxidant use. Smokers had abstained from smoking overnight. Informed consent was obtained from all subjects. The study protocol had been approved by the Senior Staff Committee of the Department.

Treatment, Follow-up and Blood Collection Protocol

Before inclusion to the study, euthyroidism in all the Graves' patients was achieved after 2-4 months (mean 2.9 months for the non-ophthalmopathy group and 2.4 months for the ophthalmopathy patients) of treatment with methimazole. The initial dose of methimazole (60 mg/day) was gradually reduced, up to the permanent dose of 15 mg/day, and L-Thyroxine was added to maintain euthyroidism. Mean cumulative methimazole doses used to achieve euthyroidism did not significantly differ between the hyperthyroid patients groups (3948 ± 421 mg for the non-ophthalmopathy group and 3533 ± 362 mg for the ophthalmopathy patients, mean ± SD). In the ophthalmopathy group, systemic corticotherapy was introduced having achieved stable euthyroidism. Initially the patients obtained 1.0 g of methylprednisolone *iv* per day for 3 consecutive days, with repetition of this 3-day cycle after 4 days. Corticotherapy was continued with prednisone *po* in a dose of 60 mg/day for 3 weeks, that along with methylprednisolone pulses constituted *an intensive phase* of the treatment. Subsequently, the prednisone dose was reduced by 10 mg/week (*a maintenance phase* of corticotherapy). After the first week of prednisone treatment, standard orbital radiotherapy with a linear accelerator [24] was performed. At the time of *the combined therapy* each orbit was irradiated with a daily dose of 2 Gy, for 5 days/week for 2 consecutive weeks (total dose of 20 Gy per orbit).

The ophthalmopathy patients underwent ophthalmological investigation before and a week after corticotherapy withdrawing, with calculation of Clinical Activity Score [23].

Venous blood samples were drawn on fasting into test tubes (heparinized and without anticoagulant) initially from all subjects. In the ophthalmopathy group blood was collected also on the first day of 50 mg/day prednisone administration and a week after corticosteroids withdrawal. After centrifugation at 1500 x g for 5 min, plasma or serum were separated and stored at -80°C until laboratory tests.

Hormonal and Immunological Thyroid Tests

All the chemicals were purchased from Sigma (St. Louis, MO, USA) and Merck (Darmstadt, Germany). Serum fT_4, fT_3 and TSH concentrations were determined using immunofluorometric assay (Delfia, Pharmacia, Upsalla, Sweden). Levels of anti TSH receptor antibodies in serum were measured by radioimmunoassay (TRAK, Brahms, Berlin, Germany).

Oxidation Products Analysis

Hydrogen peroxide (H_2O_2) concentration was assayed following the method described by Gallati and Pracht [25]. Briefly, 1 ml of plasma was mixed with 0.9 ml 1 μmol/l 3.3'.5.5'-tetramethylbenzidine and 0.1 ml horseradish peroxidase (25 U) in 0.2 M potassium citrate buffer (pH 3.95). After 30 min incubation in room temperature, 2 N sulphuric acid was added and the supernatant was read at 450 nm. A standard curve was prepared with known amounts of H_2O_2, using the same procedure.

Plasma lipid hydroperoxides (ROOH) levels were determined by the FOX II assay (ferrous oxidation in xylenol orange) [26], with a reagent PeroXOquant (lipid compatibile formulation) commercially available from Pierce (Rockford, IL, USA). This reagent was obtained by mixing of reagent A (25 mM ammonium ferrous(II) sulfate, 2.5 M H_2SO_4) with reagent C (4 mM butylated hydroxytoluen, 125 μM xylenol orange in methanol) in the proportion 1:100. Aliquots of plasma (90 μl) were transferred to vials and Tris (2-carboxyethyl) phosphine hydrochloride (TCEP) in methanol (10 μl of a 10 mM solution) was added to some vials, to remove hydroperoxides. Methanol (10 μl) was added to the remaining tubes to generate test samples. After incubation at 20°C for 30 min, 900 μl of the PeroXOquant reagent was added and the vials were left for a further 30 min. After centrifugation at 12,000*g* for 10 min, the supernatant absorbance was measured at 560 nm. The hydroperoxides were determined by the difference between the absorbance of samples with, and without, the elimination of ROOH by TCEP. A standard curve was produced with a working reagent, using known amounts of hydrogen peroxide.

Thiobarbituric acid-reacting substances (TBARS) concentration was evaluated by the use of thiobarbituric acid assay, according to Buege and Aust [27]. Briefly, 0.2 ml of serum was mixed with thiobarbituric acid reagent (consisting of 0.375% thiobarbituric acid and 15% trichloroacetic acid in 0.25 N HCl). The reaction mixture was placed in a boiling water bath for 15 min, cooled and centrifuged. Absorbance of the supernatant was evaluated at 532 nm. A standard curve was prepared with known amounts of 1.1.3.3.-tetraethoxypropane.

Antioxidant Markers Analysis

Superoxide dismutase (SOD) activity was determined by the method of Roos *et al.* [28], based on inhibition by plasma of O_2^- catalysed reduction of ferricytochrome C in comparison to known standards. For a standard curve, mixture consisting of 0.675 ml (20 mmol/l Na_2CO_3, 0.1 mmol/l EDTA, 1 mmol/l NaN_3, pH 10.0), 0.1 ml of xantine (50 μmol/l), 0.1 ml of ferricytochrome C (5 μmol/l) and 0.1 ml of a SOD standard was incubated for 5 min and absorbance was determined at 550 nm. The reaction was started by adding 0.025 ml of xantine oxidase (0.025 U/ml). The samples were read again after 5 min. For tested samples, the SOD standard was substituted with 0.1 ml of plasma.

Catalase (CAT) activity was determined spectrophotometrically by the method of Goth [29]. Briefly, 0.2 ml of plasma was incubated with 1 ml of substrate (65 μmol/ml hydrogen peroxide in 60 mmol/l sodium phosphate/potassium phosphate buffer, pH 7.4), in 37°C for 60 sec. The enzymatic reaction was stopped with 1 ml of 32.4 mmol/l ammonium molybdate and yellow complex of molybdate and hydrogen peroxide was read at 405 nm.

Glutathione peroxidase (GPx) activity was assessed by the assay available from OXIS International (Portland, OR, USA). The principle of this method is decrease in absorbance at 340 nm, as the result of the oxidation of NADPH to $NADP^+$. A plasma sample was added to a solution containing glutathione, glutathione reductase and NADPH. The enzyme reaction was initiated by adding the substrate, tert-butyl hydroperoxide. The rate of decrease in the absorbance at 340 nm was directly proportional to the glutathione peroxidase activity in the sample.

Plasma glutathion reductase (GR) activity was evaluated by the commercially available assay (OXIS International, Portland, OR, USA), based on the oxidation of NADPH to $NADP^+$ catalysed by glutathione reductase. The reduction of GSSG was determined indirectly by the measurement of the consumption of NADPH, as demonstrated by decrease in absorbance at 340 nm, as a function of time.

Ceruloplasmin (CP) was determined by oxidation of *p*-phenylodiamine, according to method of Ravin [30]. Briefly, 0.05 ml of plasma was added to 0.7 ml of substrate (7.95 mmol/l *p*-phenylodiamine in 0.43 M acetic buffer, pH 5.6) and absorbance was read at 546 nm, after 15 min incubation at 37°C. Control samples contained additionally 0.2 ml of sodium azide (460 mmol/l).

Statistical Methods

Statistical analysis was carried out using the Statistica 6.0 for Windows PL package. The results obtained were expressed as mean ± SD. Since not all data showed normal distribution (when checked by Shapiro-Wilk W test), differences among groups were tested with nonparametric tests (with $P < 0.05$ selected as a significance level). Comparison between the both Graves' patients groups (the non-ophthalmopathy group and the ophthalmopathy group before corticotherapy), as well as between all the patients subgroups and the control group was made using unpaired Kruskal-Wallis test, followed by Dunn test in case of significant difference. In the ophthalmopathy group, mean group values of the patients under treatment were compared with paired Wilcoxon test.

Results

Average antithyroid treatment period was similar in both patients groups. In all blood samples of Graves' disease patients fT_4 and fT_3 levels were not significantly different from controls (Table 1). In the non-ophthalmopathy group and in the patients with infiltrative ophthalmopathy before corticotherapy TSH level did not differ from the control subjects and decreased markedly having introduced corticosteroids. In all patients groups a level of anti TSH receptor antibodies was elevated in a similar degree.

Table 1. Thyroid hormones, TSH and anti-TSH receptor antibodies (Anti-TSHR) levels in serum from Graves' disease patients without and with infiltrative ophthalmopathy during treatment

	Control (n = 24)	Graves' disease without ophthalmopathy (n = 25)	Infiltrative Graves' ophthalmopathy (n = 20)		
			1	2	3
FT4 (pmol L^{-1})	12.6 ± 2.6	13.1 ± 3.9	12.7 ± 3.5	13.6 ± 3.4	13.3 ± 4.0
FT3 (pmol L^{-1})	7.4 ± 2.1	6.5 ± 1.8	6.9 ± 1.5	6.5 ± 1.4	6.4 ± 1.7
TSH (mU L^{-1})	1.58 ± 0.43	1.72 ± 0.51	1.66 ± 0.52	$0.04 \pm 0.01^{*,\#}$	$0.05 \pm 0.02^{*}$
Anti-TSHR	5.2 ± 3.4	$54.7 \pm 20.8^{*}$	$55.9 \pm 23.0^{*}$		

1 - before treatment, 2 - after intensive corticotherapy, 3 - a week off treatment

Results are expressed as mean ± SD.

Significant differences ($P < 0.05$): * vs. the control group, $^{\#}$ vs. the ophthalmopathy group previous assessment point.

Table 2. Hydrogen peroxide (H_2O_2) and lipid hydroperoxides (ROOH) levels in plasma and thiobarbituric acid-reacting substances (TBARS) levels in serum from Graves' disease patients without and with infiltrative ophthalmopathy during treatment

	Control (n = 24)	Graves' disease without ophthalmopathy (n = 25)	Infiltrative Graves' ophthalmopathy (n = 20)		
			1	2	3
H_2O_2 (nmol mL^{-1})	6.92 ± 1.85	7.20 ± 1.88	$12.07 \pm 1.56^{*,\circ}$	$13.53 \pm 3.19^{*}$	$7.62 \pm 2.02^{\#}$
ROOH (μmol L^{-1})	11.83 ± 3.41	13.22 ± 3.49	$16.81 \pm 4.35^{*,\circ}$	$15.88 \pm 4.75^{*}$	$13.17 \pm 4.23^{\#}$
TBARS (nmol mL^{-1})	6.23 ± 1.54	6.87 ± 1.88	$7.99 \pm 2.23^{*,\circ}$	$6.31 \pm 0.90^{\#}$	6.28 ± 1.75

1 - before treatment, 2 - after intensive corticotherapy, 3 - a week off treatment

Results are expressed as mean ± SD.

Significant differences ($P < 0.05$): * vs. the control group, $^{\circ}$ vs. the Graves' non-ophthalmopathy group, $^{\#}$ vs. the ophthalmopathy group previous assessment point.

In the individuals with infiltrative Graves' ophthalmopathy before corticosteroid treatment clinical investigation revealed high values (5.1 ± 1.1, mean ± SD) of Clinical Activity Score (CAS), which dropped significantly (2.5 ± 0.8, mean ± SD) once the therapy was completed.

The free radical activity markers levels before treatment are shown in Table 2. In the Graves' patients without ophthalmopathy H_2O_2, ROOH, and TBARS concentrations were not significantly different from controls. In the ophthalmopathy patients before therapy H_2O_2, ROOH, and TBARS levels were higher in comparison to the Graves' disease subjects without infiltrative eye changes. Intensive corticosteroid treatment combined with radiotherapy led to a TBARS level decrease, not changing H_2O_2 and ROOH concentrations. After completing corticotherapy all markers were found to be normalized a week off treatment.

Table 3. Activities of superoxide dismutase (SOD), catalase (CAT), glutathione peroxidase (GPx) and glutathione reductase (GR) and concentration of ceruloplasmin (CP) in plasma of Graves' disease patients without and with infiltrative ophthalmopathy during treatment

	Control (n = 24)	Graves' disease without ophthalmopathy (n = 25)	Infiltrative Graves' ophthalmopathy (n = 20)		
			1	2	3
SOD (U mL^{-1})	17.35 ± 4.76	18.56 ± 4.96	23.31 ± 6.66^{*,o}	22.06 ± 4.83*	18.54 ± 4.62$^{\#}$
CAT (U mL^{-1})	21.85 ± 5.99	23.01 ± 6.22	30.06 ± 9.81^{*,o}	34.34 ± 4.55$^{*,\#}$	24.04 ± 5.75$^{\#}$
GPx (mU mL^{-1})	5.84 ± 1.60	5.86 ± 1.65	5.02 ± 1.07^{*,o}	4.29 ± 0.99$^{*,\#}$	6.46 ± 0.97$^{\#}$
GR (mU mL^{-1})	12.58 ± 2.96	11.65 ± 3.09	8.37 ± 2.23^{*,o}	8.84 ± 2.06*	12.86 ± 2.94$^{\#}$
CP (mg dL^{-1})	15.86 ± 3.99	15.77 ± 4.22	18.59 ± 3.22^{*,o}	21.99 ± 5.10$^{*,\#}$	13.18 ± 2.84$^{*,\#}$

1 - before treatment, 2 - after intensive corticotherapy, 3 - a week off treatment

Results are expressed as mean ± SD.

Significant differences ($P < 0.05$): * vs. the control group, ^{o} vs. the Graves' non-ophthalmopathy group, $^{\#}$ vs. the ophthalmopathy group previous assessment point.

Table 3 summarizes a status of the extracellular antioxidant system components before treatment. In the non-ophthalmopathy group SOD, CAT, GPx and GR activities and CP level did not change in comparison to the control subjects. In the ophthalmopathy patients prior to corticosteroid treatment SOD and CAT activities and CP concentration were significantly higher, whereas GPx and GR activities were lower than in the Graves' patients without ophthalmopathy. The intensive phase of combined therapy produced an increase of CAT activity and CP level, a decrease of GPx activity and no change of SOD and GR activities. All enzymes activities normalization and CP level suppression were noted after completing the therapy.

Conclusion

Thyroid hormones accelerate the basal metabolic rate and oxidative metabolism by induction of mitochondrial enzymes. Hyperthyroidism enhances ROS generation and produces changes in antioxidant systems of various tissues [31,32]. There are also conflicting reports on the immunosuppressive and free radical scavenging properties of antithyroid drugs

[9,33,34]. To eliminate the influence of abnormal levels of thyroid hormones, the Graves' patients with stable euthyroidism achieved by use of the same antithyroid drug and treatment protocol were included to the study. Recorded by us suppression of TSH concentration with normal levels of free thyroid hormones after corticosteroids introducing is a typical phenomenon observed in the course of corticotherapy.

The changes of the extracellular indices of ROS metabolism in the patients with infiltrative Graves' ophthalmopathy despite euthyroidism achievement (the increase of H_2O_2, ROOH, TBARS and CP levels, the increase of SOD and CAT activities and the decrease in GPx and GR activities) suggest the presence of oxidative stress, presumably connected with the orbital inflammatory process [35]. Similarly, papers concerning various types of local inflammation report oxidative stress peripheral markers (ROOH, malonyldialdehyde, chemiluminescence) to be on the increase [36,37,38,39,40].

Blood antioxidant enzymes activities are described to be either increased [36,41] or decreased [37] in localized inflammatory processes. It is possible, that these contradictory data regarding the state of antioxidant defence may be due to a different evolution period of the disease. In acute inflammation, an initial increment of the antioxidant enzymes indicates that the system reacts to accelerated ROS generation [36,41]. In longer periods of evolution, there may be consumption of the antioxidant system elements, necessary for neutralizing the oxidative damage [37,41]. The last phenomenon develops *in situ* [38], and can be also seen on the periphery [37,41].

In our research, serum SOD activity was enhanced in the ophthalmopathy patients before treatment, possibly secondary to increased ROS generation. Since SOD activity should increase H_2O_2 production, protection against ROS would be conferred by coordinated increase in CAT activity [42]. In accordance with this principle, we have observed CAT activity to be increased in the ophthalmopathy group. On the other hand, experimental investigations of erythrocytes of several species show SOD may be constitutively present only at low levels, but highly inducible under oxidative stress, whereas GPx is normally abundant and less inducible [43]. Taking this into consideration we can speculate that in our patients GPx (and similarly GR) was used up most rapidly and we found its activity decrease before treatment.

High dose glucocorticoids and low dose radiotherapy are principal methods of medical treatment of infiltrative Graves' ophthalmopathy [4]. The favourable effect of corticosteroids alone is reported to be less frequent than in the case of corticotherapy combined with orbital irradiation [44]. Patients selection for the therapy is usually based on clinical evaluation of infiltrative eye changes, with calculation of Clinical Activity Score (CAS) [23]. In this chapter, high values of CAS before corticotherapy suggest a presence of orbital inflammation. Completing the treatment ophthalmological investigation shows a marked decrease in CAS, and therefore documents suppression of inflammatory changes.

Several papers document corticosteroid treatment influence on normalization of ROS metabolism peripheral markers, changed by inflammatory diseases, for example in bronchial asthma [16] or glomerular disorders [40]. In an earlier study we showed intensive corticotherapy alone results in normalization (partial for ROOH) of the changed peripheral oxidative stress markers in the patients with infiltrative ophthalmopathy. However, after withdrawal of corticosteroids the marked restoration of the increased oxidative stress indices was observed, along with activation of antioxidant defence systems (statistical significance was not found only for CAT activity) [45].

Experimental studies suggest high dose radiation induces oxidative stress, probably associated with local inflammation development [46]. Contrary, low dose irradiation beneficial effect is observed in inflammatory and autoimmune diseases (eczema, psoriasis, abscess, insertion tendinitis, ankylosing spondylitis) [21], but its influence on ROS generation and scavenging has not been studied yet. In our patients the changes suggesting oxidative stress aggravation were found just after radiotherapy, in spite of concurrent corticosteroid treatment. However, longer follow up revealed the ROS metabolism markers normalization in the individuals off combined therapy.

Our current evidence indicates that orbital irradiation combined with corticosteroids causes peripheral oxidative stress suppression in patients with infiltrative Graves' ophthalmopathy. What else, the effect persists despite the treatment completing, contrary to the use of corticosteroids alone discussed by us in the previous work.

Acknowledgements

The present study was supported by grant from the Polish Scientific Research Committee (No. 4 PO5B 073 18).

References

[1] Mariotti, S; Pinchera, A. Role of the immune system in the control of the thyroid function. In: Greer MA, editor. *The Thyroid Gland*. New York: Raven Press; 1990; 45-60.

[2] Bahn, RS; Garrity, JA; Bartley, GB; Gorman, CA. Diagnostic evaluation of Graves' ophthalmopathy. *Endocrinol Metab Clin North Am* 1988, 17, 527-545.

[3] Bahn, RS; Dutton, CM; Natt, N; Joba, W; Spitzweg, C; Heufelder, AE. Thyrotropin receptor expression in Graves' orbital adipose/connective tissues: potential autoantigen in Graves' ophthalmopathy. *J Clin Endocrinol Metab* 1998, 83, 998-1002.

[4] Perros, P; Kendall-Taylor, P. Thyroid-associated ophthalmopathy: pathogenesis and clinical management. *Baillière's Clin Endocrinol Metab* 1995, 9, 115–135.

[5] Korducki, JM; Loftus, SJ; Bahn, RS. Stimulation of glycosaminoglycan production in cultured human retroocular fibroblasts. *Invest Ophthalmol Vis Sci* 1992, 33, 2037-2042.

[6] Bahn, RS; Heufelder, AE. Pathogenesis of Graves' ophthalmopathy. *N Engl J Med* 1993, 329, 1468-1475.

[7] Halliwell, B; Gutteridge, JM. Role of free radicals in human disease: an overview. *Methods Enzymol* 1990, 186, 1-85.

[8] Ahsan, H; Ali, A; Ali, R. Oxygen free radicals and systemic autoimmunity. *Clin Exp Immunol* 2003, 131, 398-404.

[9] Weetman, AP; Holt, ME; Campbell, AK; Hall, R; McGregor, AM. Methimazole and generation of oxygen radicals by monocytes: potential role in immunosuppression. *Br Med J (Clin Res Ed)* 1984, 288, 518-520.

[10] Burch, HB; Barnes, S; Nagy, EV; Sellitti, D; Burman, KD; Bahn, RS; *et al.* Immunodetection of manganese superoxide dismutase in cultured human retroocular

fibroblasts using sera directed against the thyrotropin receptor. *J Endocrinol Invest* 1998, 21, 48-55.

[11] Burch, HB; Lahiri, S; Bahn, RS; Barnes, S. Superoxide radical production stimulates retroocular fibroblast proliferation in Graves' ophthalmopathy. *Exp Eye Res* 1997, 65, 311-316.

[12] Heufelder, AE; Wenzel, BE; Bahn, RS. Methimazole and propylthiouracil inhibit the oxygen free radical-induced expression of a 72 kilodalton heat shock protein in Graves' retroocular fibroblast. *J Clin Endocrinol Metab* 1992, 74, 737-742.

[13] Barnes, PJ. Anti-inflammatory actions of glucocorticoids: molecular mechanisms. *Clin Sci (Lond)* 1998, 94, 557-572.

[14] Whitehouse, MW; Cleland, LG. Reactive oxygen species and drug therapy for inflammatory disease. *Agents Action* 1985, 17, 173-177.

[15] Szefler, SJ; Norton, CE; Ball, B; Gross, JM; Aida, Y; Pabst, MJ. IFN-gamma and LPS overcome glucocorticoid inhibition of priming for superoxide release in human monocytes. Evidence that secretion of IL-1 and tumor necrosis factor-alpha is not essential for monocyte priming. *J Immunol* 1989, 142, 3985-3992.

[16] Majori, M; Vachier, I; Godard, P; Farce, M; Bousquet, J; Chanez, P. Superoxide anion production by monocytes of corticosteroid-treated asthmatic patients. *Eur Respir J* 1998, 11, 133-138.

[17] Umeki, S; Soejima, R. Hydrocortisone inhibits the respiratory burst oxidase from human neutrophils in whole-cell and cell-free systems. *Biochim Biophys Acta* 1990, 1052, 211-215.

[18] Youssef, AA; Baron, DN. Leucocyte superoxide dismutase in rheumatoid arthritis. *Ann Rheum Dis* 1983, 42, 558-562.

[19] Hildebrandt, G; Seed, MP; Freemantle, CN; Alam, CA; Colville-Nash, PR; Trott, KR. Mechanisms of the anti-inflammatory activity of low-dose radiation therapy. *Int J Radiat Biol* 1998, 74, 367–378.

[20] Bhuvarahamurthy, V; Balasubramanian, N; Govindasamy, S. Effect of radiotherapy and chemoradiotherapy on circulating antioxidant system of human uterine cervical carcinoma. *Mol Cell Biochem* 1996, 158, 17-23.

[21] Hildebrandt, G; Seed, MP; Freemantle, CN; Alam, CA; Colville-Nash, PR; Trott, KR. Effects of low dose ionizing radiation on murine chronic granulomatous tissue. *Strahlenther Onkol* 1998, 174, 580-588.

[22] Werner, SC. Modification of the classification of the eye changes of Graves' disease: recommendations of the ad hoc committee of the America Thyroid Association. *J Clin Endocrinol Metab* 1977, 44, 203-204.

[23] Mourtis, M; Koorneef, L; Wiersinga, WM; Prummel, MF; Berghout, A; Gaag, RD. Clinical criteria for the assessment of disease activity in Graves' ophthalmopathy: a novel approach. *Brit J Ophthalmol* 1989, 73, 639-644.

[24] Kahaly, GJ. Radiotherapy for Graves' ophthalmopathy. In: Prummel MF, editor. *Recent developments in Graves' ophthalmopathy*. Boston: Kluwer Academic Publishers; 2000, 115-17.

[25] Gallati, H; Pracht, I. Horseradish peroxidase: kinetic studies and optimization of peroxidase activity determination using the substrates H_2O_2 and 3,3',5,5'-tetramethylbenzidine. *J Clin Chem Clin Biochem* 1985, 23, 453-460.

[26] Nourooz-Zadeh, J; Tajaddini-Sarmadi, J; Wolff, SP. Measurement of plasma hydroperoxide concentrations by the ferrous oxidation-xylenol orange assay in conjunction with triphenylphosphine. *Anal Biochem* 1994, 220, 403-409.
[27] Buege, JA; Aust, SD. Microsomal lipid peroxidation. *Methods Enzymol* 1978, 52, 302-310.
[28] Roos, D; Weening, RS; Voetman, AA; van Schaik, ML; Bot, AA; Meerhof LJ; *et al.* Protection of phagocytic leukocytes by endogenous glutathione: studies in a family with glutathione reductase deficiency. *Blood* 1979, 53, 851-866.
[29] Goth, L. A simple method for determination of serum catalase activity and revision of reference range. *Clin Chim Acta* 1991, 196, 143-151.
[30] Ravin, HA. An improved colorimetric enzymatic assay of ceruloplasmin. *J Lab Clin Med* 1961, 58, 161-168.
[31] Fernandez, V; Barrientos, X; Kiperos, K; Valenzuela, A; Videla, LA. Superoxide radical generation, NADPH oxidase activity and cytochrome P-450 content of rat liver microsomal fractions in an experimental hyperthyroid state: Relation to lipid peroxidation. *Endocrinology* 1985, 117, 496-501.
[32] Bednarek, J; Wysocki, H; Sowiński, J. Oxidation products and antioxidant markers in plasma of patients with Graves' disease and toxic multinodular goiter: effect of methimazole treatment. *Free Radic Res* 2004, 38, 659-664.
[33] Wilson, R; Buchanan, L; Fraser, WD; Jenkins, C; Smith, WE; Reglinski, J; *et al.* Evidence for carbimazole as an antioxidant? *Autoimmunity* 1998, 27, 149-153.
[34] Ozdem, S; Aliciguzel, Y; Ozdem, SS; Karayalcin, U. Effects of propylthiouracil treatment on antioxidant activities in blood of toxic multinodular goiter patients. *Pharmacology* 2000, 61, 31-36.
[35] Bednarek, J; Wysocki, H; Sowiński, J. Oxidative stress peripheral parameters in Graves' disease: the effect of methimazole treatment in patients with and without infiltrative ophthalmopathy. *Clin Biochem* 2005, 38, 13-18.
[36] Koltuksuz, U; Uz, E; Ozen, S; Aydinc, M; Karaman, A; Akyol, O. Plasma superoxide dismutase activity and malondialdehyde level correlate with the extent of acute appendicitis. *Pediatr Surg Int* 2000, 16, 559-561.
[37] Orem, A; Yandi, YE; Vanizor, B; Cimsit, G; Uydu, HA; Malkoc, M. The evaluation of autoantibodies against oxidatively modified low-density lipoprotein (LDL), usceptibility of LDL to oxidation, serum lipids and lipid hydroperoxide levels, total antioxidant status, antioxidant enzyme activities, and endothelial dysfunction in patients with Behcet's disease. *Clin Biochem* 2002, 35, 217-224.
[38] Satici, A; Guzey, M; Gurler, B; Vural, H; Gurkan, T. Malondialdehyde and antioxidant enzyme levels in the aqueous humor of rabbits in endotoxin-induced uveitis. *Eur J Ophthalmol* 2003, 13, 779-783.
[39] Oldenburg, B; van Kats-Renaud, H; Koningsberger, JC; van Berge Henegouwen, GP; van Asbeck, BS. Chemiluminescence in inflammatory bowel disease patients: a parameter of inflammatory activity. *Clin Chim Acta* 2001, 310, 151-156.
[40] Das, UN; Mohan, IK; Raju, TR. Effect of corticosteroids and eicosapentaenoic acid/docosahexaenoic acid on pro-oxidant and anti-oxidant status and metabolism of essential fatty acids in patients with glomerular disorders. *Prostaglandins Leukot Essent Fatty Acids* 2001, 65, 197-203.

[41] Perrin-Nadif, R; Auburtin, G; Dusch, M; Porcher, JM; Mur, JM. Blood antioxidant enzymes as markers of exposure or effect in coal miners. *Occup Environ Med* 1996, 53, 41-45.

[42] Clemens, MC; Waller, HD. Lipid peroxidation in erythrocytes. *Chem Phys Lipids* 1987, 45, 251-268.

[43] Maral, J; Puget, K; Michelson, AM. Comparative study of superoxide dismutase activity, catalase and glutathione peroxidase levels in erythrocytes of different animals. *Biochem Biophys Res Commun* 1997, 77, 1525-1535.

[44] Bartalena, L; Marcocci, C; Chiovato, L; Laddaga, M; Lepri, G; Andreani, D; *et al.* Orbital cobalt irradiation combined with systemic corticosteroids for Graves' ophthalmopathy: Comparison with systemic corticosteroids alone. *J Clin Endocrinol Metab* 1983, 56, 1139-1144.

[45] Bednarek, J; Wysocki, H; Sowiński, J. Peripheral parameters of oxidative stress in patients with infiltrative Graves' ophthalmopathy treated with corticosteroids. *Immunol Lett* 2004, 93, 227-232.

[46] Benderitter, M; Maingon, P; Abadie, C; Assem, M; Maupoil, V; Briot, F; *et al.* Effect of in vivo heart irradiation on the development of antioxidant defenses and cardiac functions in the rat. *Radiat Res* 1995, 144, 64-72.

Index

A

B

C

D

E

H

I

J

K

L

M

N

O

P

Q

R

S

T

U